METHODS IN NEUROTRANSMITTER RECEPTOR ANALYSIS

Methods in Neurotransmitter Receptor Analysis

Editors

Henry I. Yamamura, Ph.D.

Departments of Pharmacology,
Biochemistry, and Psychiatry
College of Medicine
The University of Arizona
Health Sciences Center
Tucson, Arizona

S. J. Enna, Ph.D.

Nova Pharmaceutical Corporation
Baltimore, Maryland

Michael J. Kuhar, Ph.D.

Neuroscience Branch
National Institute on
Drug Abuse
Addiction Research Center
Baltimore, Maryland

Raven Press New York

Raven Press, Ltd., 1185 Avenue of the Americas, New York, New York 10036

Made in the United States of America

Library of Congress Cataloging-in-Publication Data

Methods in neurotransmitter receptor analysis / editors, Henry
   I. Yamamura, S.J. Enna, Michael J. Kuhar.
      p.   cm.
   Companion v. to: Neurotransmitter receptor binding. 2nd ed.
   Includes bibliographical references.
   ISBN 0-88167-609-8
   1. Neurotransmitter receptors—Research—Laboratory manuals.
 I. Yamamura, Henry I. II. Enna, S. J. III. Kuhar, Michael J.
 IV. Neurotransmitter receptor binding.
   [DNLM: 1. Neuroregulators—analysis—laboratory manuals.
 2. Radioligand Assay—laboratory manuals. 3. Synaptic Receptors—
analysis—laboratory manuals.   QV 25 M592]
 QP364.7.M47 1990
 599'.0188—dc20
 DNLM/DLC
 for Library of Congress   89-70134
                                             CIP

9 8 7 6 5 4 3 2 1

Preface

The development of new analytical tools and methodologies is the driving force for advances in science. An excellent illustration of this principle has been the emergence of neurobiology as a scientific discipline. Prior to the 1950s, the tools available for studying brain architecture, chemistry, and function could provide little more than generalized descriptions of this complex organ. This situation has changed dramatically during the past 30 years with improvements in analytical instrumentation, developments in radiochemistry and molecular biology, and refinements in *in vitro* methodologies. These advances made it possible to seek answers to questions that had not even been formulated in earlier times. With these tools, theories concerning the existence of neurotransmitters and neurotransmitter receptors were confirmed. Concepts relating to the manner in which neurotransmitters are synthesized, stored, released, conserved, and distributed, as well as those pertaining to the ionic and molecular events associated with synaptic transmission, have surfaced in a relatively short period of time because of the development of new analytical devices and methods.

One procedure that helped revolutionize neuroscience research was the receptor binding assay. Because of its potential impact, in 1978 we prepared a monograph describing this technique and its uses. This volume, *Neurotransmitter Receptor Binding*, was published by Raven Press. Because the demand for this volume exceeded our expectations, the fact that the number of binding assays expanded, that the technology was being refined and its applications multiplying, we published a second edition in 1985.

One reason for the popularity of these volumes was that the chapters were designed to be used as guides for establishing these assays in the reader's laboratory. Since publication of the second volume, the assays and the analysis of binding data have been refined further. However, because the basic principles remain unchanged, it seemed redundant to publish a third volume in the previous format. Rather, it was decided that the most appropriate course of action would be to prepare a manual that would highlight the laboratory procedures and could serve as a companion volume for *Neurotransmitter Receptor Binding*.

Readers familiar with the earlier volumes will notice that some topics covered in this manual were not addressed in them. In preparing this volume, we decided to include additional assays because of the importance of correlating binding data with receptor function. Thus, included in this manual are assay procedures for studying receptor-mediated second messenger production and accumulation. In addition, we have included chapters on the use of cultured cells for defining receptor systems and *in situ* hybridization for producing these membrane components.

Whereas the basic theories relating to the generation and analysis of binding data can be found in *Neurotransmitter Receptor Binding*, an effort has been made to incorporate into the manual theoretical issues on assays not covered in the book.

Our aim in preparing this laboratory guide is to provide the reader with the basic information, including lists of supplies and protocols, necessary for establishing these assays. We believe that by having a single source for this information, the task of assay development will be simplified as compared with the more arduous procedure of extracting details from an assembly of primary source material. In all cases, the authors have had extensive experience with these assays and, in many instances, were leaders in developing these procedures. Besides procedural matters, the strengths and weaknesses of each assay are delineated as well as some of the more common difficulties associated with their execution and data analyses. Our hope is that by simplifying the development of these assays, more investigators will take advantage of them in designing their programs, thereby expanding their research capabilities. As in the past, such an application of technologies should lead to more rapid advances in the field.

H. I. Yamamura
S. J. Enna
M. J. Kuhar

Contents

Contributors

David B. Bylund   *Department of Pharmacology, University of Nebraska, Omaha, Nebraska 68105*

Ronald S. Duman   *Department of Psychiatry, Yale University School of Medicine, New Haven, Connecticut 06510*

S. J. Enna   *Nova Pharmaceutical Corporation, 6200 Freeport Center, Baltimore, Maryland 21224*

Stephen J. Hill   *Department of Physiology and Pharmacology, Medical School, Queen's Medical Centre, Clifton Boulevard, Nottingham, NG7 2UH, United Kingdom*

Morley D. Hollenberg   *Endocrine Research Group, Department of Pharmacology and Therapeutics, University of Calgary, Faculty of Medicine, 3330 Hospital Drive N.W., Calgary, Alberta, Canada T2N 1N4*

David A. Kendall   *Department of Physiology and Pharmacology and Department of Medicine, Medical School, Queen's Medical Centre, Clifton Boulevard, Nottingham NG7 2UH, United Kingdom*

William J. Kinnier   *Nova Pharmaceutical Corporation, 6200 Freeport Center, Baltimore, Maryland 21224*

Michael J. Kuhar   *Neuroscience Branch, Addiction Research Center, National Institute on Drug Abuse, Baltimore, Maryland 21224*

Michael A. Pfenning   *Departments of Psychiatry and Pharmacology, Mayo Foundation, Rochester, Minnesota 55905*

Elliott Richelson   *Departments of Psychiatry and Pharmacology, Mayo Foundation, Rochester, Minnesota 55905*

Samuel J. Strada   *Department of Pharmacology, University of South Alabama College of Medicine, Mobile, Alabama 36688*

George R. Uhl   *Laboratory of Molecular Neurobiology, Addiction Research Center, National Institute on Drug Abuse, Baltimore, Maryland 21224 and the Departments of Neurology and Neuroscience, Johns Hopkins University School of Medicine, Baltimore, Maryland 21205*

James R. Unnerstall   *Departments of Neurology and Pharmacology, Case Western Reserve University School of Medicine and The Alzheimer Center, University Hospitals of Cleveland, Cleveland, Ohio 44106*

Henry I. Yamamura   *Departments of Pharmacology, Biochemistry, and Psychiatry, College of Medicine, The University of Arizona Health Sciences Center, Tucson, Arizona 85724*

METHODS IN NEUROTRANSMITTER RECEPTOR ANALYSIS

Methods in Neurotransmitter Receptor Analysis,
edited by Henry I. Yamamura, et al.
Raven Press, Ltd., New York © 1990.

1

Methods for Receptor Binding

*David B. Bylund and **Henry I. Yamamura

*Department of Pharmacology, University of Nebraska,
Omaha, Nebraska 68105; and
**Departments of Pharmacology, Biochemistry, and Psychiatry,
University of Arizona, Tucson, Arizona 85724

During the past 15 years, the radioligand-binding technique has become an important tool in many disciplines in the biological sciences, both in academic and indus-
trial laboratories. The most frequently used assay based on this technique is the
membrane receptor assay. It is the purpose of this chapter to give detailed procedures for the four basic experiments that are done using the membrane assay
system: saturation experiments, inhibition experiments, association kinetic experiments, and dissociation kinetic experiments. These methods are applicable to most
known neurotransmitter and hormone receptor systems, and there are literally hun-
dreds of radioligands available so that nearly any system can be profitably studied.
(For a more in-depth discussion of the ideas presented in this chapter, particularly of
a theoretical nature, the reader is referred to the chapter by Bennett and Yamamura,
entitled "Neurotransmitter, Hormone, or Drug Receptor Binding Methods" in ref.
1.) In this chapter, general considerations that are applicable to all four of the types
of experiments will be covered first, and then the details of each of the experiments
will be given. Table 9 includes a list of suggested conditions for binding assays of
some of the more well-known receptors.

GENERAL CONSIDERATIONS

Radioligand

Choice of Radioligand

For any given receptor system there are generally several radioligands available
commercially, and the investigator must make a decision as to which radioligand to
use. The factors to be considered in choosing the radioligand include the characteristics of the radioligand, the scientific question that is to be answered using radio-

ligand-binding assay, the facilities available, and the experience and personal preference of the investigator.

Characteristics of the Radioligand

The first characteristic of the radioligand to be considered is whether it contains ^{3}H or ^{125}I as the radioisotope. One of the advantages of ^{3}H is that the radioligand can be left unaltered and thus biologically indistinguishable from the unlabeled compound. By contrast, the addition of an iodine atom to a compound may alter its biological activity. A second advantage of ^{3}H is its longer half-life of about 12 years as opposed to 60 days for ^{125}I. Because of its short half-life, iodinated radioligands are usually purchased or prepared every 4 to 6 weeks. The main advantage of the iodinated radioligands is their higher specific activity which can be up to 2200 Ci/mmol as opposed to ^{3}H-radioligands which are usually in the range of 30 to 100 Ci/mmol. Radioligands containing ^{125}I, but not those containing ^{3}H, can be prepared in the investigator's laboratory if desired, thereby reducing the cost.

A second characteristic to be considered is the affinity of the radioligand for the receptor. As a general rule, the higher the affinity, the better. This is because a lower concentration of the radioligand can be used with a resulting lower level of nonspecific binding. Furthermore, the higher the affinity of the ligand, the slower the rate of dissociation, which in turn usually provides for a more convenient assay. However, a high specific activity must go hand in hand with a high affinity. Neither a radioligand of very high affinity with low specific activity nor one of high specific activity and low affinity is particularly useful. For iodinated radioligands, the affinities should be in the pM range, whereas ^{3}H-radioligands generally have affinitities in the nM range.

Finally, one needs to consider the ratio of specific to nonspecific binding and will generally choose the radioligand with the lower nonspecific binding since this improves the quality of the assay. The percent of the total binding which is specific binding is a useful index of the relative amount of nonspecific binding. A value of 50% is considered barely adequate; 70% is good, and 90% is excellent.

Considerations Related to the Question Being Asked

Two important characteristics to be considered are whether the radioligand is an agonist or an antagonist and what is the selectivity of the radioligand for receptor types and subtypes. Agonist radioligands may label only a portion of the total receptor population, the so-called high affinity state for receptors coupled to G-proteins, whereas antagonist ligands generally label all available receptors. On the other hand, an agonist radioligand may reflect more accurately receptor alterations of biological significance, since it is agonists that are biologically active in producing an effect.

Although no radioligand is completely selective for any given receptor, some are better than others. For example, the radioligand spiroperidol labels dopamine receptors in the corpus striatum but serotonin receptors in the cerebral cortex. Some α-adrenergic radioligands label both α-1 and α-2 adrenergic receptors, whereas others are selective for one or the other subtype. The β-adrenergic antagonist cyanopindolol also can label 5-hydroxytryptamine (serotonin) receptors (5-HT$_{1B}$). Thus, if you wish to study both α-1 and α-2 adrenergic receptors, a ligand that labels both receptors with similar affinities might be the best choice. Cyanopindolol might be a good choice for labeling 5-HT$_{1B}$ receptors in a tissue that does not contain β-adrenergic receptors.

Facilities

The choice of whether a ^{3}H- or ^{125}I-radioligand will be used may depend in part on the availability of scintillation counters. ^{125}I-Ligands can be quantitated using either a γ-counter or liquid scintillation counter, whereas the use of ^{3}H-ligands necessitates access to a liquid scintillation counter. One advantage of using a γ-counter is cost, since a liquid scintillation cocktail, which can be fairly expensive, is not needed.

Storage and Dilution of Radioligand

Most radioligands are stored in an aqueous solution that often contains an organic solvent such as ethanol. The solutions should be stored cold but not frozen, since freezing of the solution tends to concentrate the radioligand locally and increase the amount of radiolytic destruction of the ligand. Commercially available radioligands generally come as a solution with a concentration of 1 μCi/μl. For diluting the radioligand, an aqueous solution containing a small amount of acid (e.g., 5 mM HCl) works very well. The rationale for using the acid is that it tends to reduce the amount of nonspecific binding of the radioligand to the test tubes that are used to make the dilutions. For some radioligands, if an aqueous solution buffered at neutral pH is used, about 25% of the radioligand may be bound to the test tube. Since such stock solutions are usually diluted 50-fold (20 μl to 1.0 ml) in the final assay mixture, the small amount of acid which is carried over into the assay mixture is not sufficient to alter the pH.

Tissue

Preparation

Preparation of the tissue that contains the receptor of interest is usually fairly easy. A standard procedure is to homogenize the tissue in a hypotonic buffer using either a Polytron (Brinkmann Instruments) or a Tissumizer (Tekmar), which breaks cells and membranes into small pieces. This homogenate is then centrifuged at high speed, generally as fast as possible without using an ultracentrifuge (i.e., $50,000 \times g$) for about 10 min. Centrifugations are routinely carried out at 4°C, although for many receptors this is probably not necessary. Following centrifugation, the pellet is rehomogenized in the same buffer and centrifuged again. The resulting tissue preparation is variously called a crude particulate fraction or a membrane fraction. The purpose of the two centrifugation steps is to remove any soluble interfering substances such as endogenous neurotransmitters and guanine nucleotides which may interfere with the radioligand-binding assay. The choice of buffer for the homogenization is generally not critical; any buffer at neutral pH appears to be sufficient for most receptor preparations. For some receptor assays it is recommended that either ethylenediaminetetraacetate (EDTA) be added to the homogenization buffer and/or an incubation (20 min at 37°C) be done after the second homogenization (but before the second centrifugation) in order to more completely remove endogenous substances.

Storage

Most receptor preparations are stable to freezing and can be stored at $-20°C$ or $-80°C$ for extended periods of time. They can be stored either as the original tissue or after the first homogenization/centrifugation, as a pellet. Experience indicates that some receptors and small pieces of tissue (less than 5 mg) do not store well, and thus in these particular cases, the assay should be run on fresh tissue.

Tissue Concentration

Within reason the higher the tissue (receptor) concentration, the better the binding. It is also likely that increasing the receptor concentration will increase the ratio of specific to nonspecific binding, since a large portion of the nonspecific binding is to the glass fiber filter. However, too much tissue can lead to artifacts, and the rule of thumb is that if more than 10% of the added radioligand is bound, then the tissue concentration is too high. Furthermore, the amount of specific binding should be linearly related to the tissue concentration. A useful control experiment is to determine specific binding at several different tissue concentrations, plot the results, and then use a tissue concentration on the linear portion of the curve for future experiments (Fig. 1). For most receptor assays, a tissue concentration in the range of 2 to 10 mg, original wet weight, of tissue/ml is used. For many tissues, this corresponds to about 100 to 500 µg of membrane protein/ml.

Definition of Specific Binding

One of the most important considerations in any radioligand-binding assay is the determination of specific binding. Conceptually, specific binding can be defined as

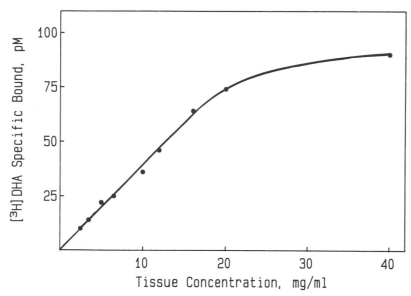

FIG. 1. Tissue concentration curve. In this experiment, a preparation of rat brain cerebral cortex at the indicated concentrations (original wet weight/ml) was incubated with 0.4 nM [³H]DHA in a final volume of 1.0 ml, and specific binding was determined. This experiment can be thought of as a saturation experiment in which the radioligand concentration is held constant, and the receptor concentration is increased.

binding to the receptor of interest. Nonspecific binding is any other observed binding. Operationally, nonspecific binding is the observed binding in the presence of an appropriate excess of unlabeled drug to block fully the receptors of interest. Nonspecific binding includes binding of the radioligand to glass fiber filters, absorption to the tissue, and dissolution in the membrane lipids. Specific binding is calculated as the difference between the total binding and nonspecific binding. Characteristically, nonspecific binding attains steady state more rapidly than specific binding and does not saturate as the concentration of radioligand is increased. As a rule of thumb, concentration of unlabeled drug should be 100 to 1000 times its concentration required to displace 50% of ligand binding (IC_{50}) at the concentration of radioligand used. For a simple, well-behaved binding system, a concentration of unlabeled ligand 100 times IC_{50} will occupy 99% of the receptor binding sites. It is important that the concentration of drug used to define nonspecific binding not be too high, since high concentrations of the drug may also inhibit nonspecific (nonreceptor) binding. Inhibition experiments (see "Inhibition Experiments") will provide a good check on the definition of nonspecific binding since all unlabeled ligands should inhibit to the nonspecific binding level.

In choosing a drug to determine nonspecific binding it is best to use a drug that is chemically dissimilar from the radioligand. This is due to the possibility of the drug inhibiting specific but nonreceptor binding sites. There are many examples in the literature in which a poor choice of the drug or concentration to determine non-specific binding has led to inadequate data and wrong conclusions.

Assay Conditions

Time of Incubation

For saturation and inhibition experiments, the theoretical model used is one of equilibrium. Thus, the time of incubation needs to be sufficient to assure that equilibrium has been reached. Since it is difficult to demonstrate that a true equilibrium has been attained, most investigators find it sufficient to demonstrate that steady state has been achieved. It is important to remember that the time to reach steady state is dependent upon the radioligand concentration used. Thus, in determining the appropriate incubation time, a low concentration of radioligand should be used. Many radioligands appear to reach steady state at room temperature within 20 min to 1 hr. A simple experiment to check that steady state has been reached is to incubate for various times, for example 10, 20, 30, 40, and 60 min. If the binding is constant between 20 and 60 min, then a 30-min incubation for additional experiments would be appropriate.

Temperature

It is most convenient to perform the assay at room temperature (about 22°C) although some investigators think that a physiological temperature (37°C) is better. In addition, some assays are run on ice (about 4°C) because it has been found empirically that the data are more reproducible at this temperature. Possible reasons for this more reproducible binding at low temperatures are decreased degradation of the radioligand, lower nonspecific binding in some cases, and the fact that some radioligands have higher affinity for the receptor at lower temperatures.

Buffer and pH

Generally, the pH should be in the physiological range between pH 7 and 8. [Tris(hydroxymethyl)aminomethane] (Tris) buffer is often used but it is not necessarily the best, and it is often advantageous to try other buffers in order to obtain optimum binding. A major reason for the popularity of Tris buffers is convenience, since they can be purchased at a preset pH, and thus pH adjustment is not needed.

Ions and Guanosine 5'-Triphosphate (GTP)

Monovalent cations such as Na^+ and divalent cations such as Mg^{2+} are often added to the incubation buffer in various assays, depending on both the radioligand

and receptor system. These ions can either enhance or inhibit the binding of the radioligand and can either increase or decrease the affinity of competing ligands for the receptor site. Similarly, guanyl nucleotides such as GTP (or the nonhydrolyzable analogue guanyl-5′-yl imidodiphosphate [Gpp(NH)p] are frequently added to incubation buffers at a concentration of about 100 μM. GTP generally decreases the affinity of agonists for the receptor and may convert a complex (biphasic) inhibition curve to a simple (single site) inhibition curve. As a general rule, it is probably best not to include these components in the incubation mixture unless their effect is known and that effect is wanted in a particular assay.

Separation of Bound Radioligand from Free Radioligand

Filtration

A crucial component of the receptor binding assay is the separation of bound radioligand from free radioligand. In carrying out the separation, it is important to prevent significant dissociation of the receptor-radioligand complex, since this is the parameter that is measured. This can be done by reducing the temperature in order to slow the rate of dissociation and by performing the separation as rapidly as possible. For membrane-binding assays, the technique most often used is vacuum filtration through glass fiber filters. The membrane fragments that contain the radioligand-receptor complex are retained by the filter, and the free radioligand passes through the filter.

A second goal is to minimize the amount of nonspecific binding. Thus, the membranes and the filter are washed with large amounts of buffer which preferentially reduce nonspecific binding. In addition, the filter may be prerinsed with certain solutions (e.g., 0.1% aqueous polyethylenimine) that are designed to decrease nonspecific binding to the filter. In certain assays, the choice of the filter material may be very important.

The advantages of the filtration assay are that it is rapid and convenient. Its disadvantages are that it can generally be used only with radioligand-receptor complexes having affinities higher than about 10 nM and that the majority of the nonspecific binding is frequently to the filter itself rather than to the tissue preparation.

Centrifugation

For assays in which the affinity of the radioligand for the receptor is in the 10 nM to 1 μM range or in cases in which nonspecific binding to the filter is prohibitively high, centrifugation techniques are often used. For receptor-radioligand systems in which the dissociation is too rapid to allow the use of filtration, the centrifugation technique can be used since the extent of dissociation is minimal. Centrifugation assays are frequently conducted in microcentrifuge tubes, and the tip of the tube containing the membrane preparation is simply cut off with a razor blade following a superficial rinsing of the tube and the surface of the pellet to lower nonspecific binding. In some assays, the membrane fragments are centrifuged through a layer of sucrose or "oil" in order to decrease nonspecific binding. The density of this "wash" solution is critical since it must be greater than the incubation mixture but less than that of the membranes. Alternatively, 12-ml centrifuge tubes can be used and the membranes centrifuged in a high-speed centrifuge.

Additional Considerations for Peptides

In binding assays that use a peptide radioligand, there may be some additional technical difficulties to be overcome as compared with using other compounds as radioligands. Peptides are more apt to bind nonspecifically to test tubes, plastic pipette tips, and filters and are frequently more sensitive to degradation during the assay. In order to minimize the amount of nonspecific radioligand binding to test tubes, several different types of plastic tubes should be screened, and attempts should be made to coat glass test tubes with various solutions. Frequently, an organosilane such as Prosil is used. An additional trick for basic peptides is to precoat the tubes with a mixture of 1% (v/v) polyethylenimine and 1% (v/v) Prosil (2). The tubes are rinsed once with distilled water, dried at 80°C, and then rinsed three more times and allowed to dry.

In order to prevent the degradation of peptides, various protease inhibitors are often included in peptide-binding assays. The exact combination of inhibitors to be used must be determined for each peptide. Care must be taken to ensure that each component is actually useful, as some protease inhibitors have been found to inhibit specific binding in certain assay systems.

LIST OF SUPPLIES

We have chosen to give detailed protocols for a fairly simple binding assay: β-adrenergic receptor binding in rat brain cerebral cortex using the ^{3}H-radioligand, dihydrolalprenolol or [^{3}H]DHA (3). This basic protocol can be modified for other ligands, receptors, and tissues according to the published literature and/or the experience of the investigator.

Solutions

Fifty Millimolar Tris Buffer, pH 8 (at 25°C)

This is prepared by dissolving 7.09 g of Trizma 8.0 (Sigma) in 1 liter of distilled water.

Tris Wash Buffer

Fifty-five grams of Tris base and 86 g of Tris acid are dissolved in 20 liters of distilled water. This will result in a 50 mM Tris buffer with a pH of about 8. The exact pH and the concentration of Tris are not critical, i.e., at 25 mM, pH 7.2, buffer would be fine.

Five Millimolar HCl

This is prepared by adding 5 ml of 1 M HCl to 995 ml of distilled water.

Filters and Tubes

Filters

Whatman GF/B glass fiber filters, either as circles or strips, which will fit the filter machine to be used are needed.

Glass Test Tubes

Borosilicate glass tubes (12×75 mm) are used to prepare dilutions of radioligand and unlabeled ligands.

Polypropylene Test Tubes

Polypropylene (12×75 mm) is used for the incubation tubes.

Centrifuge Tubes

Fifty-milliliter centrifuge tubes for an SS34 Sorvall or similar rotor are used.

Scintillation Cocktail

For lipophilic ligands such as [^{3}H]DHA, a nonaqueous scintillation cocktail can be used. For ligands that are less lipophilic, a more expensive aqueous cocktail must be used. A supply of plastic scintillation vials either, 20 or 7 ml, is also needed.

Tissue Preparation

1. About 500 mg of rat cerebral cortex is homogenized in approximately 35 ml of wash buffer using a Polytron (PT10-35 generator with PT10/TS probe) at setting 7 for 20 sec. The actual amount of tissue used should be recorded.
2. Centrifuge at 20,000 rpm ($48,000 \times g$) in a Sorvall RC2-B using a SS34 rotor for 10 min at 4°C.
3. Decant the supernatant, and repeat the homogenization and centrifugation.
4. Decant the supernatant; add 20 volumes of distilled water (10 ml/500 mg, original wet weight of tissue) and homogenize as before for 10 sec.
5. Take three 20- µl aliquots of this tissue suspension and use to determine protein concentration.
6. Add ice-cold incubation buffer to the suspension to dilute it to 130 volumes (a final volume of 66 ml/500 mg, original wet weight of tissue).

Ligands

Radioligand

[^{3}H]DHA (approximately 100 Ci/mmol, Du Pont-New England Nuclear) is used.

Unlabeled Ligands

(−)-Propranolol and (−)-norepinephrine (Sigma) are used.

SATURATION EXPERIMENTS

Principles

If a receptor preparation is incubated together with a radioactive ligand for a period of time, some amount of a radioligand-receptor complex will form. This can be represented by

$$L + R \rightleftarrows RL$$

In a saturation experiment, the amount of radioligand-receptor complex is measured as a function of the free radioligand concentration. The parameters obtained from this type of an experiment are the affinity, usually expressed as the dissociation constant, K_D, and the number of binding sites, B_{max}. The mathematical equation that relates the concentration of the radioligand-receptor complex (RL, also called B for bound) and the free radioligand concentration (L, also called F for free) is:

$$B = B_{max} \cdot F/(K_D + F) \tag{1}$$

(This equation describes a rectangular hyperbola and is mathematically equivalent to the Michaelis-Menten equation of enzyme kinetics.) A particularly useful point on the saturation curve is where the free radioligand concentration is equal to the K_D. At this point, the bound radioligand is simply equal to one-half the B_{max}. In other words the K_D is the concentration of radioligand that results in half-maximal specific binding.

It should be noted that the free radioligand concentration is the value needed in this equation, whereas it is the total radioligand concentration that is generally known. The free radioligand concentration can be approximated by subtracting the bound concentration from the total concentration. Since the bound concentration should be less than 10% of the total radioligand concentration, this is usually a fairly good approximation.

It is best to use at least a 100-fold concentration range for the radioligand in saturation experiments, particularly if the intent is to show that only a single class of binding sites is labeled. Ideally, one should go from a concentration ten-fold below the K_D to a concentration ten-fold above the K_D.

Procedure

1. Prepare tissue as described above (see "Tissue Preparation").
2. Radioligand dilutions. Six microliters of [^{3}H]DHA (1 μCi/μl) is diluted into 550 μl of 5 mM HCl in a glass test tube. This solution is thoroughly mixed, and a 200-μl aliquot is added to 300 μl of 5 mM HCl. Successive dilutions are prepared in the same manner by adding 200 μl of each dilution to 300 μl of 5 mM HCl to get the next lower dilution until six different concentrations of radioligand have been prepared. This is sufficient radioligand for three saturation curves. Table 1 shows how various concentration ranges of radioligand can be prepared.
3. Set up a rack of 24 polypropylene incubation tubes, six tubes across and four tubes deep.
4. Prepare a set of 12 uncapped scintillation vials with GF/A glass fiber filter discs on top. Duplicate 20-μl aliquots of each of the six concentrations of radioligand will be pipetted directly onto the filter paper to determine the total added radioactivity. (GF/B filters can be used for this purpose, but GF/A filters are less expensive.)
5. To the 12 tubes on the last two rows add 10 μl of a 10 mM norepinephrine solution. This solution is prepared by adding 3.2 mg of (−)-norepinephrine to 1.0 ml of 5 mM HCl.
6. To all 24 tubes add 970 μl of the tissue preparation.
7. Twenty microliters of the most dilute radioligand solution (tube 1) is added to the first column of four tubes and the two filter papers for the determination of total added radioactivity. The next most dilute solution (tube 2) is then added to the next of four tubes and two filter papers, and so on, up through radioligand tube 6.

TABLE 1. *Preparation of radioligand dilutions*

µl Radioligand	600	550	500	400	333	300
µl Diluent	400	450	500	600	667	700
Tube No.			Relative concentration			
1	1	1	1	1	1	1
2	1.7	1.8	2	2.5	3	3.3
3	2.8	3.3	4	6.2	9	11
4	4.6	6	8	16	27	37
5	7.7	11	16	39	81	123
6	13	20	32	98	243	
7	21	36	64	244		
8	36	66	128			
9	60	120	256			
10	100	217				

This table can serve as a guide for preparing appropriate dilutions of radioligand. First, choose the number of concentrations wanted and the concentration range to be covered. For example, assume that six concentrations over a 100-fold range are desired. For 6 concentrations, the fifth column of the table indicates a 98-fold range. The concentrations are prepared by adding an aliquot of a stock radioligand solution (the amount added will determine the actual concentrations) to tube, 6, which contains diluent, to give a final volume of 1.0 ml. This solution is thoroughly mixed, and a 400-µl aliquot is added to tube 5, which already contains 600 µl of diluent. After mixing, 400 µl of tube 5 is added to tube 4, which contains 600 µl of diluent. This procedure is repeated for tubes 3, 2, and 1.

8. The tubes are vortexed and then incubated at room temperature for 45 min.
9. The contents of the tubes are filtered and washed twice with 5 ml of ice-cold wash buffer.
10. The filters are placed into 20-ml scintillation vials, and 10 ml of scintillation cocktail is added.
11. The scintillation vials are shaken gently for 1 hr or left at room temperature overnight and then counted in a liquid scintillation counter.

Calculations

Initial Data Analysis

The first step in calculating the results of a saturation experiment is to determine the mean of the duplicate cpm values obtained from the scintillation counter. Three columns of six numbers are obtained. The first column is "total added"; the second column is "total binding," which is the binding to the membranes in the absence of norepinephrine; and column 3 is "nonspecific binding" or the binding in the presence of norepinephrine. Data from a typical experiment are shown in Table 2. The next step is to subtract nonspecific binding (column 3) from total binding (column 2) to obtain "specific binding" (column 4). The final step in the initial data reduction is to determine the amount of "free" radioligand concentration (column 5) by subtracting the specific binding (column 4) from the total added (column 1).

TABLE 2. *Data and calculations for a typical saturation experiment*

Experimental data					Calculated values		
Total added	Total binding	Nonspecific binding	Specific binding	Free	Specific binding	Free	Bound/ Free
1	2	3	4	5	6	7	8
		cpm				*pM*	
2,625	436	176	260	2,365	3.04	28	0.110
6,168	886	312	574	5,594	6.71	65	0.103
15,111	1,629	424	1,205	13,906	14.1	162	0.087
36,569	3,004	767	2,237	34,332	26.2	401	0.065
90,326	5,449	2,345	3,104	87,222	36.3	1,018	0.036
226,729	10,483	6,541	3,942	222,787	46.1	2,600	0.018

Saturation Plot

Although this plot is not routinely constructed, it is instructive from time to time to plot the data in this way in order to visualize the relationship between specific and nonspecific binding. A typical saturation plot is made by plotting the amount of bound radioactivity (total bound, nonspecific bound, and specifically bound) on the ordinate and the free concentration of the radioligand on the abscissa (using an arithmetic scale) as is shown in Fig. 2. As can be seen from the figure, the nonspecific binding is a straight line that will be parallel to the total binding curve at high concentrations of radioligand. The specific binding curve tends to level off or saturate at high radioligand concentration.

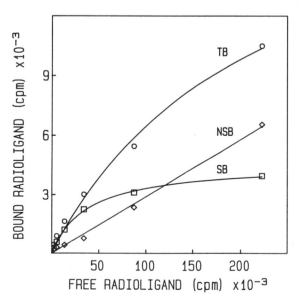

FIG. 2. Saturation plot. Total (*TB*), specific (*SB*), and nonspecific binding (*NSB*) are plotted as a function of free radioligand concentration using the data in Table 2.

Since a large concentration range of free radioligand is frequently used, it may be more convenient to plot the data on a semilogarithmic plot. As shown in Fig. 3, the specific binding is plotted on the ordinate versus the free radioligand concentration plotted on a logarithmic scale on the abscissa. In a semilogarithmic plot of saturation data, the curve typically has an S shape if the radioligand is labeling a single class of binding sites.

The data can be plotted as cpm, as was done in Fig. 2 and 3, or as pM by converting the cpm values to the concentrations. In order to do this, the cpm value is multiplied by a factor f which takes into account the specific activity of the radioligand, the incubation volume, and the efficiency of the scintillation counter

$$f = \frac{1}{\text{specific activity}} \cdot \frac{1}{\text{volume}} \cdot \frac{1}{\text{efficiency}} \cdot \frac{\text{Ci}}{2.2 \times 10^{12} \text{ dpm}} \qquad [2]$$

The final number in this equation is simply the definition of a Curie in terms of dpm. For our experiment, the specific activity of [^{3}H]DHA was 95 Ci/mmol, the incubation volume was 1.0 ml, and the efficiency of the scintillation counter was 41%; f is calculated as follows:

$$f = \frac{\text{mmol}}{95 \text{ Ci}} \cdot \frac{1}{1 \text{ ml}} \cdot \frac{\text{dpm}}{0.41 \text{ cpm}} \cdot \frac{\text{Ci}}{2.2 \times 10^{12} \text{ dpm}}$$

$$f = 1.17 \times 10^{-14} \frac{\text{mmol}}{\text{ml}} \cdot \frac{1}{\text{cpm}} = 0.0117 \text{ pM/cpm}$$

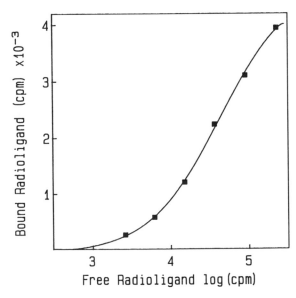

FIG. 3. Semilog saturation plot. Specific binding is plotted as a function of the log of free radioligand concentration using the data in Table 2.

Using this factor, then one can calculate the concentration of specifically bound radioligand in pM (column 6) by multiplying the values in column 4 by the factor. Similarly, the concentration of free radioligand pM (column 7) is determined by multiplying the values in column 5 by the factor.

Rosenthal (Scatchard) Analysis

With the data plotted according to Eq. 1 as shown in Fig. 2, it is difficult to determine K_D and B_{max} values since the relationship is nonlinear. However, this equation can be transformed to give a linear relationship. For binding studies, the most frequently used linear transformation is the Rosenthal equation or plot (4). The Rosenthal equation is generally given as

$$\frac{B}{F} = \frac{-1}{K_D} B - \frac{B_{max}}{K_D} \qquad [3]$$

This equation is graphically presented in Fig. 4. In a Rosenthal plot, the ratio of bound to free radioligand is plotted versus the bound radioligand. The K_D is the negative reciprocal of the slope, and the B_{max} is the intercept on the x-axis. It should be noted that this equation is of the form $y = mx + c$, where y is equal to B/F, m is equal to $-1/K_D$, x is equal to B, and c is equal to B_{max}/K_D. Thus, B_{max} and K_D can be determined either by plotting the data as shown in Fig. 4 or by performing linear regression analysis using a calculator or computer.

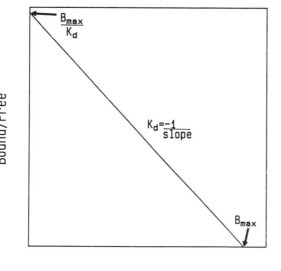

Bound

FIG. 4. Graphic representation of the Rosenthal equation.

METHODS FOR RECEPTOR BINDING

For the typical experiment being considered, the B/F is given in column 8 of Table 2. (The values in column 8 can be calculated by dividing column 4 by column 5 or by dividing column 6 by column 7). The data are graphed as a Rosenthal plot in Fig. 5. The K_D calculated by linear regression is 0.46 nM, and the B_{max} is 54 pM. Once the B_{max} value is determined, the density of binding sites can be calculated in either pmol/g, wet weight of tissue or fmol/mg of protein by simply dividing by the tissue concentration or protein concentration in the assay. Thus for our example

$$B_{max} = \frac{54 \text{ pmol}}{1} \cdot \frac{0.066 \text{ l}}{0.5 \text{ g tissue}} = 7.1 \text{ pmol/g tissue}$$

In this experiment, the protein concentration in the incubation tube was 0.34 mg/ml. Thus,

$$B_{max} = 54 \text{ pmol/l} \times \text{ml/0.34 mg} = 160 \text{ fmol/mg protein}$$

In a saturation experiment plotted according to the Rosenthal equation, the data points will be fairly evenly distributed from the ordinate to the abscissa, if the appropriate concentration range was chosen for the radioligand.

This transformation is commonly called a Scatchard plot. This name is incorrect since the Scatchard derivation assumes that the molecular weight and concentration of the receptor are known. The Rosenthal derivation does not make these assumptions. Nevertheless, in the literature Rosenthal plots are often incorrectly designated as Scatchard plots.

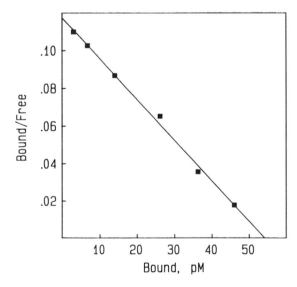

FIG. 5. Rosenthal plot of saturation data. Specific binding divided by free radioligand concentration is plotted versus specific binding using the data in Table 2.

Additional Comments

It is also possible to plot the data in units of fmol/mg of protein rather than in units of pM. This is particularly useful for comparing several different experiments that were done at different protein concentrations. In order to do this, the bound concentration column 6 is simply divided by the protein concentration, then bound over free is calculated from this new value of specific binding.

Saturation experiments sometimes turn out to be more complex than the simple case just described. For example, consider the possibility of two classes of binding sites rather than just one class. For purposes of illustration, assume there is a higher affinity site that has a K_D of 1.0 and a B_{max} of 1.0 and a lower affinity site that has a K_D of 20 and a B_{max} of 5. If these two sites are independent, then the total binding observed will simply be the sum of the binding at each of the two sites. When the data from such an experiment are graphed, a curvilinear Rosenthal plot results as shown in Fig. 6. Also shown on the graph are two straight lines each representing one of the two binding sites. One nice feature of the Rosenthal plot is that the sum of these two lines gives the curve of the data points. Thus, for any line drawn through the origin (i.e., any free concentration of radioligand), the sum of the distances to the lines representing the two sites is equal to the distance to the curve.

If a curvilinear Rosenthal plot is attained, and the decision is made to analyze the data as two independent binding sites, it is best to use a computer to determine the two K_D and B_{max} values (see Chapter 2). However, it is still a good idea to check the values obtained by simply substituting them back into the two-site equation to see how closely the original data are reproduced.

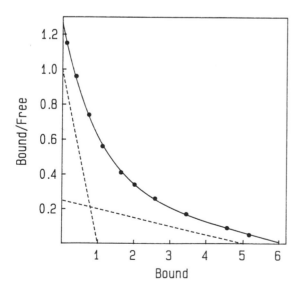

FIG. 6. Curvilinear Rosenthal plot. These are hypothetical data generated using Eq. 4 with $K_D^1 = 1.0$, $K_D^2 = 20$, $B_{max}^1 = 1.0$, and $B_{max}^2 = 5$. The steeper line represents the higher affinity site ($K_D^1 = 1$), and the shallower line is the lower affinity site ($K_D^2 = 20$).

$$B = B^1 + B^2 = \frac{B_{max}^1 \cdot F}{K_D^1 + F} \cdot \frac{B_{max}^2 \cdot F}{K_D^2 + F} \qquad [4]$$

It should be emphasized that there are many possible reasons for curvilinear Rosenthal plots. The existence of two independent classes of binding sites is only one of the possible interpretations. Other possible reasons include negative cooperativity and a variety of incorrect assay procedures.

INHIBITION EXPERIMENTS

Principles

For an inhibition experiment, the receptor concentration, the radioligand concentration, and time are all constant, whereas the concentration of the unlabeled or inhibiting drug is variable. When the inhibitor concentration is zero, a fraction of the receptors will be bound with radioligand. However, as the inhibitor concentration is increased, the inhibitor will compete with the radioligand for the receptor binding site. This will decrease the concentration of free receptor and thus the concentration of radioligand-receptor complex. The equation relating the concentration of bound radioligand to the inhibitor concentration (I) is:

$$B = \frac{B_{max} \cdot F}{F + K_D (1 + I/K_i)} \qquad [5]$$

In this equation, K_i is the inhibition constant and is the affinity of the inhibitor for the receptor. Inhibition data are generally visualized by plotting the amount of bound radioligand on the ordinate and the logarithm of the concentration of the inhibitor on the abscissa. It is useful to define a parameter that is called the inhibitory concentration 50 or the concentration of the competing drug that inhibits 50% of the specific binding. This IC_{50} is the experimentally determined parameter and is always greater than or equal to the K_i.

In the simplest case, as the concentration of inhibitor is increased over a 100-fold range from one-tenth the IC_{50} to ten times the IC_{50}, the amount of radioligand specifically bound decreases from approximately 90 to 10% of the binding in the absence of inhibitor. This provides a good method for checking quickly whether the data are consistent with a simple one-site model. Simply check tenfold below and tenfold above the IC_{50} to determine if binding is approximately 90 and 10%, respectively. Note that IC_{50} is dependent upon the concentration of radioligand used in the experiment, whereas K_i is independent of radioligand concentration. A useful rule is that when the concentration of radioligand is equal to its K_D, the K_i for the inhibitor will be one-half of the IC_{50}.

The incubation time needs to be sufficiently long so that the binding of the unlabeled or competing drug as well as the radioligand is at steady state. It is important to realize that high-affinity competing ligands may take longer to reach steady state than the radioligand.

Procedure

1. Prepare tissue as described above under "Tissue Preparation."
2. Radioligand: The radioligand concentration used in an inhibition experiment should be less than its K_D value. The concentration of tissue and/or the incubation volume should be adjusted so that less than 10% of the radioligand is bound. Add 4 μl of stock [^{3}H]DHA (1 μCi/μl) to 3.2 ml of 5 mM HCl. This is sufficient radioligand for six inhibition experiments.
3. Inhibitor or competing ligand: Various concentrations of the inhibitor are prepared with an equal number of concentrations above and below the IC_{50} value. Typically, approximately nine concentrations of the inhibitor are used. A concentration spacing of half-log units is frequently appropriate. Since the inhibitor will be diluted 100-fold in the assay, the stock solutions are made up 100-fold more concentrated. For example, 1.0 and 0.3 mM solutions of the inhibitor can be prepared, and then each of these can be sequentially diluted tenfold in 5 mM HCl to give the appropriate concentrations as is shown in Table 3.
   Prepare a 1.0 mM solution of (−)-propranolol by dissolving 3.0 mg of (−)-propranolol in 10 ml of 5 mM HCl. Dilute 0.3 ml of this solution with 0.7 ml of 5 mM HCl to give a 0.3 mM solution. Prepare 100 μM, 10 μM, 1 μM, 100 nM, 10 nM, and 1 nM solutions by sequentially diluting 100 μl of the previous solution (i.e., tenfold higher concentration) with 900 μl of 5 mM HCl. Similarly, prepare 30 μM, 3 μM, 300 nM, and 30 nM solutions from the 0.3 mM solution.
4. Set up 24 assay tubes in two rows of 12. The first and last pairs of tubes receive 10 μl of the diluent, and the 11th pair of tubes receives 10 μl of 10 mM (−)-

TABLE 3. *Dilution of inhibitor*

Concentration of inhibitor in stock solution	Concentration of inhibitor in assay
1 mM	10 μM
0.3 mM	3 μM
100 μM	1 μM
30 μM	300 nM
10 pM	100 nM
3 μM	30 nM
1 μM	10 nM
300 nM	3 nM
100 nM	1 nM
30 nM	0.3 nM
10 nM	0.1 nM
3 nM	0.03 nM
1 nM	0.01 nM

norepinephrine (3.2 mg in 1 ml of 5 mM HCl) as a check on nonspecific binding (see Table 4). Pairs of tubes 2 through 10 receive 10 μl of the appropriate dilution of the inhibitor.

5. Tissue preparation (970 μl) is added to each of the 24 tubes.
6. [³H]DHA (20 μl) is added to the tubes to start the incubation. The total added radioactivity is also determined by pipetting 20 μl of the [³H]DHA solution onto duplicate GF/A glass fiber filter discs.
7. The assay is incubated for 45 min at room temperature.
8. The contents of the tubes are filtered and washed twice with 5 ml of ice-cold wash buffer.
9. The filters are placed into 20-ml scintillation vials, and 10 ml of scintillation cocktail is added.
10. The scintillation vials are gently shaken for 1 hr or left at room temperature overnight and then counted in a liquid scintillation counter.

Calculations

The calculations for an inhibition experiment are somewhat simpler than that for saturation experiments. The first step is to determine the mean of the duplicate cpm values. These values can then be directly plotted on a semilog plot to give a typical inhibition curve (Fig. 7). Note that it is total binding that has been plotted and not specific binding. As with the saturation data, this initial plot is curvilinear and thus is not well suited to determining IC_{50}.

One useful way of linearizing the data is called a logit-log plot. The data are first calculated in terms of percent bound (P) where 100% is the amount specifically bound in the absence of the competing drug. This is done by first taking the mean of the diluent tubes (tubes 1 and 12) and subtracting the mean of the nonspecific values (NSB; in this case, tubes 10 and 11). This is the 100% value, or B_0. For tubes 2 through 9, P is calculated by subtracting the nonspecific binding from the amount bound (B); dividing by B_0, and multiplying by 100:

$$P = \frac{B - NSB}{B_0} \times 100$$

The logit transformation is the natural logarithm (ln) of the ratio of percent bound to 100 minus the percent bound.

$$\text{logit} = \ln [P/(100 - P)]$$

The IC_{50} is 50% binding, and the logit of 50% [ln(1)] is 0. Thus, the IC_{50} can be determined either by linear correlation or by plotting the data and graphically determining the IC_{50}. Special logit graph paper is available (Team, Box 25, Tamworth, NH 03886) which allows one to plot the data directly as percent bound (see Fig. 8). In this example, the IC_{50} is 1.0 nM. From the slope of the logit plot one can determine the Hill coefficient (n_H). The slope is determined either from the linear regres-

TABLE 4. *Inhibition assay*

Tube no. (in duplicate)	Addition (10 µl)	Final concentration	Abbreviated notation[a]	Tube no. (in duplicate)	Addition (10 µl)	Final concentration	Abbreviated notation[a]
		nM				*nM*	
1	Diluent			7	1 µM propranolol	10	1–8
2	1 nM propranolol	0.01	1–11	8	3 µM propranolol	30	3–8
3	10 nM propranolol	0.1	1–10	9	10 µM propranolol	100	1–7
4	30 nM propranolol	0.3	3–10	10	100 µM propranolol	1µM	1–6
5	100 nM propranolol	1.0	1–9	11	10 mM norepinephrine	100µM	1–4
6	300 nM propranolol	3	3–9	12	diluent		

[a]The abbreviated notation is simply an indication of the final concentration: 1–6 means 1×10^{-6} M or 1 µM. Total binding (tube receiving diluent) is determined twice as a control for the start versus end of the assay and because it will be used to express the other values.

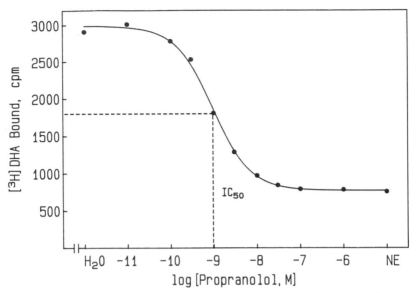

FIG. 7. Inhibition curve. For this experiment, the total added [³H]DHA was 41,682 cpm, and the estimated free radioligand, F, is total added $- B_o$ (41,682 $-$ 2,258) $=$ 39,424. By multiplying by the factor $f = 0.0117$ pM/cpm (see "Saturation Plot," above), the free concentration is 0.46 nM.

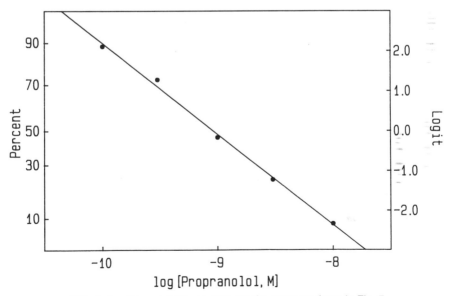

FIG. 8. Logit-log plot. These data are the same as those in Fig. 7.

sion using a calculator or a computer or graphically by determining the logit of the amount bound at two concentrations Cl and C2 of inhibitor that are two orders of magnitude apart. The equation for determining the n_H is $n_H = $ (logit [Cl] − logit [C2])/2(2.3). For the illustrated experiment with Cl = 0.1 nM and C2 = 10 nM, $n_H = [2.22 - (2.43)]/4.6 = 1.01$. The logit-log plot and the Hill plot are identical except that the natural logarithm is used in the former whereas the common logarithm is used in the latter. Thus, a slope of 2.3 on the log plot would be a slope of 1.0 on the Hill plot, since ln is equal to 2.303 log.

For a simple binding system with n_H equal to 1, the K_i value can be calculated from the IC$_{50}$ by the following equation (5, 6)

$$K_i = \frac{IC_{50}}{1 + F/K_D} \qquad [6]$$

where F is the free radioligand concentration and K_D is the affinity of the radioligand for the receptor. Using the example illustrated in Fig. 7 and 8, IC$_{50}$ = 1.0 nM; $F = 0.46$ nM (see legend to Fig. 7) and $K_D = 0.46$ nM. The K_D is determined in a separate saturation experiment such as that illustrated in Fig. 5. Thus, $K_i = 1.0/(1 + 0.46/0.46) = 1.0/2 = 0.5$ nM.

For more complex binding systems, this equation is not strictly valid, but often investigators will make this correction to give an apparent K_i in order to adjust for the concentration of radioligand used.

Additional Comments

Another method for plotting inhibition data is indicated in Fig. 9. Although this plot is not yet widely used, it has some advantages over the logit-log plot. In this plot, the amount of bound radioligand is plotted on the ordinate, and the inhibitor concentration is multiplied by the bound radioligand on the abscissa (7). The slope of this line is the negative reciprocal of the IC$_{50}$, and the intercept of the ordinate is B_o or the amount of binding in the absence of inhibitor. This plot is similar to the Rosenthal plot in that the negative reciprocal of the slope is the affinity. A major advantage of this plot over the logit-log plot is the data are not transformed into percent binding.

In inhibition experiments it is not unusual to obtain data that can be interpreted as indicating two independent classes of binding sites. This is similar to the two-site binding data considered previously in saturation experiments. For some hypothetical data, logit-log plot and a plot of bound versus bound × inhibitor are presented in Fig. 10. In a logit-log plot, the existence of the two classes of binding sites is often not readily apparent, whereas the bound versus bound × inhibitor plot clearly indicates the presence of two binding sites. The straight lines in the plot in Fig. 10 (*right panel*) represent the two binding sites. When data such as these are obtained experimentally, it is best to determine the four constants using computer programs. However, this type of plot provides a useful visualization of the data.

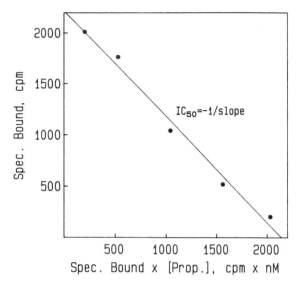

FIG. 9. Bound versus bound × inhibition plot. These data are the same as those in Fig. 7 and 8.

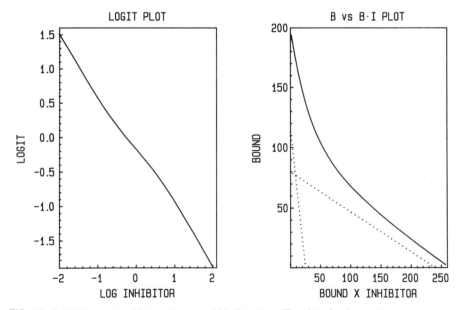

FIG. 10. Inhibition plots with two classes of binding sites. The data for these plots were generated by assuming two classes of independent binding sites, IC_{50} values of 0.2 and 3.0 nM, with 60% of the sites having the higher affinity and 40% the lower affinity. The plot on the *left* is a logit-log plot, whereas the one on the *right* is a plot of bound versus bound × inhibitor concentration (see ref. 7). Note that the presence of two classes of sites is more apparent in the plot on the *right*.

A simple inhibition curve (as in Fig. 6) does not indicate whether the inhibition is competitive or noncompetitive. One method for determining the type of inhibition is to do several saturation experiments in the presence of several concentrations of the inhibitor. A change in K_D but no change in B_{max} is indicative of competitive inhibition; a change in B_{max} but no change in K_D suggests noncompetitive inhibition.

A special case of inhibition experiments is when the inhibitor is identical to the radioligand. In this case then, inhibition and saturation experiment are really the same.

KINETIC EXPERIMENTS: ASSOCIATION

Principles

In association experiments, the amounts of receptor and radioligand are constant, and the concentration of radioligand bound to receptor is determined as a function of time. The rate of association or the rate of formation of R (the radioligand-receptor complex) is defined as dB/dt and is equal to $k_{+1} \cdot F \cdot R$ where k_{+1} is the forward rate constant or the association rate, F is the concentration of free radioligand, and R is the concentration of free receptor. This is called a second-order rate equation since two reactants are involved (radioligand and receptor).

There are two main uses for association experiments. The first is determining the time when steady state has been reached so that saturation and inhibition experiments may be properly performed. It is important to realize that the time required to reach equilibrium is dependent not only on the rate constant but also on the concentrations of radioligand and receptor. Thus, the lower the concentration of either receptor or radioligand, the longer the time that will be needed to reach steady state.

The second reason for doing association experiments is to determine the k_{+1}. Since K_D is equal to k_{-1}/k_{+1} (where k_{-1} is the dissociation rate constant), kinetic experiments provide an independent estimate of the equilibrium dissociation constant and thus provide a check on the internal consistency of the receptor-radioligand system being studied.

Procedure

1. Prepare tissue as described above (see "Tissue Preparation").
2. Radioligand: The concentration of radioligand should be reasonably low. For experiments determining the rate constant, a concentration at or below the K_D is reasonable, whereas for determining time to steady state, concentration $^1/_5$ to $^1/_{10}$, the K_D would be appropriate, if good data can still be obtained at that low a concentration.

   Dilute 4 μl of [^{3}H]DHA (1 μCi/μl) into 3.2 ml of diluent, which will give about 30,000 cpm/20 μl. This is sufficient radioligand for six 24-tube assays.

3. Prepare a 10 mM solution of (−)-norepinephrine in the diluent (3.2 mg in 1 ml).
4. Set up a rack of 12 duplicate incubation tubes. Add 10 μl of the norepinephrine solution to duplicate tubes 3, 7, and 11. These tubes will be used to determine nonspecific binding.
5. Add 970 μl of tissue to all 24 tubes.
6. Add 20 μl of radioligand to the tubes at the times indicated in Table 5. A stopwatch should be started at the time that radioligand is added to duplicate tubes 12, and all incubation tubes are filtered at 45.0 min. Total added radioligand is determined by adding 20 μl of the [^{3}H]DHA solution to duplicate GF/A glass fiber filter discs.
7. The filters are removed and counted as described as for saturation and inhibition experiments.

The above procedure assumes that a filter machine is available which will filter the 24 tubes simultaneously. If this is not the case, then the time that the radioligand is added has to be adjusted to allow for individual filtering of the samples. One sample every 15 sec is a reasonable interval.

Calculations

The first step in the calculations after averaging the duplicate values is to determine nonspecific binding. Data from a typical experiment are given in Table 6. The nonspecific binding values from the three data points (tubes 3, 7, and 11) can be averaged, plotted, or fit to a line using a linear regression program on a calculator or computer. Nonspecific binding will likely change very little during the time of the assay. The mean of the nonspecific binding values or individual values for each time point (interpolated either mathematically by linear regression or graphically)

TABLE 5. *Timed addition of radioligand for association experiments*

Tube no.	Time radioligand added	Time of incubation
	min	
1	44	1
2	43	2
3 (+NE[a])	42	3
4	41	4
5	39	6
6	37	8
7 (+NE)	36	9
8	35	10
9	25	20
10	15	30
11 (+NE)	1	44
12	0	45

[a] +NE, presence of norepinephrine.

TABLE 6. *Data and calculations for a typical association experiment*

Time of incubation	Total binding	Specific binding[a]	$\dfrac{B_e}{B_e - B}$	$\ln \dfrac{B_e}{B_e - B}$
min	*cpm*			
1	1044	301	1.23	0.210
2	1318	575	1.57	0.449
4	1430	687	1.76	0.566
6	1875	1132	3.48	1.246
8	1991	1248	4.66	1.536
10	1996	1253	4.73	1.554
20	2292	1549	39.73	3.682
30	2345	1602		
45	2319	1576		

[a]The specific binding was calculated by subtracting the mean of the three nonspecific binding estimates (tubes 3, 7, and 11 were 688, 789, and 753 cpm, respectively; mean, 743) from the total binding. Free radioligand was 35,700 cpm or 0.42 nM. B_e was determined by taking the mean of the 30- and 45-min time points (1,589 cpm).

are subtracted from each total binding to give specific binding at each time point. These values then are plotted as a function of time as shown in Fig. 11. If the purpose of the experiment is to confirm steady state, this can be done visually from the plot. If the curve has not become parallel with the *x*-axis, then longer time points need to be done.

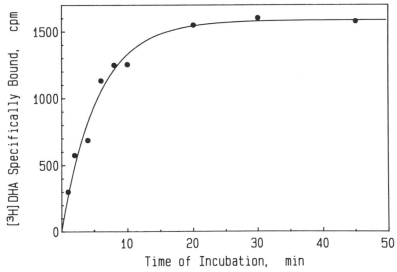

FIG. 11. Association curve. The data for this plot are given in Table 6. Using a nonlinear regression program (Graph Pad, ISI Software, Philadelphia, PA) the k_{obs} was 0.182 min^{-1} nM^{-1}, and $B_e = 1584$ cpm. Using this k_{obs}, and a $k_{-1} = 0.081$ (Fig. 14), k_{+1} was found to be 0.24 min^{-1} nM^{-1} and $K_D = 0.34$ nM.

For the calculation of k_{+1} the pseudo first-order method is used. This method assumes that the radioligand concentration is constant, which is a reasonable assumption if less than 10% of the radioligand is bound. Preferably, the data should be fit by nonlinear regression techniques (for example, see legend to Fig. 11). Alternately, the natural logarithm of the ratio of the amount of radioligand bound at steady state (B_e) divided by the difference between the radioligand bound at steady state and the amount bound at time t (B) is plotted versus time according to the equation:

$$\ln \frac{B_e}{B_e - B} = (k_{+1} \cdot F + k_{-1})t + k_{obs} \cdot t \qquad [7]$$

The graph for a typical experiment is given in Fig. 12. The parameter k_{obs} (k observed) is the slope of the plotted line). The k_{obs} from the data in Fig. 12 is 0.194 min^{-1}. If k_{-1} is known from independent experiments (see "Kinetic Experiments: Dissociation"), then k_{+1} can be calculated:

$$k_{+1} = (k_{obs} - k_{-1})/F \qquad [8]$$

For a typical dissociation experiment (see Fig. 14; the k_{-1} was found to be 0.081 min^{-1}. Thus, $k_{+1} = (0.180 - 0.081)0.42 = 0.24$ min^{-1} nM^{-1}. The K_D value can be calculated from $K_D = k_{-1}/k_{+1}$. For our typical experiment, $K_D = 0.081/0.24 = 0.34$ mM, which is in good agreement with the K_D calculated from the saturation experiment (0.45 nM, see "Rosenthal (Scatchard) Analysis").

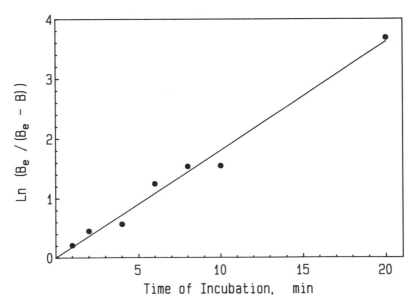

FIG. 12. Pseudo first-order association plot. The data for this plot are given in Table 6. The slope, which is k_{obs}, is 0.180 min^{-1}.

Additional Comments

It is possible to calculate both k_{+1} and k_{-1} from association experiments. This is done by determining k_{obs} at three or more different concentrations of radioligand. These concentrations should cover at least a 10-fold range. By rearranging Eq. 8, we get:

$$k_{obs} = k_{+1} \cdot F + k_{-1}$$

This equation is of the form $y = mx + b$, and thus a graph of k_{obs} versus F will have a slope of k_1 and an y-intercept of k_{-1}.

An alternate method for calculating k_{+1} is to use the second-order rate equation:

$$k_{+1} = \frac{1}{t(F - B_{max})} \ln \frac{B_{max}(F - B)}{F(B_{max} - B)}$$

where F and B_{max} are the initial (i.e., $t = 0$) free radioligand and receptor concentrations, and B is the concentration of radioligand bound to receptor at time, t. In practice, this equation is not particularly useful if less than 10% of the radioligand is bound (i.e., normal conditions for a radioligand-binding assay) since the term $F - B$ will be prone to a large error.

KINETIC EXPERIMENTS: DISSOCIATION

Principles

The dissociation rate constant, k_{-1}, can generally be determined in a relatively easy manner. The radioligand is incubated with the receptor for a period of time in order to obtain a sufficient amount of radioligand-receptor complex. Although it is not necessary to reach steady state, the assay is more convenient if conducted under steady state conditions. Further binding of radioligand to the receptor is prevented by either a 50-fold or greater dilution of the incubation mixture or the addition of excess unlabeled drug in order to occupy all the free receptors. (For example, if a 1.0 ml reaction is added to 49 ml of buffer, the rate of association would be $^{1}/_{50} \times {}^{1}/_{50}$ or $^{1}/_{2500}$ of what it was previously since the concentrations of both the radioligand and the receptor have been decreased 50-fold. An excess of unlabeled drug is defined as $100 \times$ the concentration that will occupy 50% of the sites, i.e., $100 \times IC_{50}$.) In either case, association is effectively prevented so that only the dissociation reaction is measured. The dissociation is generally a first-order process. (Radioactive decay is another example of a first-order process.)

Procedure

1. Prepare tissue as described above (see "Tissue Preparation").
2. Set up a rack of 24 assay tubes in two rows of 12.

3. Prepare a 10 mM norepinephrine solution (3.2 mg of $(-)$-norepinephrine in 1.0 ml of 5 mM HCl). Add 10 μl of this solution to the duplicate tubes 12.
4. Add 970 μl of tissue to each of the 24 tubes.
5. Dilute 4 μl of [^{3}H]DHA into 3.2 ml of diluent. This is sufficient radioligand for six 24-tube assays. Add 20 μl of this radioligand solution to each of the 24 tubes.
6. Let the tubes incubate for 30 min until steady state is reached. (A shorter incubation time can be used, but if a steady state has not been reached, then the addition of radioactivity must be timed so that all assay tubes are incubated for the identical time period.)
7. Add 10 μl of the norepinephrine solution to duplicate tube 11, start a stopwatch, and then continue to add norepinephrine as detailed in Table 7. Forty-five minutes later, the incubations are filtered, washed, and counted.

Calculations

1. The mean of the duplicate cpm values is determined. Nonspecific binding (tubes 12) is assumed to be constant and is subtracted from the total binding values. Data and calculations from a typical experiment are given in Table 8. If amount bound at the longer time points is the same as nonspecific binding, then dissociation has been complete. However, it is not necessary to obtain complete dissociation in order to estimate the k_{-1}. A dissociation curve for the typical experiment is illustrated in Fig. 13.
2. These data can be fit directly by nonlinear regression techniques to determine k_{-1}. Alternately, divide the amount bound (B) at each time point by the value obtained from tubes 1 (this is the B_0 value, or the value at time zero). The ln of B/B_0 is determined and plotted versus time (see Fig. 14), or the data can be fit by a linear regression program. The slope of this line is $-k_{-1}$; k_{-1} is also

TABLE 7. *Timed addition of competing drug for dissociation experiment*

Tube no.	Time competitor added	Time of dissociation
	min	
1	Diluent	0
2	44	1
3	43	2
4	41	4
5	39	6
6	37	8
7	35	10
8	30	15
9	25	20
10	15	30
11	0	45
12	Before radioligand	

TABLE 8. *Data and calculations for a typical dissociation experiment*

Time of dissociation	Total binding	Specific binding[a]	B/B_o	log B/B_o
min	*cpm*			
0	2326	1763	1	0
1	2036	1473	0.836	−0.180
2	1879	1316	0.746	−0.292
4	1723	1160	0.658	−0.419
6	1545	982	0.557	−0.585
8	1363	800	0.454	−0.790
10	1264	701	0.398	−0.922
15	1096	533	0.302	−1.197
20	935	372	0.211	−1.556
30	790	277	0.129	−2.050
45	602	39	0.037	−3.811

[a]The specific binding was calculated by subtracting the nonspecific binding (tube 12, 563 cpm) from the total binding.

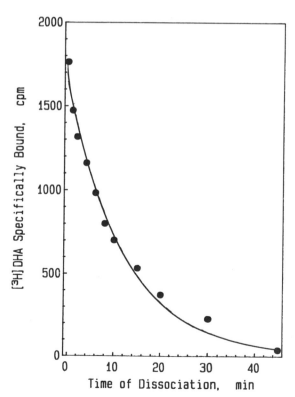

FIG. 13. Dissociation curve. The data for this plot are given in Table 8. Using a nonlinear regression program (Graph Pad) the k_{-1} was 0.081 min^{-1}.

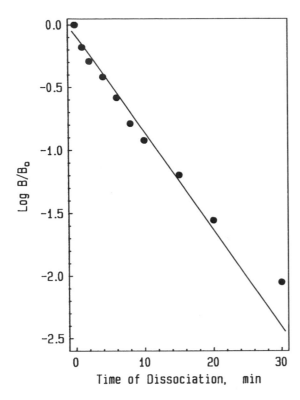

FIG. 14. Semilogarithmic plot of dissociation data. The natural logarithm (ln) of B/B_o (see Table 8) is plotted as a function of time. The slope of this line, which is k_{-1}, is 0.078 min^{-1}.

equal to $0.693/t_{1/2}$, where $t_{1/2}$ is the time at which B is equal to one-half of B_0 (ln $0.5 = 0.693$). For our typical experiment, $k_{-1} = 0.078$ min^{-1} and $t_{1/2} = 8.9$ min.

Additional Comments

An alternate procedure for dissociation experiments, particularly if a filter machine is not available, is to use one reaction mixture of 25 ml and then filter 1.0 ml aliquots at the appropriate time. Radioligand and tissue are incubated together for 30 min, and then starting at time zero, norepinephrine (100 μM final concentration) is added, and aliquots are removed at the appropriate times and filtered. This procedure would require two additional 1.0 ml tubes for the determination of nonspecific binding.

SUGGESTED CONDITIONS FOR RADIOLIGAND BINDING ASSAYS

Table 9 is a listing of the basic conditions for some of the more popular receptor binding assays. No attempt has been made to make the listing complete but rather to

TABLE 9. *Conditions for radioligand-binding assays*

Receptor	Radioligand	Agonist or antagonist	Definition of nonspecific binding	Incubation Buffer	pH	Time	Temperature
						min	°C
Adenosine							
A$_1$	[³H]Cyclohexyladenosine	Agonist	10 µM 2-CADO	50 mM Tris-HCl	7.4	120	25
A$_2$	[³H]NECA	Agonist	10 µM 2-CADO	50 mM Tris-HCl	7.4	125	25
Adrenergic							
α-1	[³H]Prazosin	Antagonist	100 µM Norepinephrine	25 mM Glycylglycine	7.4	30	25
	¹²⁵I-HEAT	Antagonist	100 µM Norepinephrine	25 mM Glycylglycine	7.4	45	25
α-2	[³H]Rauwolscine	Antagonist	10 µM Norepinephrine	25 mM Glycylglycine	7.4	45	25
	[³H]UK 14,304	Agonist	100 µM Norepinephrine	25 mM Glycylglycine	7.4	60	25
β	[³H]Dihydroalprenolol	Antagonist	100 µM Norepinephrine	25 mM Glycylglycine	8.0	45	25
	¹²⁵I-Pindolol	Antagonist	100 µM Norepinephrine	50 mM Tris-HCl	8.0	60	25
Benzodiazepine	[³H]Flunitrazepam	Agonist	1 µM Clonazepam	50 mM Na/KPO$_4$	7.4	75	4
Cholinergic							
Muscarinic	[³H](−)QNB	Antagonist	1 µM Atropine	50 mM Na/KPO$_4$	7.4	120	25
M$_1$	[³H]Pirenzepine	Antagonist	1 µM Atropine	10 mM Na/KPO$_4$	7.4	60	25
M$_2$	[³H]AF-DX 116	Antagonist	1 µM Atropine	50 mM Na/KPO$_4$	7.4	60	25
Dopamine							
D$_1$	[³H]SCH 23,390	Antagonist	1 µM SCH 23,390	50 mM Tris-HCl[a]	7.4	60	37
D$_2$	¹²⁵I-Sulpiride	Antagonist	30 µM Apomorphine	50 mM Tris-HCl[b]	7.4	30	30
GABA-A	[³H]Muscimol	Agonist	1 mM GABA	50 mM Tris citrate	7.4	90	25
Histamine							
H$_1$	[³H]Pyrilamine	Antagonist	2 µM Pyrilamine	50 mM Tris-HCl	7.4	60	25
Opioid							
δ	[³H]DPDPE	Agonist	1 µM Naltrexone	50 mM Tris-HCl	7.4	240	25
ϰ	[³H]U 69,593	Agonist	1 µM Naltrexone	50 mM Tris-HCl	7.4	60	25
µ	[³H]PL 17	Agonist	1 µM Naltrexone	50 mM Tris-HCl	7.4	60	25
Serotonin							
5-HT$_{1A}$	[³H]8-OH-DPAT	Agonist	10 µM Serotonin	25 mM Tris-HCl[c]	7.4	30	25
5-HT$_{1B}$	¹²⁵I-Cyanopindolol	Agonist	10 µM Serotonin +30 µM Isoproterenol	25 mM Tris-HCl	8.0	20	25

(Table continues)

TABLE 9. Continued.

Receptor	Radioligand	Agonist or antagonist	Definition of nonspecific binding	Incubation			
				Buffer	pH	Time	Temperature
5-HT$_2$	[^{3}H]Ketanserin	Antagonist	10 µM Serotonin	25 mM Tris-HCl	7.4	20	25
Angiotensin	^{125}I-Ser^{1}Isoleu^8, Ang. II	Agonist	1 µM Angiotensin II	50 mM Na/KPO$_4$	7.4	240	25
Bradykinin	[^{3}H]Bradykinin	Agonist	1 µM Bradykinin	25 mM TES^d	6.8	100	25
Neuropeptide Y	^{125}I-NPY	Agonist	0.3 µM NPY	50 mM Tris-HCl^e	7.4	90	37
Neurotensin	[^{3}H]Neurotensin	Agonist	1 µM Neurotensin	10 mM TES-KOH^f	7.4	60	20
Somatostatin	^{125}I-CGP 23,996	Agonist	1 µM Trp^8-SRIF	50 µM Tris-HCl^g	7.4	60	25
TRH	[^{3}H]MeTRH	Agonist	10 µM MeTRH	20 mM K$_2$HPO$_4$	7.4	360	4
VIP	^{125}I-VIP	Agonist	0.3 µM VIP	25 mM glycylglycine	8.0	20	25

The abbreviations used are: CADO, Chloradenosine; NECA, 5′N-ethylcarboxamidoadenosine; [^{125}I]HEAT, β-3-iodo-[^{125}I]-4-hydroxyphenyl-ethyl-aminomethyl-tetralone; UK, 14,304, 5-bromo-6-[2-imidazolin-2yl- amino]quinoxaline; QNB, quinuclidinylbenzilate; AF-DX-116, (11[[2-[(diethylamino) methyl]-1-piperidinyl]acetyl]-5,11-dihydro-6H-pryrido [2,3-b][1,4]benzodiazepine-6-) one; SCH-23390, 7-Chloro-8-hydroxy-3-methyl-1-phenyl-2,3,4,5-tetrahydro-1H-3-benzazepine; GABA, γ-aminobutyric acid; DPDPE, [D-Pen^2,D-Pen^5]-enkephalin; U69,593, 5α, 7α, 8β-(-)-N-methyl-N-[7-(1-pyrrolidinyl)-1-oxaspiro(4,5) dec-8-yl]-phenyl-benzene acetamide; PL 17, [NMe-Phe^3-D-Pro^4]morphiceptin; [^{3}H]8-OH-DPAT, (±)-8-hydroxy-2-(di-n-propylamino)tetralin hydrobromide; Ser, serine; Isoleu, isoleucine; Ang, angiotensin; TES, N-tris[hydroxymethyl]methyl-2-aminoethamesulfonic acid; NPY, Neuropeptide y; CGP 23996, (desamino)Cys-Lys-Asn-Phe-Trp-Lys-Thr-Tyr-Thr-Ser-Cys; Trp, tryptophan; SRIF, somatotropin release-inhibiting factor (somatostatin); MeTRH, methy TRH; VIP, Vasoactive intestinal polypeptide.

^{a}Plus 5 mM MgSO$_4$, 0.5 mM EDTA, 0.02% ascorbic acid.

^{b}Plus 120 mM NaCl, 5 mM KCl, 1 mM CaCl$_2$, 1 mM MgCl$_2$, 5.7 mM ascorbic acid, 10 µM hydroxyquinoline.

^{c}Plus 10 µM pargyline, 0.1 mM ascorbic acid.

^{d}Plus 1 mM 1, 10 phenanthroline, 1 mM dithiothreitol, 2 µM captopril, 140 µg/ml bacitracin, 0.1% bovine serum albumin.

^{e}Plus 5 mM MgCl$_2$, 0.1 mg/ml soybean trypsin inhibitor, 0.1% bovine serum albumin, 0.25 mg/ml bacitracin.

^{f}Plus 1 mM EGTA, 1 mM benzamide, 0.02% bacitracin, 0.002% soybean trypsin inhibitor.

^{g}Plus 20 µg/ml bacitracin.

give some general information to use as a guide. Both ^{3}H- and ^{125}I-radioligands are included where appropriate. It should be emphasized that the listing only provides a starting point, and that the final conditions must be carefully validated in each laboratory.

REFERENCES

1. Yamamura HI, Enna SJ, Kuhar MJ, eds. *Neurotransmitter receptor binding*, 2nd ed. New York: Raven Press, 1985.
2. Turner JT, Bylund DB. *J Pharmacol Exp Ther* 1987;242:873–881.
3. Bylund DB, Snyder SH. *Mol Pharmacol* 1967;12:568–580.
4. Rosenthal HE. *Anal Biochem* 1967;20:525–532.
5. Cheng YC, Prusoff WH. *Biochem Pharmacol* 1973;22:3099–3108.
6. Chou TC. *Mol Pharmacol J* 1974;10:235–247.
7. Bylund DB. *Anal Biochem* 1986;159:50–57.

BIBLIOGRAPHY

Boulton AA, Baker GB, Hrdina PD, eds., *Neuromethods 4: Receptor binding*. Clifton NJ: Humana Press, 1986.

Methods in Neurotransmitter Receptor Analysis,
edited by Henry I. Yamamura, et al.
Raven Press, Ltd., New York © 1990.

2

Computer-assisted Analysis of Binding Data

James R. Unnerstall

*Departments of Neurology and Pharmacology, Case Western Reserve University School of
Medicine and The Alzheimer Center, University Hospitals of Cleveland,
Cleveland, Ohio 44106*

Whenever one uses receptor binding techniques to address an experimental question, the ultimate goal is the accurate determination of the affinity of a ligand for a defined binding site and the relative number of these sites. In the not too distant past, the assessment of these measurements was deceptively simple. Linear transformations of bound ligand as a function of the concentration of radiolabeled ligand or unlabeled competitor, such as Rosenthal or Hill plots, provided adequate measurements of these binding parameters. However, as the technology and our understanding of the molecular interactions between hormones or transmitters and their receptors improved, the seemingly simple linear transformations of binding data began to yield more complex results.

We now know that these apparent anomalies represent important information concerning the varying selectivity of ligands for multiple classes of receptors and the molecular nature of ligand-receptor interactions. In order to utilize binding experiments adequately to measure these complex interactions, we have been required to revamp our thinking in both the design of the binding experiment and the analysis of the data. Issues involved in experimental design are discussed in the other chapters of this volume. Although some of these principles will be reiterated in this chapter, the focus here will be on the principles underlying the analysis of binding data using computer-assisted nonlinear curve-fitting techniques.

Although the mathematical models and statistical principles that underlie the nonlinear analysis of equilibrium binding data have been understood for several years, these tools have, in general, been underutilized. Now, personal computers (PCs)are generally available to most laboratories, and inexpensive to moderately priced software designed specifically for binding analysis is available for the PC. Thus, there is now no excuse for analyzing complex binding data without the use of mathematically appropriate techniques.

Although mathematical concepts will be presented to highlight certain principles, the focus of these discussions will be on the underlying logic of the principles so that one can apply these techniques sensibly to a particular experimental problem. If one chooses to use multipurpose statistical software to perform the analysis of binding data, there are sources available which describe the appropriate mathematical derivations. Since all of the software packages discussed in this chapter have adequate documentation and descriptions of the basic procedures, this chapter will not be a tutorial for any given program. However, in the discussion and presentation of examples, the nomenclature and procedures developed by Munson and Rodbard (1) in their program "SCAFIT" (also adapted by McPherson, ref. 2) will be utilized. Although different programs have their idiosyncracies with respect to data entering, terminology, and operating procedures, the principles established by Munson and Rodbard (1) apply to every program.

From the start, it is important to remember that these analytical procedures will not magically produce unique, correct answers. In fact, analysis of the same data set by different programs could produce different results. This fact should stimulate respect for the experimental protocol that underlies the data. With respect to differences between software, curve-fitting techniques are just that—techniques similar to any assay that one may perform. As anyone who writes software will attest, there are many paths to the solution of an equation. With respect to binding analysis, the single equaltion that is being solved has numerous variables, and at least two of these are unknowns (affinity and capacity, in the simplest case). Thus, there is an infinite number of solutions to the equation. The raw binding data will limit the number of solutions. Yet, there is always some uncertainty in the measurements. Thus, the accuracy of the final affinity and capacity estimates is directly proportional to the precision and extent of the raw data (conversely, in plain computer jargon: garbage in, garbage out).

Potential errors in measurement make it absolutely essential to analyze binding data using as powerful a mathematical and statistical method as possible. Further, an understanding of how experimental errors can affect the mathematical results can suggest approaches for increasing the confidence in the data by experimental means. Within this discussion, the strengths and limitations of computer-assisted nonlinear binding analysis should become evident.

PRINCIPLES

Curve-fitting Technique

The Binding Model

All of the available programs dedicated to binding analysis will fit data according to the law of mass action, assuming independent noninteracting binding sites that are measured at equilibrium. (This model also appears to work for intraconvertible binding sites assessed at equilibrium.) Algorithms for testing allosteric binding models are being developed for SCAFIT and can be developed using the more general statistical programs available for "mainframe" computers. Technically, the

Marquardt-Levenberg modification of the Gauss-Newtonian fitting method of "steepest descent" to reach the lowest sum of squares is used to determine the estimates of the binding parameters (dependent measures). Unless one plans to write a fitting program, understanding this algorithm is not necessary. This iterative ("trial-and-error") technique is universally accepted as the best basic technique for nonlinear least squares curve fitting.

For the ideal saturation experiment (with no nonspecific binding), we know that the plot of bound ligand as a function of the free ligand concentration will be a hyperbola described by the following occupancy equation

$$B = \frac{B_m \cdot F}{F + K_D} \qquad [1]$$

where B is bound ligand at free ligand concentration F, and K_D and B_m are the equilibrium dissociation constant and B_{max}, respectively.

If the ligand binds to more than one independent site, then the amount of ligand bound at a given concentration of free ligand simply becomes the sum of the multiple factors:

$$B = \frac{B_{m1} \cdot F}{F + K_{D1}} + \frac{B_{m2} \cdot F}{F + K_{D2}} + \cdots \qquad [2]$$

In the first idealized case, all of the binding can be attributed to a single homogenous population of sites. In this case, the nonlinear analysis will probably provide results similar to those obtained using a Rosenthal plot (assuming the analysis has been carried to saturation). The results will not be identical since the Rosenthal plot is a transformation of the original data, and the dependent variable measured (bound ligand) and all of the errors of measurement associated with this variable are represented on both axes. Further, using the Rosenthal plot, one could try to get away with a two-point analysis, since two points define a straight line. However, the raw data are nonlinear, and two dependent variables are being determined by the data. Statistically, an absolute minimum of three points is required to define the curve. This is what is meant by degrees of freedom (df) where N is the number of ligand concentrations assessed and k is the number of variables being measured:

$$df = N - k \qquad [3]$$

Of course, a three-point saturation experiment, with one degree of freedom, will leave no room for error. Moreover, there are usually more than two variables being assessed in any given data set.

Multiple Sites and Receptor Occupancy

In the second case, in which the ligand may bind to more than one site, it can be seen that even at very low concentrations of free ligand, there will be some contribution to the total binding site occupancy by the lower affinity site. Thus, linear approximations of curvilinear Rosenthal plots provide poor estimates of binding

TABLE 1. *Calculation of receptor occupancy for the two-site binding model*

[F] (nM)	[B], S1 (nM)	[B], S2 (nM)	[B], S (nM)	N	[B], T (nM)	[L], T (nM)
0.100	0.0182	0.0079	0.0261	0.0001	0.0262	0.1262
0.200	0.0333	0.0157	0.0490	0.0001	0.0491	0.2491
0.300	0.0462	0.0233	0.0695	0.0002	0.0696	0.3696
0.500	0.0667	0.0381	0.1048	0.0003	0.1050	0.6050
0.700	0.0824	0.0523	0.1347	0.0004	0.1350	0.8350
1.000	0.1000	0.0727	0.1727	0.0005	0.1732	1.1723
2.000	0.1333	0.1333	0.2667	0.0010	0.2677	2.2677
3.000	0.1500	0.1846	0.3346	0.0015	0.3361	3.3361
5.000	0.1667	0.2667	0.4333	0.0025	0.4358	5.4358
6.500	0.1733	0.3152	0.4885	0.0033	0.4917	6.9917

These data were generated using the theoretical occupancy equation as described in the text (eq. 6). The parameters that were used to generate the tabled values for the two sites are listed below. All values (except for the ratio N) are given in nM. These values are taken from those used to generate the data set analyzed in Table 3. Note that [B], T (total bound) is the sum of the specific and nonspecific binding for all the sites (S1, S2 and N, respectively) at each concentration of ligand, whereas [L], T (total ligand concentration) is the sum of the bound and free ([F]) ligand concentration. The algorithm used to estimate the parameters calculates the free ligand concentration, as well as the specific and nonspecific binding, by "subtracting" each of these components from the data provided (i.e., total ligand and total bound concentrations). Site 1: K_D, 1.0; B_{max}, 0.2; N, 0.0005. Site 2: K_D 10.0; B_{max}, 0.8.

parameters for multiple sites since the two arms of the curve are not independent. Accurate assessment of the binding parameters for each individual site requires subtracting the contribution of the binding of one site from the other (Table 1). This is the first hint of the rationale underlying *iterative* curve fitting. After the first set of estimates for the multiple sites is made, the actual amount of binding predicted for each independent site must be calculated. The two sets of figures must then be added for each concentration of free ligand. Finally, the resultant calculated curve must be compared with the actual data for "goodness of fit." Through successive iterative approximations, new estimates are tested using a defined set of rules. When the goodness of fit cannot be improved by a set percent, the iterations end, and the final estimates are provided.

These successive approximations are analogous to the swing of a pendulum. It is often educational to compare the estimates after each iteration of the computer. If the first set of estimates is reasonable but a little high, the next estimate will be low but a little closer. If for any reason the initial estimates are extremely inaccurate for the data set, this pendulum may go out of control, and totally unrealistic answers will be produced. Fortunately, each program has built-in limitations that will terminate the analysis and prompt the user for new input.

Competition Analysis

For a competition analysis, the free ligand concentration is usually held constant while the concentration of unlabeled competitor becomes the independent variable.

For a given concentration of ligand and competitor, the occupancy equation is simply an extension of Eq. 1, where the K_D of the ligand is modified by the concentration of the competitor and its affinity for the particular binding site

$$B = \frac{B_m \cdot \uparrow F}{F + K_D (1 + I/K_i)} \qquad [4]$$

where I is the concentration of the competitive inhibitor and K_I is the equilibrium dissociation constant of the competitor. For more than one independent binding site, the model is an extension of Eq. 2

$$B = \frac{B_{m1} \cdot \uparrow F}{F + K_{D1}(1 + I/K_{i1})} + \frac{B_{m2} \cdot \uparrow F}{F + K_{D2}(1 + I/K_{i2})} + \cdots \qquad [5]$$

This model can cover a host of experimental cases, e.g., a labeled and unlabeled ligand binding to two sites or both ligands having different affinities.

A situation that is often encountered is the differentiation of multiple classes of binding sites by competition of a nonselective radiolabeled ligand with selective unlabeled ligands. In these instances, the model given in Eq. 5 must be restricted so that K_{D1} and K_{D2} are not only equal but the same. Different programs have their own ways for handling this situation. For example, when using SCAFIT, the program will ask for shared parameters. In this case, one would tell the computer to share K_{D1} and K_{D2} [the actual parameters being measured by K11 and K12, which represent the equilibrium association constants for the labeled ligand designated as ligand 1 (the first digit after the K) for sites 1 and 2 (the second digit after the K)]. In this way, the program will know that the single K_D or K_A estimate given for the two sites are equal, and the two sites are chemically equivalent (at least as far as the ligand is concerned).

Model Testing

This example raises two other issues. The first is model testing. Note that the general model given in Eq. 5 can be restricted in any number of ways, e.g., the K_D values are equivalent but the K_i values are different; the K_i values are equal but the K_D values are different; all affinities are unique, and so on. There is no reason to expect that any set of binding data preferentially represents a particular model. Thus, when analyzing data, each model should be tested by restricting or sharing the different variables. If a certain model does not fit the data, the program will simply not be able to calculate an answer (rather, a message like "Ill Conditioning" will be given). In this way, a statistical evaluation of the best binding model can be obtained. Note that every restriction produces an extra degree of freedom. For example, sharing the K_D values will make one less measurement for the program to calculate. Conversely, the more complex the model, the fewer degrees of freedom and the greater the number of data points required to evaluate the data adequately.

It is important to remember that results based on a single experiment may not describe accurately the characteristics of a particular population of binding sites. An example of this situation is presented under "Final Precautions."

Simultaneous Analysis of Multiple Experiments

The second issue suggested by the general model presented in Eq. 5 revolves around the comparison of saturation and competition data. Usually, saturation and competition analyses are performed in individual experiments and analyzed separately. If a labeled ligand binds to a single site, the values for the K_D can simply be plugged into the competition analysis as a constant for the purpose of calculating K_i. The general model does suggest, however, that greater accuracy can be obtained by performing saturation experiments in the presence of varying concentrations of competitor (or conversely, competition experiments at varying concentrations of labeled ligand) and analyzing the data as a set. Normally, massive assays such as this are not performed. However, if experiments are designed in this manner, some interesting revelations can be obtained.

For example, it has been assumed that ^{125}I-pindolol or ^{125}I cyanopindolol binds with equal affinity to β_1- and β_2-adrenergic receptors. However, analysis of the competition of β_1- and β_2- selective drugs at varying concentrations of ^{125}I-pindolol or ^{125}I cyanopindolol results in different proportions of the two binding site populations as a function of the concentration of labeled ligand utilized. After complete analysis, the data indicate that the affinities of the labeled ligands for the two binding sites are slightly different (by a factor of 2 to 5) (3). Differences that subtle cannot be evaluated by saturation analysis alone (4, 5). Yet, they can make substantial changes in the estimate of the concentration of the subclasses of binding sites, particularly at low concentrations of labeled ligand.

Similarly, when both labeled and unlabeled ligand bind with different affinities to different subclasses of binding sites, there is no way that one can automatically assign the different components of the saturation and competition curves to one of the subclasses. For example, it is often assumed in the analysis of complex competition data that the radiolabeled ligand, which is held at a constant concentration, binds with equal affinity to the multiple binding sites differentiated by the unlabeled competitor. When the competition data are analyzed by themselves, the convention that was described above requires restricting K_{i1} and K_{i2} as shared constants. However, if saturation analysis of the labeled ligand reveals two binding sites, this restriction would lead to inaccurate estimates of K_i for the competing ligand. Thus, different constant values can be assigned to K_{i1} and K_{i2}. However, in order to match the high- and low-affinity components of the binding of the the two ligands accurately, the binding site occupancies for the labeled ligand at the concentration used must be known. Further, these occupancies must be matched to the proportion of binding sites displaced with different affinities by the competitor. In such complex binding situations, a statistical approach is required to make these assignments.

The best approach is to analyze saturation and competition data simultaneously.

Thus, parameter estimates, especially B_{max} estimates, can be matched for the different binding components, and random errors that could produce erroneous inflections in a single experiment can be minimized. The facility for such simultaneous analysis of multiple experiments is available with certain mainframe general statistical programs, such as MLAB on the PROPHET system (6, 7) as well as SCAFIT (1). PC-based programs will have limitations on the number of data points, parameters, and experiments which can be analyzed simultaneously. For most experimental situations, these limits will be rarely encountered. Assignment of appropriate identifiers and selection of the models are somewhat tricky and require familiarity with the software. Some examples using SCAFIT will be given in a later section.

Using similar logic, it is worthwhile to analyze replications of the same experiment simultaneously to reduce the contribution of random erroneous inflections and increase the degrees of freedom of the analysis.

Estimation of Free Ligand Concentration

All the models appropriately call for the use of free ligand concentration in calculating the binding parameters. Usually, the total amount of ligand that was added to the assay tubes is known. The programs utilize these total values and calculate the free ligand concentrations by subtracting the total amount of ligand bound for each concentration. This calculation is performed with each iteration.

This correction, which is rarely performed manually, clearly increases the accuracy of the determination. Note, however, that this method cannot account for ligand that may, for example, stick to the sides of the tube and thus decrease the real free concentration even further. If there are any doubts concerning the influence of such variables on the free ligand concentrations, assessment of tube blanks or aliquots of supernatant following pelleting of the labeled tissue by centrifugation may be required. The corrections would have to be applied to the total ligand added *before* the value is added to the data set.

Similar corrections can be applied to the free ligand concentration for estimates of nonspecific binding. More often than not, these corrections are never made in manual analysis of the data, where it is generally assumed that the free ligand concentration is the same in the total and nonspecific incubation tubes. Yet, it is not hard to imagine the free concentration of ligand in the "blanks" could be quite different from the "totals," especially if the percentage of nonspecific binding is low. In order to understand how this correction applies to the measurement of nonspecific binding, it is necessary to know how these programs actually estimate nonspecific binding.

Estimation of Nonspecific Binding

Up to now, binding models have been discussed in the ideal sense, i.e., nonselective or nonspecific binding does not exist. However, this is seldom true. The standard method for measuring nonspecific binding is to analyze parallel sets of incubation tubes, one with radiolabeled ligand and tissue alone, and a second containing an excess of unlabeled ligand or selective competing drug that saturates the binding site being studied. Since this definition has been repeatedly emphasized in our training, the concept of mathematically estimating nonspecific binding often elicits negative reactions.

The general binding model presented in Eq. 2 and 5 can be extended to include the measure of nonspecific binding:

$$B_T = \frac{B_{m1} \cdot F}{F + K_{D1}} + \frac{B_{m2} \cdot F}{F + K_{D2}} + \ldots + N \cdot \uparrow F \qquad [6]$$

where B_T is the total ligand binding at a free concentration of ligand F, and N is the proportion of the of the total binding attributed to nonspecific binding at the given free ligand concentration. N is the estimated parameter that represents nonspecific binding. According to Eq. 6, the nonspecific binding at any concentration is defined as a constant percentage (N) of the free ligand concentration. Thus, Eq. 6 simply states that adding the specific and nonspecific binding yields the total binding at a given ligand concentration.

This definition is perfectly consistent with standard criteria and assumptions concerning nonspecific binding, i.e., nonspecific binding is linearly related to the ligand concentration (Fig. 1A). The estimate of N is based on a formal definition that states that N is the ratio of bound/free at infinite free concentration (Fig. 1B) (2).

A more common sense explanation of N can be given. Take a data set where total binding is expressed as a function of free ligand concentration. If some part of that binding represents high-affinity binding to saturable and selective population of receptors that can be defined by a K_D and B_{max}, then subtraction of the binding represented by these parameters from a total binding should leave the nonspecific binding. This binding should be linearly related to the ligand concentration as defined in Eq. 6, i.e., nonspecific binding is equal to the ligand concentration times the slope factor N. With each iteration, each parameter is appropriately adjusted, and the calculated specific and nonspecific binding are summed. The residual error between calculated and actual total binding is then calculated. This process not only serves to reduce the overall error of the parameter estimates but also results in more reliable estimates of the critical binding parameters.

Does this mean that we should throw out all of the "old-fashioned" concepts concerning measurement of nonspecific binding? Certainly not! In fact, having the empirical measurement of nonspecific binding becomes more important in terms of evaluating adequately the appropriateness of the model and binding parameters that are determined mathematically. Translated into practical terms, this means that models should be tested and parameters estimated both with and without the empirical nonspecific binding being utilized in the calculations. If the parameter estimates and significant models are fairly close for the two calculations, one can be confident that the system being studied is stable and that the conditions that were utilized to perform the assay are selective. On the other hand, if any of the parameter estimates

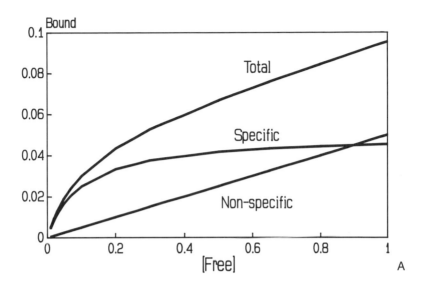

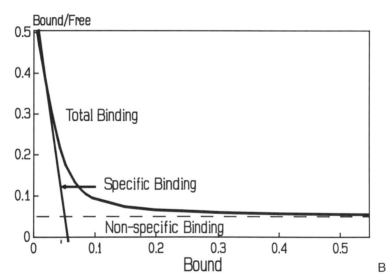

FIG. 1. Saturation and Rosenthal plots of computer-generated "ideal" binding data. The K_D was set at 0.1 nM, B_{max} at 50 pM, and N at 0.05. In **A,** note that the nonspecific binding, which is equal to N times the free ligand concentration, is linear. The Rosenthal transformation of these data is shown in **B.** Nonspecific binding is displayed as a component of the binding. The nonspecific component (*dotted line*) is parallel to the X-axis (bound) where $Y = 0.05$. The specific binding is represented by the *solid dark line*. The nonspecific binding is the asymptote of the curved plot representing total binding. Thus, by definition, the parameter N is the bound/free ratio at infinite free ligand concentrations.

are radically different (by more than a standard deviation) or if the significant model is different when the data are analyzed by these alternate methods, then something is wrong. Usually, it means that the empirically measured nonspecific binding is not linear with respect to ligand concentration, and some nonselective binding is being measured. This will often be reflected in the detection of a second site when total binding is assessed. This second site may indicate nonselective binding. Thus, an unexpected significant two-site fit of total binding may not represent the discovery of a new subclass of receptors. It could just as well be the result of the use of a nonselective ligand or competitor to define a particular receptor.

The practical problem in assessing nonspecific binding involves the incorporation of the empirical measures into the data set being analyzed. Most of the software packages that are available for nonlinear curve fitting have a "front end" program that is designed for raw data input and formatting. Different packages handle the nonspecific binding in various ways. For example, Munson and Rodbard's SCAFIT accepts direct input of nonspecific binding. However, the competitor is assumed to be chemically and/or kinetically identical to the ligand. The data are treated as an isotopic dilution (i.e., a total ligand concentration, and bound value is calculated based on an assumed dilution of the specific activity of the radiolabeled ligand). SCAFIT uses these values as if they represent total binding at infinitely high concentrations of ligand for determining the value of N (bound/free at infinitely high concentrations of ligand). This facility can be fudged to accept data obtained through the use of a chemically and kinetically distinct competitor (i.e., estimate the amount of unlabeled ligand added to be 100 to 1,000 times the K_D), but this could muddle the eventual interpretation of the parameter estimates.

The software that accompanies McPherson's adaptation of SCAFIT actually prepares a data set in which the empirical nonspecific binding is subtracted from the total binding. When the data set with background subtracted is analyzed by SCAFIT, N must be restricted and set as a constant equal to zero. This method is useful for comparative purposes but is generally inadequate. First, data and the accompanying degrees of freedom are lost, thus weakening the statistical power of the analysis. Second, the estimates of free ligand concentration may be biased, especially if the nonspecific binding is high.

The best estimates are those obtained when the nonspecific binding is a fitted parameter. These are the best values to report. If direct measures of the nonspecific binding can be incorporated into the analysis, the estimate of N will be improved. Nevertheless, it is still worthwhile to compare the parameter estimates that are obtained with and without the nonspecific binding measure incorporated into the data (either by inclusion or subtraction).

Statistical Weighting

Application of appropriate "weights" to the raw data plays an important part in the least squares analysis of nonlinear functions. When data are weighted, varying amounts of importance are placed on individual points. The weights (importance) are assigned by estimating the amount of error associated with a given measure. The smaller the error, the greater the weight carried by that measure. Since the statistical measure of variance is the standard mathematical form for evaluating the error and confidence limits associated with a given measurement, the weight assigned to a given measure will be proportional to the inverse of the variance, or

$$W = 1 / \sigma^2 \qquad [7]$$

where W is the weighting factor, and σ^2 is the estimate of the population variance.

Most users accept the default weighting factors provided by the application software without too much thought. It is important to understand the basis of the derivation, especially since different programs utilize different models for deriving these weighting factors.

The major problem for understanding the use of the weighting factors centers on the assumptions utilized for estimating the variance associated with a given measure. The first model is theoretically derived from the binomial theorem. Measurements of bound ligand are usually obtained by using nuclear counting techniques. Since radioactive disintegrations are discrete events, the distribution of an infinite number of observed disintegrations/min, (dpm) for a sample having true dpm equal to a value m will follow the binomial distribution that has a mean of m and a variance equal to the mean. If this model of variance is utilized, then the weighting factor for each measurement will be equal to the reciprocal of the average dpm. It follows that the lower the dpm, the closer the true value will be to the measured value and thus, the greater the weight, even if the percent error in the measurement is great (see Table 2). For example, if 100 dpm are measured, the true value is probably within $+/-$ 100 dpm. If 1,000 dpm are measured, the true value would probably be within $+/-$ 1,000 dpm. This estimate of the variance best corresponds to experiments in which the samples are counted for equal lengths of time. In this case, the same number of observations (number of disintegrations in 1-min intervals) is made on each sample. Samples can be counted to a preset level of error (i.e., an equal number of disintegrations can be counted for each sample), thus minimizing this source of error.

However, we are all familiar with the fact that counting errors are not the only source of experimental variance encountered in a binding assay. When random experimental errors are taken into account, standard errors will often be a constant percentage of the radioactivity measured. Here again, the lower the dpm, the lower the variance and thus, the greater the weight. For example, with 10% error, if 100 dpm are measured, the standard deviation will be 10, and the variance will be 100; if 1,000 dpm are measured, the standard deviation will be 100, and the variance will be 10,000.

The major difference between these two models is the shape of the functional relationship between the measure and its associated variance. In the first case (binomial), the variance is linearly related to the measure. In the second case (constant percent error), the variance is exponentially related to the measure.

TABLE 2. *Variance models and calculation of weighting factors*

Bound	σ^2	A. Quadratic model Weight	σ	% Error	% Weight
y	$0.0001y^2$	$1/y^2$			
1	1E-4	10000.00	0.01	1.0	99.0000
10	0.01	100.00	0.10	1.0	0.9900
100	1.00	1.00	1.00	1.0	0.0099
1000	100.00	0.01	10.00	1.0	0.0001

Bound	σ^2	B. Linear model Weight	σ	% Error	% Weight
y	y	$1/y$			
1	1.0	1.000	1.00	100.00	90.009
10	10.0	0.100	3.16	31.62	9.001
100	100.0	0.010	10.00	10.00	0.900
1000	1000.0	0.001	31.62	3.16	0.090

These calculations are based on the general weighting model discussed in ref. 8: $\sigma^2 = A_0 + A_1Y + A_2Y^2 + A_3Y^{A4}$. For the quadratic model (part A) $A_2 = 0.0001$, and the other constants equal zero. For the linear model, $A_1 = 1$, and the other constants equal zero. For illustrative purposes, the data under "% error" are simply $\sigma/Y \cdot \uparrow 100$, and "% weight" are the weighting factors for each point/the sum of the weighting factors $\cdot \uparrow 100$. Note that for the quadratic model, the percent errors are constant, whereas for the linear model the percent errors are inversely proportional to the amount bound. When compared with the linear model, the quadratic model assigns proportionally less variance to the smaller values, thus higher weights. This is reflected in the final column. The algorithm used by these programs assumes that the total variance in the data set will be proportional to the assigned weights. Thus, to reduce the variance maximally, the algorithm will draw the line of best fit closer to the points having the higher weights, thus reducing the overall sum of squares. The linear model assigns less weight to the smaller values and hence may enable the program to fit more closely the higher points in a data set without sacrificing accuracy in measurement associated with the smaller values. However, the linear model may not describe accurately the actual variance in the data set even though the quadratic model may underestimate the variance in the smaller measurements. In the end, the choice of the variance model needs to be based on empirical evidence, and calculations should be made using both models. An example of an application of both models is given in Table 3.

In reality, which is the best model to use? Rodbard and colleagues (8) empirically analyzed an extensive set of radioimmunoassay data and tested several functions for their ability to describe accurately the relationship between the dependent measure and its associated variance. Over the range of data analyzed, no difference could be discerned between the linear, quadratic, or power functions in their abilities to describe the relationship.

Thus, for a given situation, the choice of model becomes an empirical question. However, various programs use different default values. For example, the analysis software available from Lundon Software (Cleveland, OH) uses a linear model based on the binomial theorem. The SCAFIT defaults, one the other hand, use the quadratic model based on the assumption of constant percent error.

SCAFIT provides the facility to utilize several models. A general equation is available which combines components of the linear, quadratic, and power functions. By setting the values of the various constants to either zero or some finite value, any of these functions can be utilized to define the variance. The general equation is

$$\sigma^2 = A_0 + A_1Y + A_2Y^2 + A_3Y^{A4} \qquad [8]$$

where σ^2 is the estimated variance, Y is the measure of binding at a given ligand concentration, $A_0 + A_1Y$ represents the linear component of the equation, $A_0 + A_1Y + A_2Y^2$ is the quadratic component, and A_3Y^{A4} is the power component. For the constant percent error model, A_2 is set to 0.0001 and $A_0 = A_1 = A_3 = A_4 = 0$ (equivalent to 1% constant error). For the binomial model, A_1 should equal 1 while $A_0 = A_2 = A_3 = A_4 = 0$ (Table 2). Other compromises between the linear and quadratic model have been suggested, e.g., setting $\sigma^2 = Y^{1.5}$ ($A_0 = A_1 = A_2 = 0$; $A_3 = 0.001$; $A_4 = 1.5$).

By using variance models rather than actual variance measurements, the weight given to each measurement is calculated from the binding predicted by each iteration for every concentration of ligand. The weighting function serves to assign different proportions of the total variance to different data points. Initially, the points with the high weights will appear to contribute disproportionately to the total sum of squares (Table 2). Since the goal of the curve-fitting algorithm is the reduction of the sum of all the squared differences betwen predicted and actual measures (minimization of the sum of squares), the program will tend to fit the points with higher weights more closely after each iteration in its attempt to reduce the sums of squares. Since the smaller values will have greater weights (no matter what variance model is used), these smaller values will be fitted more closely than the larger values.

The practical outcome of this manipulation can be seen when attempting to distinguish statistically between one- and two-site fits (Table 3). In a saturation analysis, the smaller measurements will represent binding to a high-affinity component. Thus, estimates of high-affinity parameters have dramatically lower standard errors of measurement than low-affinity parameters. In certain cases, the extreme weighting of small measurements will tend to produce unreasonably high estimates of the equilibrium association constant of a high-affinity site, particularly when the maximal binding corresponding to this site is a small percentage of the total number specific binding sites. This problem is more often seen when using the quadratic model, which tends to overestimate the contribution of the variance of the smaller measures to the total sums of squares. On the other hand, use of the quadratic model provides a more conservative approach to the statistical differentiation of one- and two-site models. Thus, more measures (degrees of freedom) are required for distinguishing two binding components in a given experiment. This has the advantage of increasing the accuracy of the parameter estimates. Although the linear model enables the differentiation of multiple binding components with fewer degrees of freedom, the accuracy of the estimates is reduced. On the other hand, use of the linear model minimizes the overestimation of the affinity of high-affinity binding components since proportionately less weight is given to the smaller measurements. Thus, low-affinity components are assessed more accurately.

TABLE 3. *Comparison of quadratic and linear models of variance in distinguishing multiple binding sites from a data set*

A. 10-Point curve, quadratic model

Final parameter estimates $+/-$ standard error (approximate) (one-site fit)

$K11$	=	2.752518E + 08	$+/-$	5.294547E + 07	(1/$K11$ 3.633037E-09)
$R1$	=	7.298068E-11	$+/-$	1.092683E-11	
$N1$	=	6.192524E-04	$+/-$	2.136815E-04	
$C1$	=	1			

Final parameter estimates $+/-$ standard error (approximate) (two-site fit)

$K11$	=	4.880376E + 08	$+/-$	2.59201E + 08	(1/$K11$ 2.049022E-09)
$K12$	=	2.926145E + 07	$+/-$	2.645414E + 07	(1/$K12$ 3.417466E-08)
$R1$	=	3.807435E-11	$+/-$	2.341282E-11	
$R2$	=	1.215714E-10	$+/-$	2.405212E-11	
$N1$	=	0			
$C1$	=	1			

Fit	Sum of squares	df	Mean square	F
1	876.1345	6	146.0224	5.15 ($P = 0.072$)
2	431.5256	5	86.30512	

B. 18-Point curve, quadratic model

Final parameter estimates $+/-$ standard error (approximate) (one-site fit)

$K11$	=	2.841752E + 08	$+/-$	3.742164E + 07	(1/$K11$ 3.518956E-09)
$R1$	=	7.064342E-11	$+/-$	7.085883E-12	
$N1$	=	7.653924E-04	$+/-$	1.516664E-04	
$C1$	=	1			

Final parameter estimates $+/-$ standard error (approximate) (two-site fit)

$K11$	=	4.754004E + 08	$+/-$	1.669784E + 08	(1/$K11$ 2.10349E-09)
$K12$	=	2.682836E + 07	$+/-$	1.754385E + 07	(1/$K12$ 3.727399E-08)
$R1$	=	3.959519E-11	$+/-$	1.581219E-11	
$R2$	=	1.272604E-10	$+/-$	1.860072E-11	
$N1$	=	0			
$C1$	=	1			

Fit	Sum of squares	df	Mean square	F
1	1533.023	14	109.5016	8 ($P = 0.014$)
2	949.0595	13	73.00457	

C. 10-point curve, linear model			
Final parameter estimates $+/-$ standard error (approximate) (one-site fit)			
$K11$ =	$1.994033E+08$	$+/-$	$5.938618E+07$	$(1/K11\ 5.014961E-09)$
$R1$ =	$8.733337E-11$	$+/-$	$1.492026E-11$	
$N1$ =	$4.385776E-04$	$+/-$	$1.850695E-04$	
$C1$ =	1			

Final parameter estimates $+/-$ standard error (approximate) (two-site fit)			
$K11$ =	$8.510469E+08$	$+/-$	$7.293353E+08$	$(1/K11\ 1.175023E-09)$
$K12$ =	$4.440834E+07$	$+/-$	$2.077343E+07$	$(1/K12\ 2.251829E-08)$
$R1$ =	$2.269781E-11$	$+/-$	$1.702379E-11$	
$R2$ =	$1.273679E-10$	$+/-$	$1.300458E-11$	
$N1$ =	0			
$C1$ =	1			

Fit	Sum of squares	df	Mean square	F
1	$4.604452E-12$	6	$7.674087E-13$	$11.25\ (P=0.02)$
2	$1.417072E-12$	5	$2.834143E-13$	

The estimates shown in this table are taken directly from the final output obtained using the program SCAFIT (1). The data utilized to produce these fits were computer generated using Lotus 1,2,3. Initial occupancy values were derived using Eq. 2 based on K_D values of 1 and 10 nM and B_{max} values of 200 and 800 pM for the high- and low-affinity sites, respectively. N was set at 0.005. Random error (15%) was introduced into the data entered into SCAFIT. This program compares all fits on a given data set and statistically compares the various sets of estimates (these are presented after the two-site fit for each case). The F and p values provide the information required to determine which model is better (in this case, the one- or two-site fit). Note (in set A) that the two-site fit with 5 df does not reach significance ($p=0.07$) when the quadratic variance model is used. When the linear variance model is used on the same data (in set C), the two-site fit is now significantly better than the one-site fit ($p=0.02$). Also note that the standard errors for the high-affinity site are better when using the quadratic model, whereas the standard errors for the low-affinity site are better when using the linear model. In situations in which the difference in affinities approaches two orders of magnitude, the estimate for the high-affinity site will tend to become exaggerated when the quadratic model is used. Note that in this case the parameter estimates obtained using the linear model come a bit closer to the "true" values of the site which were used to generate the data. Also note that in this case the nonspecific binding was "lumped" with the low-affinity site (i.e., set to zero), tending to inflate the B_{max} of the low-affinity site. This suggests that the low-affinity site may not be statistically distinguishable from nonspecific binding, and more experiments are required to determine whether the low-affinity binding component is specific binding.

SUPPLIES

Hardware

In order to perform computer-assisted binding analysis, you obviously need a computer. Although most of the available programs were originally written for mainframe computers (e.g., DEC 10), there are now several versions that can be used on the personal computer, particualrly the IBM or IBM clone variety (that use DOS 2.0 or higher as the computer operating system). Although the PC versions will have limitations on the number of experiments or experimental measurements that can be analyzed (when compared with mainframe versions), these limitations are seldom a problem for routine analyses. Further, the calculations are identical in either mainframe or PC versions.

The speed of the analysis increases exponentially with the upgrades on the microprocessor. Thus, the use of Intel 8088-based computers (IBM-PC-XT varieties) is far faster than performing the calculations by hand, whereas the Intel 80286 computers (PC-AT varieties) are extremely fast, and the Intel 80386-based computers perform the calculations at speeds indistinguishable from a VAX or DEC 10-type computer. Installation of the program on a hard disk is recommended, as well as the use of a math coprocessor (Intel 8087, 80287, or 80387). These programs also run on the newer PS2 systems if DOS 2.0 or greater is used as the operating system. However, a 5 1/4-inch disk drive is necessary to copy the programs to either a hard disk or 3 1/2-inch diskette. The computer should have a minimum of 256K RAM, with 512K being preferred.

Data files should be stored in subdirectories on the hard disk, or better yet, on a floppy disk. Experience dictates that routine use of the software by one or several investigators will rapidly generate an unmanageable collection of small data and graphics files which can become lost on a hard disk if some basic disk organization is not maintained.

Software

LIGAND

The original LIGAND program (1) is available for a nominal charge (one letter and two blank 5 1/4-inch double-sided high-density diskettes) from the National Institutes of Health. Although this PC version has severe data-handling limitations when compared with the original version on the NIH DEC 10, this program provides an economical and expeditious means for performing routine data analysis.

The set of routines in the package includes not only SCAFIT (the actual nonlinear curve-fitting routine) but also other routines for entering the raw data and transforming the data to a format suitable for SCAFIT. Although the data-entering routines are not as user friendly as those packaged with commercially available software, the procedures utilized with this program have some advantages, particularly in regard to the entering of actual raw nonspecific binding data. SCAFIT will automatically supply initial estimates of the binding parameters which are usually quite accurate. The graphics are basic, and lines representing various binding components are not shown. However, confidence limits are graphed, as well as rudimentary plots of the residuals (i.e., how the actual data fall along the curve of best fit). The photocopied documentation is extensive and accurate, although it is sometimes hard to follow and assumes some prior understanding of the basics of the analytical procedure. To obtain the PC version of LIGAND, write to Dr. Peter J. Munson, Laboratory of Theoretical and Physical Biology, National Institute of Child Health and Human Development, NIH, Bld. 10 Room 6C101, Bethesda, MD 20892. You will be sent a form to return with two blank floppy disks.

EBDA

A little more sophisticated adaptation of SCAFIT by Grant McPherson (2) is available from Elsevier-Biosoft for approximately $250. The package includes SCAFIT and a front-end program, EBDA, which is used for raw data entering and editing, determination of initial parameter estimates, and data formatting. Other routines are available for the nonlinear analysis of kinetic binding data and protein determinations. The present version of EBDA has a reasonably easy method for entering the raw data and full-screen editing capabilities. However, data must be organized, since the program requires that the data be entered in a specific order (e.g., competitor concentration, total binding, nonspecific binding, total ligand added).

EBDA is organized to facilitate the entry of data from different experimental procedures, i.e. "hot" saturations (the concentration of the radiolabeled ligand is varied); "cold" saturations (the concentration of the radiolabeled ligand remains constant while the concentration of unlabeled and chemically identical ligand is varied; and "drug" competitions (the concentration of radiolabeled ligand remains constant while the concentration of unlabeled and chemically distinct competitor is varied). "Linear" parameter estimates are made, and basic Rosenthal, Hill, log-dose and Eadie-Hofstee plots are presented. Estimates of multiple sites can be made from the Rosenthal or Eadie-Hofstee plots by a linear interpolation method, i.e., pick points that appear to represent linear components of the data and perform linear regression on that subset of points. When using this method for the determination of initial parameter estimates, the minimal number of points that appear to represent the *asymptotes* of the binding components best should be chosen. These values can then be used in SCAFIT as initial parameter estimates. The SCAFIT routine in this package does not automatically supply initial parameter estimates.

Although raw nonspecific binding data are entered into the calculation, they are not handled as a directly fitted variable as in LIGAND. Instead, EBDA will produce two SCAFIT files: one in which the nonspecific binding is subtracted from the total binding; and one in which only the total binding is used. As discussed in a previous section, this method could affect the accuracy of the determinations since, in the first case, the specific binding data cannot be adjusted for nonspecific binding, and in the second case, *only* theoretical nonspecific binding is estimated. In this case, it is best to analyze both sets of data. Although fitting the data without the nonspecific binding will provide the superior estimate, it should be determined whether major discrepancies exist between the estimates obtained with the two different data sets. Another disadvantage of this program is that coefficients of the variance model are preset. With this package, the quadratic model is used as a default. This is not serious since this is the most preferred model, and this default eliminates one variable that could be confusing to the inexperienced user. If one wishes to change the defaults, a text editor or word-processing program is required.

Graphic presentations of the original and fitted Rosenthal and competition curves are far better than those available with LIGAND. The facilities exist within the software for plotting the graphics to a Hewlitt-Packard pen plotter.

Versions for both the PC and Apple Macintosh, which come with easy to read and understand documentation, are available for $249 from BIOSOFT, P.O. Box 580, Milltown, NJ 08850; 201-613-9013.

Lundon I and II

A more recent addition to the list of programs available for binding analysis comes from Lundon Software, Inc. These are by far the easiest software packages to use, especially for the computer-shy individual. These unique software packages have very accessible data entry and editing procedures and excellent graphics. Further, the user is not required to jump from different subroutines to make initial parameter estimates and complete the analysis. The software uses nomenclature that is more familiar to the average investigator. The documentation is clear and readable. The same basic algorithms used in the SCAFIT programs are used in these packages. The linear variance model is used as the default.

Their ease of use, however, restricts some functionality. Lundon I and Lundon II are individual modules designed to analyze saturation and competition data individually. Thus, simultaneous analysis of multiple experiments, especially simultaneous analysis of saturation and displacement data, are difficult to perform. Further, the coefficients of the variance model are difficult to change. Thus, some of the powerful advantages of the SCAFIT software are lost. Nevertheless, for routine data analysis by individual investigators, this program is a very useful alternative to the more complex SCAFIT programs.

Another advantage of the Lundon software is the growing list of vendors who are supporting Lundon hardware. For example, the Data Capture software available from Beckman Instruments for use with their scintillation and γ-counters will support the direct transfer of raw data to the Lundon package. Similarly, the MCID image analysis system available from Imaging Research, Inc. (Brock University, St. Catherines, Ontario, Canada) will also support the direct formatting and transfer of data to the Lundon software. (The Beckman Data Capture software, as well as many other image analysis packages, supports the transfer of data to Lotus 1,2,3 and/or ASCII format. By using a spread sheet program such as Lotus 1,2,3, these data can be easily sorted and transformed to the SCAFIT format.)

Lundon I and II can be obtained for $450 each from Lundon Software, Inc., P.O. Box 21820, Cleveland, OH 44121; 216-371-6220

PROPHET

If you are member of a research group that has access to either VAX/Ultrix systems (Digital Equipment Systems) or Sun Microsystems Terminals and have available an individual who is experienced in mathematical and computer analysis, the PROPHET package should be considered as an alternative to these others. This is particularly true if your research requires analysis of complex biochemical systems that do not easily lend themselves to analysis by basic binding models. Although expensive when compared with the PC packages, the PROPHET system is extremely powerful and flexible and can be adapted to a variety of statistical tasks that are required in the laboratory.

Softward development for PROPHET is under contract by the NIH with Bolt, Beranek and Newman, Inc., of Cambridge, MA. Information concerning the PROPHET system can be obtained from Bolt, Beranek and Newman, Inc., 10 Molton St., Cambridge, MA 02115; 617-873-3000.

PROCEDURES

No one protocol can be described for performing the data analysis since the procedures will be dependent upon the software package that is utilized. Further, the documentation that is available with each package will be the most useful source for describing data entry and procedures required to make initial parameter estimates.

On the other hand, providing some examples of an analytical procedure should help clarify some the issues discussed in previous sections. In the next section, an actual data analysis session using the program SCAFIT as adapted by Grant McPherson will be described. Before doing this, it may be wise to review some of the symbolic nomenclature used in SCAFIT. Although the terminology is unique to SCAFIT, it shares commonalities with other software packages. In addition, an understanding of the symbolic language used with SCAFIT will easily translate to the terminology used by other programs.

Binding Parameters

Ligand affinities are always reported as equilibrium association constants (K_A). The shorthand used by SCAFIT is simply K. Each K is coded with two identifiers.

The first numerical code is used to identify the ligand; the second is used to identify the binding site.

When preparing the data set for SCAFIT analysis, it is necessary to code the labeled ligand and the varying ligand. For example, in a saturation analysis, in which only one ligand is used, both the labeled ligand and the varying ligand will be given the code *1* since by definition, in a saturation experiment, the concentrations of the labeled ligand will be varied. The affinity constants will be coded *K11* (ligand one, site one), *K12* (ligand one, site two), and so on. Under normal circumstances, ligand code *1* is reserved for the labeled ligand. In a competition analysis, the labeled ligand is usually still coded *1*, while the competing ligand that is unlabeled (and whose concentration is varied) is coded *2*, i.e., *K21* (ligand two, site one), *K22* (ligand two, site two). If a one-site analysis of competition data is being performed, there will be both a *K11* and a *K21*. When performing a two-site fit, there will be a *K11* and *K12*, as well as a *K21* and a *K22*.

There may be instances in which this rule of thumb will be reversed. Such a situation was described by Munson and Rodbard (1). To give a simple example, in the first pair of experiments, saturation analysis of radiolabeled ligand A was performed, as well as competition of radiolabeled A by unlabeled drug B. When the data files were compiled from both experiments, ligand A was given the code *1* (varying ligand and labeled ligand in the saturation analysis), whereas B was coded *2* (varying ligand in the competition analysis, while A, the labeled ligand, was still coded *1*). In the second pair of experiments, the paradigm was reversed. Now B was labeled and A became the competing, unlabeled ligand. In order to analyze both sets of experiments simultaneously using SCAFIT, the ligand codes needed to be maintained. Thus, when preparing the data set from the saturation analysis of ligand B, both the varying ligand and labeled ligand were assigned the code *2*. In the competition analysis, A, the varying unlabeled ligand, was given the code *1* while B, the labeled ligand, was given the code *2*.

Affinity constants are given in units of molar concentration.

B_{max} values are represented by the label R followed by the code for the site, e.g., R*1* (site one), R*2* (site two). Units are in molar concentration. To convert these units to ligand bound mg of tissue, protein, or DNA, for example, the incubation volume and amount of tissue, protein, or DNA added to each tube must be known. For example, if *R1* is 2×10^{-11} M (20pM) and the incubation volume was 1.0 ml, then there will be 20 fmol of binding site/tube. If 5 mg of protein was added/tube, then the B_{max} will be 4 fmol/mg of protein.

N1 and *N2* are the non-specific binding constants for ligand 1 and ligand 2. Since *N* is the ratio of ligand that is nonspecifically bound to total ligand added to the incubation, this parameter is unitless. If the nonspecific binding has been subtracted from the data prior to the analysis, *N* will be set as a constant equal to zero. In competition studies, in which it is impossible to measure the nonspecific binding of the unlabeled ligand, *N* for the unlabeled ligand will always be constant and equal to zero (unless a saturation experiment using that same ligand is analyzed simultaneously as described by Munson and Rodbard and McPherson in the documentation accompanying their software). Often, *N1* and *N2* is shared. This assumes that the unlabeled competitor is pharmacologically equivalent to the drug used to define empirically the nonspecific binding. This assumption limits the ability of the program to test this hypothesis directly.

C1 and *C2* are correction factors used to normalize multiple experiments that are analyzed simultaneously. This is accomplished by correcting the variances in B_{max} values obtained in different experiments due to slight differences in the amount of tissue that is added/tube in any given experiment. The numerical code corresponds to the different data sets as they are called into the SCAFIT program. Thus, the first data set listed for analysis will be coded *C1*, the second *C2*, and so on. Usually, *C1* is held constant and set equal to *1*, while the other *C* factors are allowed to vary. Thus, the other data sets will be normalized to the first experiment.

The classifications of *shared parameters* and *constant parameter* are critically important to the definition of the binding model that is to be tested. For example, in an analysis of competition data, it may be desirable to test the hypothesis that the labeled ligand binds to two different binding sites with equal affinity, whereas the competing drug binds to the two sites with different affinities. Since this question calls for the calculation of a two-site fit, there will be a *K11* and a *K12* as well as a *K21* and a *K22*. However, *K11* and *K12* will be *shared*, in other words, equal. If a saturation analysis of ligand 1 is not included in the data set, then *K11* and *K12* will also be constant. On the other hand, the labeled ligand may bind to the two sites with different affinities, while the unlabeled competitor binds to both sites with equal affinity. In this case, *K21* and *K22* will be shared but not constant. To test this hypothesis adequately, saturation data for ligand 1 should be analyzed simultaneously. If the labeled ligand binds to two sites, but the unlabeled recognizes only the corresponding high-affinity site, the *K21* would be set as constant equal to zero (here you absolutely need the saturation data for ligand 1 to test this hypothesis).

Other examples could be given. However, it is essential to remember that this facility represents the most powerful tool available with these programs for testing different binding models. Sometimes, several models will provide statistically equivalent results. To discriminate among the possibilities, additional experiments designed around the model described by Munson and Rodbard (1) may be required. In some cases, common sense and a literature review may dictate the best model from several. In other instances, the program may not be able to fit a model, no matter how you adjust or manipulate the parameters. In these cases, you can assume that the model just does not fit the data.

EXAMPLES

The following examples are taken from the output of actual analysis sessions using the adaptation of SCAFIT by Grant McPherson. In these examples, saturation analysis of the relatively nonselective β-adrenergic antagonist ^{125}I-pindolol and competition analysis of the β_1-selective antagonist ICI89,406 in human cortical membranes will be performed. The saturation data were generated using Lotus 1,2,3 using parameters reported by Neve et al. (3) for ^{125}I-pindolol binding to β_1- and β_2-adrenergic binding sites. Comments will be presented in parentheses. User entries will be underlined. Study these examples, and refer to the previous discussions as an aid in understanding the ongoing process.

EBDA/LIGAND V3.0   15:01:08 04-03-1988

IBM PC version including PLOT by G.A. McPherson (1985)

Number of ligands: ? 1
Type the data file name(s) (no extension), [CR] to continue . . .
File 1: ? IPNSAT *(computer code for generated data file)*
Title: IPIN SATURATION IN HUMAN CTX THEORETICAL
Curve file name: IPNSAT.CRV
Weighting parameters   0   0   .0001   0   0
Varying ligand code: 1 labeled ligand code: 1
Number of sites: ? 1 *(one site fit will be tested . . . should always be done!)*
Weight points according to replicate number (Y/N): ? N *(The data files include the number of replicates analyzed at a given concentration, even though the average value will be used. This facility may increase the accuracy of results if widely varying replicates were used to generate the averages. Usually, the answer here will be "NO".)*
Do you want the same shared groups as before (Y/N) [Y]: ? Y *(If a possible answer appears in brackets, hitting the [ENTER] key will supply this answer as a default. When the program is first started, there are no previously defined shared parameters. For simple saturation analyses, there are no shared groups, so you will want the same shared groups as before!)*
Input constant parameters [C1]: ?
C1 = [1]: ?
Initial estimate for parameter K11 [0]: ? 1E10
Initial estimate for parameter R1 [0]: ? 1E-11
Initial estimate for parameter N1 [0]: ? .014 *(If you are using the NIH version of SCAFIT, the program will prompt you with its own initial parameter estimates. In this version, these estimates are usually taken from the initial analyses performed in EBDA. When additional analyses are performed on the same data set, the most recent parameter estimates will appear in the brackets. The value entered for N1 is a "cheater's estimate" since this was the value used to generate the data set!)*

IT.	K11	R1	N1	C1	RES.VAR.
0	1E + 10	1E-11	.014	1	11220.94

(The final value is the average sum of squares associated with these estimates. If the initial residual variance is an exponential, there usually is something critically wrong with these estimates. Perform your initial iterations one at a

time to make sure that the parameter values do not go to an unreasonable extreme. If any of the values appear extreme, e.g., K11 approaches 1E + 20, stop the process and reset the extreme value.)

Number of additional iterations: ? <u>10</u> *(If you want to reset your estimates, type "0".)*

1   8.47795E + 09   7.112661E = 13   5.098438E-03   1   6925.694

(after seven more iterations . . .)

Final parameter estimates $+/-$ Standard error (approximate)

K11 = 7.388975E + 09 +/− 1.037645E + 09   (1/K11 1.353368E-10)
R1   = 4.253121E-13   +/− 5.640424E-14
N1   = 3.052775E-04   +/− 5.447962E-05
C1   = 1

Curve	Sum of squares	D.F.	Mean square	F	Residuals (+) (−)		Runs
IPNSAT	1108.449	15	73.89658		9	9	7 (P> .05)
TOTAL	1108.449	15	73.89658		9	9	

(The "run test" is a nonparametric assessment of the goodness of fit. If the actual data clump in sequences on either side of the curve of best fit, the runs test will be significant, suggesting that the errors are not randomly distributed on either side of the curve. Thus, a two-site fit would be appropriate.)

Another fit (Y/N) [N]: ? <u>N</u>

Graphics data in IPNSAT.GRF

(In the next session, this same data will be analyzed simultaneously with the competition data.)

Number of ligands: ? <u>2</u>

Type the data file name(s) (no extension), kCRl to continue . . .

File 1: ? <u>IPNSAT</u>

Title: IPIN SATURATION IN HUMAN CTX THEORETICAL

Curve file name: IPNSAT.CRV

Weighting parameters   0   0   .0001   0   0

Varying ligand code: 1 labeled ligand code: 1

File 2: ? <u>ICI89406</u>

Title: ^{125}I-PINDOLOL DISPLACEMENT BY ICI89 IN HUMAN CORT. HOM.

Curve file name: ICI89406.CRV

Weighting parameters   0   0   .0001   0   0

Varying ligand code: 2 labeled ligand code: 1

Number of sites: ? <u>1</u> *(Always try the one-site fit first so that you can determine statistically whether the two-site fit is better than the one-site fit.)*

Weight points according to replicate number (Y/N): ? <u>N</u>

Do you want the same shared groups as before (Y/N) [Y] : ? <u>Y</u>

Input constant parameters [C1]: ? <u>N2 C1</u>

N2 = [0]: ?

C1 = [1]: ? *(The default values are used for N2 and C1 as discussed previously.)*

Initial estimate for parameter K11 [0]: ? <u>1E10</u> (*^{125}I-Pindolol*)

Initial estimate for parameter K21 [0]: ? 1E7 *(ICI89406)*
Initial estimate for parameter R1 [0]: ? 1E-11
Initial estimate for parameter N1 [0]: ? .014
Initial estimate for parameter C2 [1]: ? *(The default value is used. If the same basic protocol is used for both experiments, the final estimate for C2 should be very close to 1, the value set for C1.)*
(After five iterations . . .)
Final parameter estimates +/− Standard error (approximate)
K11 = 1.130618E + 10 +/− 1.16946E + 09   (1/K11 8.844717E-11)
K21 = 4.305514E + 07 +/− 8069327   (1/K21 2.322603E-08)
R1   = 1.102637E-11   +/− 7.83625E-13
N1   = 1.597204E-02   +/− 7.595673E-04
N2   = 0
C1   = 1
C2   = .9442555   +/− 4.035104E-02

Curve	Sum of squares	D.F.	Mean square	F	Residuals (+) (−)		Runs
IPNSAT	910.3499	15.5	58.73225	.51 (P = .174)	9	9	8 (P>.05)
ICI89406	2478.069	21.5	115.259	1.96 (P = .184)	12	12	4 (P<.01)

(Note the significant runs test on the displacement data.)

| TOTAL | 3388.419 | 37 | 91.57888 | | 21 | 21 | |

Another fit (Y/N) [N]: ? Y
Number of sites: ? 2
Weight points according to replicate number (Y/N): ? N
Do you want the same shared groups as before (Y/N) [Y]: ? N *(A new model will be tested.)*
Input a group of shared parameters: ? K11 K12 *(the hypothesis that the labeled ligand binds with equal affinity to the two sites will be tested.)*
Input a group of shared parameters: ? *(No other shared parameters required.)*
Input constant parameters [C1]: ? N2 C1
N2 = [0]: ?
C1 = [1]: ?
Initial estimate for parameter K11 [0]: ? 1E10
Initial estimate for parameter K21 [0]: ? 1E9
Initial estimate for parameter K22 [0]: ? 1E7
Initial estimate for parameter R1 [0]: ? 7E-12
Initial estimate for parameter R2 [0]: ? 5E-12
Initial estimate for parameter N1 [0]: ? .014
Initial estimate for parameter C2 [1]: ?
(After two iterations . . .)
Final parameter estimates +/− standard error (approximate)
K11 = 9.701475E + 09 +/− 6.67532E + 08   (1/K11 1.030771E-10)
K12 = 9.701475E + 09 +/− 6.67532E + 08   (1/K12 1.030771E-10)

K21 = 6.555397E + 08 +/− 2.889093E + 08 (1/K21 1.525461E-09)
K22 = 9724336 +/− 2928287 (1/K22 1.028348E-07)
R1 = 7.274491E-12 +/− 8.625555E-13
R2 = 5.56522E-12 +/− 7.675414E-13
N1 = 1.369111E-02 +/− 5.619549E-04
N2 = 0
C1 = 1
C2 = 1.049626 +/− 3.918903E = 02

Curve	Sum of squares	D.F.	Mean square	F	Residuals (+) (−)		Runs
IPNSAT	1106.367	14.5	76.3012	6.55 (P = 0)	9	9	7 (P>.05)
ICI89406	238.9322	20.5	11.65523	.15 (P = 0)	9	15	12 (P>.05)
TOTAL	1345.3	35	38.43713		18	24	

Fit	Sum of Squares	D.F.	Mean square	F
1	3388.419	37	91.57888	26.58 (P = 0)
2	1345.3	35	38.43713	—

(The significant F test indicates that the two site fit is statistically better than the one site fit.)

Another fit (Y/N) [N]: ? Y

(Another model will be tested. This time the hypothesis that both the labeled and unlabeled ligand binds with different affinities to the two sites will be tested.)

Number of sites: ? 2

Weight points according to replicate number (Y/N): ? N

Do you want the same shared groups as before (Y/N) [Y]: ? N

Input a group of shared parameters: ? *(This time, no parameters are equal.)*

Input constant parameters [N2 C1]: ?

N2 = [0]: ?

C1 = [1]: ?

Initial estimate for parameter K11 [9.701475E + 09]: ? 4E9

Initial estimate for parameter K12 [9.701475E + 09]: ? 1.4E10

Initial estimate for parameter K21 [6.555397E + 08]: ?

Initial estimate for parameter K22 [9724336]: ?

Initial estimate for parameter R1 [7.274491E-12]: ?

Initial estimate for parameter R2 [5.56522E-12]: ?

Initial estimate for parameter N1 [1.369111E-02]: ?

Initial estimate for parameter C2 [1.049626]: ?

(After three iterations . . .)

Final parameter estimates +/− Standard error (approximate)

K11 = 3.792986E + 09 +/− 1.068518E + 09 (1/K11 2.636445E-10)
K12 = 2.058409E + 10 +/− 3.502665E + 09 (1/K12 4.858122E-11)

```
K21  =  4.985515E + 08  +/-  1.979123E + 08    (1/K21 2.005811E-09)
K22  =  1.60281E + 07   +/-  4076153           (1/K22 6.239043E-08)
R1   =  1.184669E-11    +/-  2.086014E-12
R2   =  4.18434E-12     +/-  6.109826E-13
N1   =  1.287585E-02    +/-  6.36689E-04
N2   =  0
C1   =  1
C2   =  1.106684        +/-  .049094
```

Curve	Sum of squares	D.F.	Mean square	F	Residuals (+) (−)		Runs
IPNSAT	990.4316	14	70.74512	6.73 (P = 0)	9	9	7 (P > .05)
ICI89406	210.0831	20	10.50415	.15 (P = 0)	10	14	13 (P > .05)
TOTAL	1200.515	34	35.30925		19	23	

Fit	Sum of Squares	D.F.	Mean square	F
1	3388.419	37	91.57888	17.21 (P = 0)
2	1345.3	35	38.43713	0 (P = 0)
3	1200.515	34	35.30925	—

(The third fit is not statistically different from the second fit. This says that either model fits the data. Based on more extensive experimentation, it is known that the model tested in fit 3 is the better model. Thus, these parameter estimates should be chosen as the ones that best describe the data. The K_D for ^{125}I-pindolol are not that far off from those used to generate the data set, namely 211 and 67 pM for the β_1 and β_2 sites, respectively.)

Another fit (Y/N) [N]: ? N

Graphics data in IPNSATB2.GRF *(see Fig. 2)*.

FINAL PRECAUTIONS

One fact cannot be overemphasized: computer-assisted analysis of binding data is not the magic solution for binding data analysis. It must be remembered that the answers given by the various programs do not necessarily represent the final truth. Many variables influence the results that are obtained. As has been discussed, some of these are technique dependent. These include the use of different variance models, the testing of various binding models, and the inclusion/exclusion of non-specific binding.

Many more variables are data dependent. These include the actual variability of the data, the number of measurements made, the range of concentrations utilized in an experiment, and the accuracy of initial parameter estimates.

One final example, illustrated in Table 4, highlights some of these variables. Table 4 lists the final parameter estimates derived from data obtained in three differ-ent "theoretical" experiments. These theoretical data are computer-generated satura-

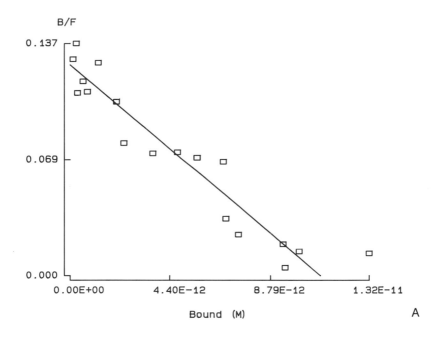

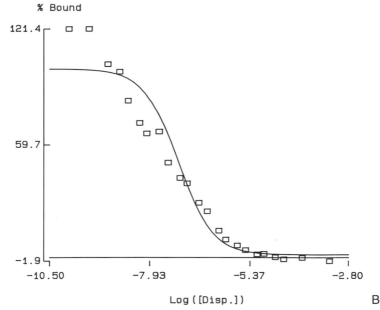

FIG. 2. Computer-generated plots representing the curves of best fit for the ^{125}I-pindolol saturation and ICI89406 competition data analyzed simultaneously. The Rosenthal transformation shown in **A** represents the fit generated using the one-site model, and **B** shows the corresponding fit of the competition data. **Panel B** exemplifies what is meant by a significant runs test. Note that the first four points lie above the curve of best fit, the next seven lie below the curve, the next six above the curve, and the final six below the curve. It is clear from this visual inspection that the points do not fall randomly around the curve.

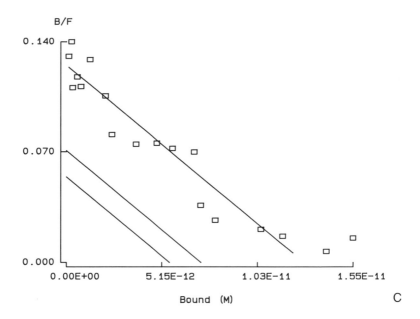

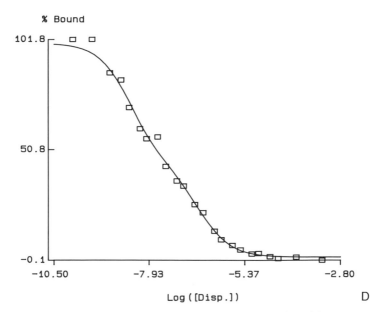

FIG. 2. *Continued.* **Panel C** represents the Rosenthal transformation of the saturation data fit by the two-site model in which the labeled ligand binds with equal affinity to both sites. The *diagonals* in the *lower lefthand* corner represent the binding components attributable to the two sites. The corresponding competition data are shown in **panel D.**

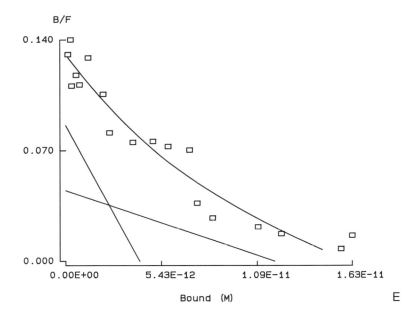

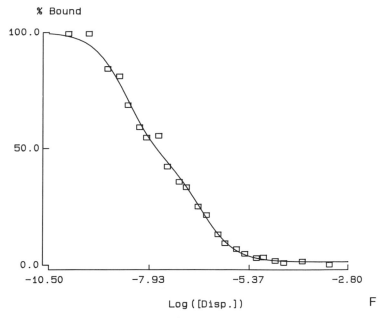

FIG. 2. *Continued.* **Panel E** is the same saturation data, but fit to a two-site model in which the labeled ligand does not bind with equal affinity to the two sites. The two binding components are represented by the *diagonals*. The corresponding competition data are shown in **panel F.** These plots were generated on a Hewlitt-Packard ColorPro plotter using the *Plot* subroutine in the McPherson adaptation of SCAFIT. See the text for details.

tion plots. The parameters used to generate the data are listed in Table 4 (note that the "true" K_D values are 0.1 and 10 nM for the high- and low-affinity sites). The difference between the three data sets is the range of ligand concentrations used in the experiments.

In experiment 1, the ligand concentrations ranged from 0.1 to 100 nM, and the significant two-site fit ($p = 0.048$) provided K_D estimates of 0.78 and 100 nM for the high- and low-affinity sites, respectively. Notice that the investigator did not run off to publish these significant results (Table 4A). The problem lies in the fact that the highest ligand concentration utilized was equal to the low-affinity K_D. In order to measure this site accurately, concentrations of ligand eight to ten times higher than the K_D need to be utilized.

Thus, the experiment was repeated, and the previous data were used to adjust the range of ligand concentrations (0.09 to 1000 nM). In this experiment, the investigator performed a centrifugation assay to separate bound from free ligand (remember that ligand will dissociate from binding sites too rapidly for accurate use of filtration separation if the K_D is greater than 10 nM; see ref. 9.). This time, K_D values of 0.12 and 12 nM were obtained (Table 4B). These values are quite different from those obtained in the first experiment (but very close to the "true" values). Further, the ligand concentrations used in this experiment were not low enough to measure the high-affinity site accurately. The investigator did analyze the two experiments simultaneously and obtained parameter estimates close to those in the second experiment.

Yet, to be sure that this second set of results represented some measure of reality, the investigator went back to the bench and repeated the experiment, this time using ligand concentrations that varied from 0.01 to 1000 nM. K_D values of 0.09 and 7.1 nM were obtained (Table 4C). These values are very close to those obtained in experiment 2 and are appropriately bracketed by the range of ligand concentrations used in this experiment. When all three experiments were analyzed simultaneously, the results obtained in the second and third experiments were confirmed (Table 4D). These estimates are reasonably close to the values used to generate the data.

The take-home message from this example is this: do not trust the first set of measurements that are calculated. Use common scientific sense when evaluating the appropriateness of the results. Repeat the experiments, varying the range of ligand concentrations utilized and when necessary, the methods used to perform the experiment.

Further, when analyzing a data set, repeat the data analysis, varying the initial estimates to be sure that the final estimates are reasonably close. Anomalies in the data can produce different final estimates that are dependent upon the initial estimates provided. If the initial parameter estimates are unreasonable (usually by more than a factor of ten in any two of the estimates), the computer will not be able to calculate final estimates. In addition, the greater the number of replicate experiments analyzed, the harder it will be to give the computer grossly inaccurate initial estimates.

TABLE 4. *Effects of ligand concentration range on the estimation of binding parameters*

A. Experiment 1: Ligand concentration varies from 0.1 to 100 nM			
Final parameter estimates +/− standard error (approximate)			
$K11$	=	1.274614E + 09 +/−	2.985066E + 08 (1/$K11$ 7.845511E-10)
$K12$	=	9143786 +/−	1.683986E + 07 (1/$K12$ 1.093639E-07)
$R1$	=	5.461935E-10 +/−	9.668152E-11
$R2$	=	3.844733E-09 +/−	7.644947E-09
$N1$	=	1.156066E-02 +/−	1.847713E-02
$C1$	=	1	

B. Experiment 2: Ligand concentration varies from 0.09 1000 nM			
Final parameter estimates +/− standard error (approximate)			
$K11$	=	8.715378E + 09 +/−	3.099988E + 09 (1/$K11$ 1.147397E-10)
$K12$	=	8.565826E + 07 +/−	2.654465E + 07 (1/$K12$ 1.16743E-08)
$R1$	=	5.635568E-11 +/−	1.037684E-11
$R2$	=	4.857798E-10 +/−	7.326603E-11
$N1$	=	5.579941E-03 +/−	3.906785E-04
$C1$	=	1	

C. Experiment 3: Ligand concentration varies from 0.01 to 1000 nM			
Final parameter estimates +/− standard error (approximate)			
$K11$	=	1.111293E + 10 +/−	3.604E + 09 (1/$K11$ 8.998529E-11)
$K12$	=	1.407259E + 08 +/−	6.555869E + 07 (1/$K12$ 7.106012E-09)
$R1$	=	4.358502E-11 +/−	1.086998E-11
$R2$	=	4.178213E-10 +/−	1.141189E-10
$N1$	=	5.860598E-03 +/−	1.786153E-03
$C1$	=	1	

D. Simultaneous analysis of the three experiments			
Final parameter estimates +/− standard error (approximate)			
$K11$	=	8455067E + 09 +/−	1.690801E + 09 (1/$K11$ 1.182723E-10)
$K12$	=	1.145494E + 08 +/−	2.583521E + 07 (1/$K12$ 8.729858E-09)
$R1$	=	1.635407E-10 +/−	2.237989E-11
$R2$	=	1.31529E-09 +/−	1.440508E-10
$N1$	=	.0185873 +/−	1.422651E-03
$C1$	=	1	
$C2$	=	.3200255 +/−	1.188461E-02
$C3$	=	.3251131 +/−	1.240825E-02

These data sets were generated from a common set of parameters using Lotus 1,2,3. 15% random error was introduced into the data for analysis by SCAFIT. The quadratic variance model was used for this analysis. High-affinity site: K_D, 0.1 nM; B_{max}, 50 pM; N, 0.005. Low-affinity site: K_D, 10 nM; B_{max}, 500 pM.

Analysis of Autoradiographic Data

Application of these tools to receptor autoradiographic data is becoming increasingly popular. These procedures are perfectly applicable to "slide-binding" data (with one caveat). In fact, it is essential that kinetic, saturation, and competition experiments are carried out in slide-mounted tissue sections prior to the autoradiography experiment (10), since knowledge of binding site occupancy is essential to interpretation of autoradiography data that are commonly obtained using a single concentration of ligand or drug. In these preliminary experiments, we know the incubation volume, the amount of ligand added, and the number of replicates in a Coplin jar or mailer. These can be entered directly into the data analysis. Radioactivity concentrations determined from aliquots taken from individual incubations must be adjusted for the total incubation volume (e.g., 1,000 dpm in a 100-μl aliquot is 100,000 dpm in a 10-ml incubation). Use aliquots obtained prior to the incubation, since total ligand is used to calculate the binding parameters. For autoradiography experiments, if small volumes of ligand are applied directly to the slide, use the dpm added; for incubations performed in large volumes, use ligand measurements taken after the incubations, and enter the appropriately large volume. In this way, the measures of bound ligand will minimally alter the program estimates of free ligand concentrations. Further, binding concentrations measured in discrete areas will bias the free ligand estimations less if large incubation volumes are entered into the calculations.

REFERENCES

1. Munson PJ, Rodbard D. *Anal Biochem* 1980;107:220–239.
2. McPherson GA *J Pharmacol Methods* 1985;14:213–228.
3. Neve KA, McGonigle P, Molinoff PB. *J Pharmacol Exp Ther* 1986;238:46–53.
4. DeLean A, Hancock AA, Lefkowitz RJ. *Mol Pharmacol* 1982;21:5–16.
5. Molinoff PB, Wolfe BB, Weiland GA. *Life Sci* 1981;29:427–433.
6. Abramson SN, Mcgonigle P, Molinoff PB. *Mol Pharmacol*1987;31:103–111.
7. McGonigle P, Neve KA, Molinoff PB *Mol Pharmacol* 1986;30:329–337.
8. Rodbard D, Lenox RH, Wray HL, Ramseth D. *Clin Chem* 1976;22:350–358.
9. Bennett JP Jr, Yamamura HI. In Yamamura HI, Enna SJ, Kuhar MJ, eds. *Neurotransmitter receptor binding* ed 2. New York: Raven Press, 1985;61–89.
10. Young WS III, Kuhar MJ *Brain Res* 1979;179:255–270.

BIBLIOGRAPHY

Klotz IM. *Science* 1982;217:1247–1249.
McGonigle P. In: Tallarida RJ, Williams M, eds. *Receptor site analysis in pharmacology*. Springer-Verlag, New York:1988.
Motulsky HJ, Ransnas LA. *FASEB J* 1987;1:365–74.
Munson PJ In: Marangos PJ, Campbell IC, Cohen RM, eds. *Brain receptor methodologies*. New York: Academic Press, 1988.
Norby JH, Ottolenghi P, Jensen J. *Anal Biochem* 1980;102:318–320.
Rodbard D. In: Rodbard D, and Forti G, eds. *Computers in endocrinology*. New York: Raven Press, 1984.

Methods in Neurotransmitter Receptor Analysis,
edited by Henry I. Yamamura, et al.
Raven Press, Ltd., New York © 1990.

3

Measurement of [³H]Inositol Phospholipid Turnover

David A. Kendall and Stephen J. Hill

*Department of Physiology and Pharmacology, Medical School, Queen's Medical Centre,
Nottingham NG7 2UH United Kingdom*

In recent years, there has been a growing awareness of the mechanisms by which cells recognize chemical signals and translate them into intracellular responses. This awareness has transformed our understanding of chemical transmission in the central nervous system. It is possible to divide neurotransmitter receptors into two broad groups on the basis of their associated transduction systems. Some receptors are linked to ion channels and produce changes in membrane potential by directly controlling the opening of ion gates [e.g., γ-aminobutyric acid ($GABA_A$), nicotinic cholinergic receptors), whereas others generate intracellular signals, so-called second messengers, when activated. This latter group can be subdivided into receptors that are linked (positively or negatively) to adenylate cyclase and produce their effects via control of cyclic adenosine monophosphate (AMP) formation, and those that increase intracelluar calcium ion concentration when stimulated (e.g., muscarinic, α_1-adreno-, histamine H_1-receptors). The purpose of this chapter is to describe some of the methods available for investigating the function of these calcium-mobilizing receptors within the central nervous system.

It is now widely accepted that stimulation of calcium-mobilizing receptors accelerates the hydrolysis of phosphatidylinositol 4,5-bisphosphate (PIP_2) within the plasma membrane, by the enzyme phospholipase C (*PLC*, Fig. 1). This process is analogous to that generating cyclic AMP in that it is under the control of a guanosine 5'-triphosphate (GTP)-binding protein. Hydrolysis of the phospholipid initiates a second messenger cascade consisting of inositol 1,4,5-trisphosphate (Ins-1,4,5-P_3), which directly mobilizes bound calcium from intracellular stores; inositol 1,3,4,5-tetrakisphosphate (Ins-1,3,4,5-P_4), which appears to be involved in the gating of extracellular calcium; and diacyglycerol, which activates the ubiquitous protein kinase C (see Fig. 1). Often, but not inevitably associated with inositol phospholipid hydrolysis is the activation of guanylate cyclase and cyclic guanosine 5'-monophosphate (GMP) formation.

This chapter will deal mainly with the methods available for monitoring the pro-

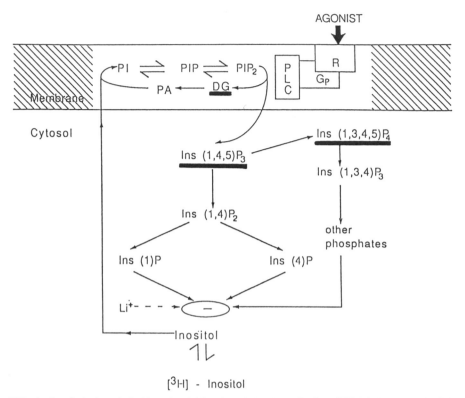

FIG. 1. Inositol phospholipid cycle. *PLC*, phospholipidase C; Gp, GTP binding protein; PA; phosphotidic acid: R, receptor.

duction of inositol phosphates, which can be used as an index of receptor activation. The level of technical sophistication employed, however, must be tailored by the reader to the particular question that is to be addressed.

PRINCIPLES

[³H]Inositol labeling

The aim of the methods described in this chapter is to monitor the production of water-soluble (i.e., cytosolic) [³H]inositol phosphates (see Fig. 1) following pre-labeling with *myo*-[³H] inositol. The [³H]inositol is readily taken up into brain slices, mixes with the endogenous pool of free *myo*-inositol within cells, and is consequently available for incorporation into the membrane inositol-containing phospholipids, phosphatidylinositol (PI; Fig. 2), phosphatidylinositol 4-phosphate (PIP), and PIP₂ (see Fig. 1). Following activation of a membrane-bound receptor with an agonist, the enzyme phospholipase C is activated, which cleaves the polar

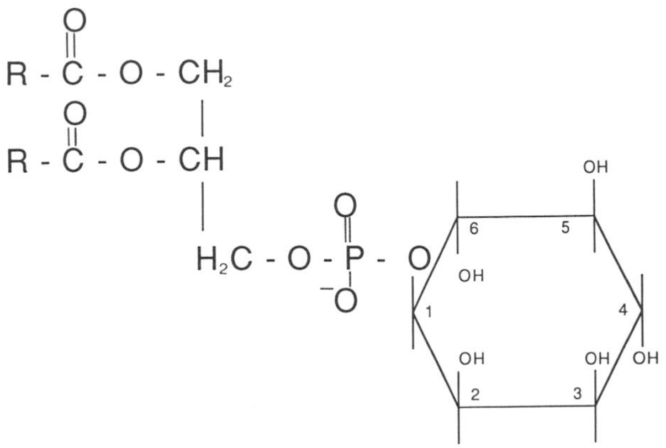

FIG. 2. Phosphatidylinositol.

inositol phosphate headgroup from PIP_2 on the inner leaflet of the plasma membrane, releasing $[^3H]Ins-1,4,5-P_3$ into the cytosol and leaving the remaining lipid-soluble diacyglycerol in the membrane (Fig. 1). The $[^3H]Ins-1,4,5-P_3$ is then metabolized by various intracellular phosphatases and kinases to yield a wide range of different $[^3H]$inositol phosphate compounds (Fig. 1). These are finally degraded to free $[^3H]$inositol, which can then be incorporated back into the membrane phospholipids. Addition of lithium ions can inhibit a number of these steps, but most importantly, it can prevent the conversion of $[^3H]$inositol monophosphates to free $[^3H]$inositol and hence produce an accumulation of $[^3H]$inositol monophosphates (Fig. 1). The cells are then lysed, and the water-soluble $[^3H]$inositol phosphates are separated from $[^3H]$inositol by anion-exchange chromatography. The amount of $[^3H]$inositol present in PI, PIP, and PIP_2 can also be determined by extraction of the phospholipids with chloroform/methanol. The phospholipids may also be deacylated (i.e., removal of the long-chain fatty acids denoted by R in Fig. 2) in mild alkaline conditions to yield glycerophosphoinositols that can be also separated by anion-exchange chromatography to give an indication of the labeling in the individual inositol phospholipids.

Anion-exchange Chromatography

The anion-exchange resin used in most studies of inositol phosphate accumulation is the strongly basic AG 1 resin, which comprises a cross-linked styrene-divinyl benzene lattice derivatized with the cationic functional group $CH_3N^+(CH_3)_3$. This is normally supplied in two ionic forms (chloride or formate) but can easily be converted from one to the other (or a completely different form) by application of an appropriate number of bed volumes of a molar solution of the required counterion (the volumes required are determined by the relative selectivities of each ion (see Table 1). The sample ion (inositol phosphate in this case) is absorbed onto the ion-

TABLE 1. *Relative affinities of counter-ions for AG 1-X8 resins*

Counter-ion	affinity for AG 1-X8 (OH$^-$ = 1.0)
OH$^-$	1.0
Formate	4.6
HPO$_4^-$	5.0
Chloride	22.0
HSO$_4^-$	85.0
Citrate	220.0

Data taken from Bio-rad 1986 catalog.

exchange column by attraction to the stationary cationic functional group on the resin. In doing this, it will displace the counter-ion already present (i.e., chloride or formate). The bound inositol phosphate ions can then be eluted by introducing competing ions. This can be done in one of two ways: (*a*) by introducing an ion with higher affinity for the exchanger; or (*b*) by introducing a larger amount of an ion with an equal or lower affinity for the resin. The relative affinities of several counter-ions for AG 1-X8 resins is given in Table 1. It should be noted that the pH of the sample and of the eluting medium may also alter the charge on the sample ion. For example, samples containing [³H]inositol phosphates are normally applied at pH 7 in order to maintain the negative charge on all of the phosphate groups and hence their attraction to the stationary positive charge on the resin. However, elution of samples with solutions containing formic acid and HCl will reduce the negative charge on the inositol phosphates in addition to providing chloride and formate counter-ions.

SUPPLIES

The major stock solutions and specialist materials required for inositol phosphate assays are listed below under the appropriate heading.

[³H]Inositol

Myo-[2-³H]Inositol (15 to 20 Ci/ mmol) can be obtained from Du Pont-New England Nuclear or Amersham International. Immediately before use, [³H]inositol should be passed through a column (0.5 ml of a 50:50 slurry in distilled water) of Dowex 1 resin 100 to 200 mesh (formate form) in order to remove radiolytic decomposition products that otherwise interfere with the determination of inositol phosphates (i.e., coelute on anion exchange).

Extraction of Inositol Phosphates

Chloroform
Chloroform/methanol (1:2, v/v)

Chloroform/methanol/10 M HCl (100:200:1, v/v)
Borax (6.25 mM)
Trichloroacetic acid (TCA) (15%, w/v)
Diethyl ether
Perchloric acid (10%, w/v)
KOH (0.15 M)
[Tris(hydroxymethyl)aminomethane] (Tris)-HCl (50 mM, pH 7.0)
Freon (1,1,2-trichlorotrifluoroethane)/tri-*n*-octylamine. (1:1)

Separation of Inositol Phosphates

Dowex 1 X-8 100 to 200 mesh (chloride form)
Dowex AG 1-X8 200 to 400 mesh resin (formate form)
Bio-rad Econo-Columns
HCl (1 M)
Ammonium formate (25 mM)
Ammonium formate (200 mM)
Ammonium formate (500 mM)/formic acid (0.1 M)
Ammonium formate (800 mM)/formic acid (0.1 M)
Ammonium formate (1 M)/formic acid (0.1 M)

Measurement of Lipid Labeling

Thin-layer Chromatography (TLC)

TLC plates (Merck high-performance Silica Gel 60)
Water/methanol (3:2) containing 1% potassium oxylate
Chloroform/acetone/methanol/acetic acid/water (40:15:13:12:8, v/v).

Deacylation

NaOH (1.2 M) in methanol/water (1:1)
Dowex 50, 200 to 400 mesh (H$^+$ form)
Ammonium formate (180 mM) + sodium tetraborate (5 mM)
Ammonium formate (300 mM) in formic acid (0.1 M)
Ammonium formate (2 M in formic acid (0.1 M).

PROCEDURES

The procedures outlined below give detailed quantities for a final incubation of 300 μl containing 50 μl of a gravity-packed suspension of cerebral cortical slices.

These amounts, however, can be scaled up or down to suit the particular experimental requirements. A number of different approaches have been detailed in the following sections, but as a general rule, only one protocol should be chosen from each section. In certain cases, a choice of one protocol (e.g., extraction protocol) determines which subsequent protocols must be followed (e.g., neutralization procedures), and where necessary this is indicated.

Preparation of Brain Slices

Brain slices can be prepared from a number of different brain regions, although some thought needs to be given to the size of the brain region under study and the tissue requirements (in bulk terms) of the proposed experiment. For example, cerebral cortex, cerebellum and hippocampus provide sufficient tissue for most experiments, but the use of small discrete nuclei would severely limit the size of any experiment. Rodents (guinea pigs, rats, and mice) are killed by cervical dislocation and decapitation. The brains are rapidly removed and dissected over ice. Brain slices are normally prepared by slicing brain regions in two directions (350×350 μm; 90° apart) on a McIlwain tissue chopper. The slices are then transferred to screw-topped bottles containing Krebs-Henseleit buffer (NaCl, 118 mM; KCl, 4.7 mM; $CaCl_2$, 2.5 mM; $MgSO_4$, 1.2 mM; KH_2PO_4, 1.2 mM; $NaHCO_3$, 25 mM; glucose, 5.5 mM) equilibrated with O_2/CO_2 (95:5) to a final pH of 7.4. A modified Krebs with a lower calcium ($CaCl_2$, 1.3 mM) and higher glucose (11.7 mM) has also been used in many experiments, particularly those using rat tissues. The slices are then gently agitated at 37°C in a shaking water bath for 1 hr with at least two intermediate changes of buffer. The slices are finally allowed to settle under gravity prior to transfer to individual incubation tubes or a low-volume incubation containing [³H]inositol.

Prelabeling with [³H]Inositol

Two methods are available for labeling tissue slices with [³H]inositol, a prelabeling method and a continuous labeling method. In the first method, all of the slices are incubated together in a single incubation containing the radioligand. This method is particularly useful if one wishes to label tissues with high levels of [³H]inositol (usually in small volumes to conserve funds!) under similar conditions and then allocate tissues to different incubations conditions (e.g., different calcium ion concentrations), following a brief wash of the slices with Krebs-Henseleit buffer. This method has proven very useful in smooth muscle preparations in which it is not possible to achieve a very homogenous slice preparation and in which depletion of the [³H]inositol in the medium can occur to differing extents if the labeling is done in individual incubation tubes. However, a large amount of free [³H]inositol remains in the slices, and it should not be assumed that no further incorporation of the ligand into the phospholipid pool is possible. The second method involves adding [³H]inositol to individual incubation tubes in which the label is present for the entire incubation procedure, and this method is included in the description of general incubation conditions below.

Prelabeling Method

After the 1-hr preincubation in Krebs-Henseleit buffer, the medium is decanted and the slices resuspended in 5 ml of Krebs-Henseleit buffer containing 40 to 120 μCi (0.5 to 1.5 μM, final concentration) in a 25-ml conical flask. The contents are then gassed with O_2/CO_2 (95:5), the flask stoppered, and the incubation continued for 1 hr in a shaking water bath at 37°C. The gassing procedure is repeated at 15-min intervals during this procedure. The prelabeled slices are then washed twice with 20 ml of normal Krebs medium and allowed to settle under gravity. If lithium chloride is to be present in the final incubation medium, lithium-containing Krebs buffer is used for the final washing procedure.

Lithium: Present or Not?

The observation that lithium inhibits inositol monophosphate phosphatase and thereby causes an accumulation of inositol monophosphate ($Ins-P_1$), stimulated interest in phospholipid hydrolysis in the CNS since it provided a means of amplifying relatively small receptor responses. This is analogous to the use of phosphodiesterase inhibitors in assays for cyclic AMP. However, workers should be circumspect in the use of lithium. If the experiment is designed to monitor receptor activation by measurement of total inositol phosphates, lithium can be included to amplify maximally the signal generated. However, since lithium has multiple effects on the generation of the separate phosphates including *inhibition* of $Ins-1,3,4,5-P_4$, more involved procedures should omit the ion.

Many investigators have employed 10 mM (final concentration in incubation) LiCl in their brain slice assays. However, this appears to be a supramaximal concentration, and a maximal enhancement of $Ins-P_1$ can be obtained with 1 to 5 mM lithium in our hands. There is no prolonged time lag in the onset of lithium's action and no apparent desensitization, so it can be added to the assay when required, e.g., at the start of the incorporation of [³H]inositol or just before the addition of agonists.

Incubation Conditions

Fifty-microliter aliquots of the gently packed slices obtained following tissue preparation or prelabeling with [³H]inositol are added to flat bottomed plastic vials (e.g., insert vials, 5-ml capacity) containing Krebs-Henseleit buffer (final volume, 300 μl). If the slices have not already been labeled with [³H]inositol as described above, then *myo*-[³H]inositol (0.3 to 1.0 μCi) would be added at this stage in 10 μl of medium. Lithium chloride (5 mM) would also normally be present in the Krebs buffer at this stage. If lithium is to be present, then the slices should be washed in Krebs buffer containing 5 mM lithium chloride immediately following prelabeling or tissue preparation. The incubation vials are then gassed by applying a stream of O_2/CO_2 (95:5) to the surface of the vial contents, capped, and incubated in a shaking water bath at 37°C for an additional 30 min. Antagonist drugs would be added at the beginning of this incubation period in 10 μl of medium. Agonists are then added in 10 μl of medium, the vials gassed again with O_2/CO_2 (95:5), capped, and incubated for an additional period (normally 20 to 45 min for most pharmacological studies) prior to stopping the reaction by one of the procedures listed below.

Termination of Incubations and Extraction of Water-soluble Inositol Phosphates

Four basic methods are available for termination of incubations and extraction of water-soluble inositol phosphates, and only one of the following methods should be chosen. The choice of which method to use depends on personal preference, although it is important to remember that *acid* conditions (i.e., the second through the fourth methods below) are required for optimal extraction of the more polar phosphates such as the bis, tris, and tetrakisphosphates (see "Comparison of Extraction Techniques"). Furthermore, if there is an interest in the cyclic inositol phosphates, then a neutral extraction procedure (e.g., the first method) will be necessary since cleavage of the cyclic ring occurs in acid media.

Chloroform/Methanol

Incubations are terminated by adding 0.94 ml of a mixture of chloroform/methanol (1:2, v/v) to each incubation tube to form a one-phase alcoholic solvent system with the aqueous contents of the incubation. The tubes are then vortexed and left to stand for 15 to 30 min. The nonpolar solvent chloroform is present in order to partition the lipids, and the polar solvent methanol is included in order to disrupt the hydrogen bonding and electrostatic forces between lipids and proteins such as lipid-degrading enzymes. This terminates the action of phospholipase C. Chloroform (0.31 ml) and water (0.31 ml) are then added, and the tubes are centrifuged at *ca.* $1,550 \times g$ for 10 min to separate the two phases. The water-soluble inositol phosphates are readily partitioned into the upper methanol water phase, and the lipids and phospholipids are left in the lower chloroform phase. A portion (0.75 ml) of the upper aqueous phase is then removed and diluted to 3 ml prior to separation of inositol phosphates by anion-exchange chromatography. No neutralization is necessary with this extraction technique. An advantage of this technique is that a portion of the chloroform phase (200 μl) can also be taken for analysis of the labeled inositol-containing phospholipids. It should be noted, however, that there are some reports that PIP is extracted into the aqueous methanol phase to a certain extent using this technique.

Acidified Chloroform/Methanol

Incubations are terminated by adding 0.94 ml of a mixture of chloroform/methanol/10 M HCl (100:200:1, v/v) to each incubation as described (under "Chloroform/Methanol") for neutral chloroform/methanol. Chloroform (0.31 ml) and water (0.31 ml) are then added to separate the phases (see "Chloroform/Methanol"); 0.75 ml of the upper phase is then removed and neutralized with 6.25 mM borax (approximately 1.2 ml, but this needs to be checked with each new stock solution), diluted to 3 ml with water, and then taken for separation of inositol phosphates. As described under "Chloroform/Methanol," a sample of the chloroform phase (200 μl) can be taken for analysis of labeled phospholipids.

TCA

Incubations are terminated by the addition of 0.25 ml of ice-cold TCA (15%, w/v) and left on ice for 15 min. This procedure completely precipitates proteins from aqueous solution by the formation of acid-insoluble salts with the protein. The tubes are then centrifuged at *ca.* 1,500 × g for 10 min to sediment the tissue and proteins. Three hundred twenty microliters of the supernatant is then taken and washed five times with 2.0 ml of diethyl ether to remove the TCA. The extract is finally neutralized with 6.25 mM borax (approximately 0.4 ml, but see comment in the preceding section) and diluted to 3 ml prior to anion-exchange chromatography.

Perchloric Acid (PCA)

Incubations are terminated with 0.1 ml of PCA (10%, w/v) and left on ice for at least 15 min. PCA precipitates proteins and hence terminates all biochemical reactions in exactly the same way as TCA (see above). The acid extract is then neutralized with 0.15 M KOH (approximately 0.7 ml) and left on ice for an additional 15 min to precipitate $KClO_4$. The $KClO_4$ is then removed by brief centrifugation at 4°C (1,500 × g for 10 min). Samples of the neutralized extract (0.7 ml) are then diluted to 3 ml with Tris buffer (50 mM, pH 7.0) and applied to anion-exchange columns. It is important that the neutralization with KOH is checked for each new stock solution of PCA and KOH. This is because an overestimate of the KOH needed for neutralization can provide sufficiently alkaline conditions for deacylation of the phospholipids (see "Measurement of Inositol Phospholipid Labeling") and hence a high background level of water-soluble inositol-containing molecules (glycerophosphoinositols).

Freon/Octylamine Neutralization for PCA- or TCA-terminated Reactions

This procedure is an *alternative* to the KOH and diethyl ether-borax neutralization procedures required following PCA and TCA addition. Following addition of

PCA or TCA, samples are left on ice for 20 min prior to centrifugation at $1,500 \times g$ for 10 min. Samples (350 μl) of the supernatant are then added to 125 μl of 10 mM ethylenediaminetetraacetate (EDTA) in 1.5-ml microcentrifuge tubes, followed by 500 μl of 1:1 Freon tri-n-octylamine. The samples are then vortexed and left to stand for 10 min prior to centrifugation ($12,000 \times g$ for 5 min) in a microcentrifuge; 350 μl of the upper aqueous phase is then taken for analysis of inositol phosphates.

Inositol Phosphate Separation

Total Inositol Phosphates

Total [³H]inositol phosphates can be separated from *mvo*-[³H]inositol and other tritiated products using Dowex 1 anion-exchange resin in either the formate or chloride form. Analytical grade resin in the formate form can be purchased from Bio-Rad, but the more economical standard commercial grade, purchased as the chloride form, is effective for this purpose.

Chloride form resin can be converted to the formate form on a suitable sized colume as follows:

$$\text{Dowex-Cl}^- + 30 \text{ volumes of 1 M NaOH} \rightarrow \text{Dowex OH}^-$$

$$\text{Dowex-OH}^- \text{ (wash with 4 volumes of water)}$$
$$+ \text{ 4 volumes of 1 M formic acid} \rightarrow \text{Dowex formate}^-$$

The formate form is finally washed with water until the pH is greater than 4.8. Two to three liters is normally required for 30 g of resin. Commercial chloride form resin is washed with 2 volumes of 1 M HCl followed by 5 volumes of water before use.

The separation procedure is as follows:

1. Apply the sample to 0.5 ml (wet bed volume) of Dowex chloride or Dowex formate resin in a Bio-Rad Econo-Column; discard the eluate.
2. Wash the column with 20 ml of water; discard the eluate. This removes free [³H]inositol.
3. Elute the total [³H]inositol phosphates into a scintillation vial with 2.5 ml of 1 M ammonium formate/100 mM formic acid (for the formate form resin) or 2.5 ml of 1 M HCl (for the chloride resin); add scintillant and count.
4. Wash the columns with an additional 5 ml of acid followed by 20 ml of water and store the columns under water.

In direct comparisons, we have found no apparent advantages in using formate form Dowex instead of the easier to prepare chloride form for total inositol phosphate separations.

Separation of Individual Inositol Phosphates

Individual [³H]inositol phosphates (but not their isomers) can be separated using simple Dowex column chromatography as follows.

1. Dilute the neutralized sample to 5 ml with 5 mM $NaHCO_3$.
2. Apply it to 1 ml of Dowex AG 1-X8 200 to 400 mesh resin (formate form) contained in glass columns (6 mm, internal diameter), and discard the eluate.
3. Wash the column with water to remove the [³H]inositol (approximately 20 ml).
4. Elute glycerophosphoinositol with 25 mM ammonium formate (approximately 12 ml).
5. Elute inositol monophosphates with 200 mM ammonium formate (approximately 14 ml).
6. Elute inositol bisphosphates with 500 mM ammonium formate/100 mM formic acid (approximately 14 ml).
7. Elute inositol trisphosphates with 800 mM ammonium formate/100 mM formic acid (approximately 14 ml).
8. Elute inositol tetrakisphosphate with 1 M ammomium formate/100 mM formic acid (approximately 16 ml).
9. Elute higher phosphates with 2 M ammonium formate/100 mM formic acid (approximately 8 ml).

Suitable aliquots of these fractions can then be transferred to scintillation vials for counting. It must be emphasized that the volumes of eluants (in parentheses) are only guidelines and that individuals must verify their separations by constructing spectra on the basis of collecting 1- or 2-ml fractions stepwise until radioactivity in each fraction has returned to background level, and by spiking samples with radioactive standards.

Before storage of columns in water, they are washed with 2 ml of 1 M formic acid followed by 8 ml of water. The columns can be reused many times, a limiting factor being growth of molds on the resin after some months.

High-Performance Liquid Chromatography (HPLC) Separation of Inositol Phosphates

It is necessary to employ HPLC techniques if a separation of the isomers of the various inositol phosphates is required. The protocol that we will describe was designed to investigate Ins-1,3,4,5-P_4 and the isomers of inositol trisphosphate (Ins-1,3,4-P_3 and Ins-1,4,5-P_3). Variations on this theme will be required if, for instance, the aim of the experiment is to examine inositol monophosphate and bisphosphate isomers. This method is based on that of Batty et al. (1), using a Beckman gradient HPLC system, with a 20-cm column packed with Whatman Partisil 10 SAX resin and a 20-cm guard column packed with silica.

In experiments using mouse cerebral cortical slices, we pool extracts from five individual incubations containing 25 μl of slices preincubated with 1.5 μCi of [³H]inositol in order to get sufficient radioactivity into the higher phosphates after short-term (1 to 10 min) incubation with receptor agonists.

Neutralized samples are filtered (Millipore, 0.45-μm pore size) before loading in a 2-ml injection loop. Samples are spiked with adenosine 5'-triphosphate (ATP) and GTP which coelute with Ins-1,3,4-P_3 and Ins-1,4,5-P_3 and serve as ultraviolet-detectable markers for the isomers when monitored at 254 nm. The eluant used is ammonium formate buffered to pH 3.7 with orthophosphoric acid. The concentration of ammonium formate is increased linearly from 0 (i.e., water) to 0.75 M over 5 min, at a flow rate of 1.25 ml/min (during which time glycerophosphoinositol is eluted) and is then held constant for 2 min. Inositol monophosphates and bisphosphates are then eluted by a linear increase over 6 min to 1.0 M ammonium formate/ phosphoric acid. After an additional 5 min at this concentration, the gradient is increased to a final concentration of 1.7 M ammonium formate over 10 min. Ins-1,3,4-P_3 and Ins-1,4,5-P_3 are sequentially eluted on this portion of the gradient. The concentration is held constant for 6 min to elute inositol tetrakisphosphate before returning to water over 2 min. Over appropriate regions of the gradient, 0.25-min fractions are collected in scintillation vials with the aid of an autosampler.

The high concentrations of ammonium formate in the eluting buffer are a potential hazard to the HPLC pumps, and particular attention to regular flushing with water and a high standard of maintenance are necessary to prolong pump life. The use of silica guard columns significantly enhances the life of the partisil analytical columns. Other gradient systems have been characterized for the separation of inositol monophosphate and bisphosphate isomers. Readers are referred to the report of Dean and Moyer (2) which details separation of the isomers of inositol monophosphate, bisphosphate and trisphosphate using ammonium phosphate (pH 3.8) as the mobile phase.

Standards

Verification of the chromatographic separations is, of course, essential. Radioactive inositol phosphate standards can be begged, bought, or made. It would therefore be unfair to suggest possible sources for obtaining standards as gifts but if funds are available [³H]Ins-P_1, [³H]inositol 1,4-bisphosphate (Ins-1,4-P_2), and [³H]Ins-1,4,5-P_3 can be purchased from Du Pont-New England Nuclear. It is not necessary to run standards for every isomer as the identity of Ins-1,4,5-P_3 for example, could be inferred as long as standard Ins-1,3,4-P_3 could be shown to elute with one of the pair of inositol trisphosphate peaks on a chromatogram.

The preparation of ³²P-labeled Ins-1,4,5-P_3 and Ins-1,4-P_2 from ³²P-labeled human erythrocytes is described by Downes et al. in ref. 3 and that of [³H]Ins-1,3,4-P_3 and Ins-1,3,4,5-P_4 from [³H]inositol-prelabeled parotid slices in ref. 4.

Measurement of Inositol Phospholipid Labeling

We have concentrated in this chapter on the production of [³H]inositol phosphates from [³H]inositol-labeled brain slices, since this is a direct measure of phospholipase C-mediated phosphoinositide hydrolysis. However, it is often valuable to measure the amount of label incorporated into the phospholipids. Some workers normalize their data by expressing amounts of inositol phosphates produced as a factor of label incorporated into the phospholipids, but this can produce very misleading results if, for instance, a particular stimulus has a direct effect on lipid incorporation as well as on the receptor-coupled breakdown process.

Total Lipid Labeling

An estimate of the incorporation of [³H]inositol into the total lipid phase can be made by simply taking an aliquot of the lower chloroform phase (of incubations stopped with chloroform/methanol/HCl), leaving it to dry at room temperature, adding scintillant, and counting. If incubations are stopped with PCA or TCA, the slices can be treated with chloroform/methanol/10 M HCl (100:200:1) after removal of the medium and the same procedure followed.

Labeling of Individual Inositol Phospholipids

If measurements of [³H]inositol incorporation into individual phosphoinositides are to be made, two basic procedures are available separation by TLC or deacylation of phospholipids followed by separation of the derived glycerophosphoinositols on anion-exchange columns.

The same extraction procedure can be used in both methods.

1. Stop incubations with 300 μl of 1.0 M TCA.
2. The incubation tubes are centrifuged, and the supernatants are discarded.
3. The slices are washed with 1 ml of 5% TCA/1 mM EDTA followed by 1 ml of water, and the supernatants are discarded.
4. Methanol:chloroform (940 μl, 2:1) containing 100 mM HCl is added, and the slices are incubated for 10 min at room temperature.
5. Chloroform (310 μl) and HCl (560 μl, 0.1 M) are added, the tubes are vortexed and centrifuged to separate the phases.
6. The lower chloroform phase is taken and dried under nitrogen; this contains the phosphoinositides and other lipids.

TLC Separations

1. The extract is redissolved in a known volume of chloroform/methanol (1:4).
2. TLC plates (Merck high-performance Silica Gel 60) are impregnated with potassium oxylate by development in water/methanol (3:2) containing 1% potassium oxylate, drying at room temperature, and activating at 110°C for 15 min.
3. Aliquots (20 μl) of the extract are spotted onto the plates along with unlabeled phospholipid standards, and one-dimensional chromatograms developed in a paper-lined chromatography chamber with chloroform/acetone/methanol/acetic

acid/water (40:15:13:12:8, v/v) or chloroform/methanol/NH$_4$OH/water (18:14:1:3).

4. Lipids are detected with iodine vapor, and the plates are divided into 5-mm strips that are scraped off and counted for radioactivity.

Typical retardation factor (R$_f$) values obtained are PI, 0.75; PIP, 0.56; PIP$_2$, 0.44.

Deacylation and Separation of Glycerophosphoinositols

Deacylation

1. The extract is redissolved in 1 ml of chloroform/methanol (1:4).
2. NaOH (50 µl, 1.2 M) in methanol/water (1:1) is added, and the tubes are incubated at 37°C for 15 min; this mild alkaline hydrolysis removes fatty acids from the phospholipids.
3. Chloroform/methanol (2 ml, 9:1) and water (2 ml) are added, and the tubes are vortexed.
4. The tubes are centrifuged to separate the phases.
5. The upper aqeous phase (2.5 ml) is applied to a small column containing 200 µl (50%, w/v, slurry) Dowex 50, 200 to 400 mesh (H$^+$ form) to remove the NaOH.
6. Glycerophosphoinositols are washed through with 1.5 ml of water, collected, and the pH adjusted to between 7 and 8 with 1 ml of 25 mM NaHCO$_3$.

Separation of Glycerophosphoinositols

1. The sample is applied to columns containing 1 ml of Dowex AG 1-X8 200 to 400 mesh in the formate form and the eluate discarded.
2. [^{3}H]Inositol (very little) is washed off in 10 ml of water.
3. GPI (glycerophosphoinositol from PI) is eluted in about 30 ml 180 mM ammonium formate + 5 mM sodium tetraborate.
4. GPIP (glycerophosphoinositol phosphate, form PIP) is eluted in about 20 ml of 300 mM ammonium formate in 0.1 M formic acid.
5. GPIP$_2$ (glycerophosphoinositol-bisphosphate, from PIP$_2$) is eluted in about 18 ml of 2 M ammonium formate in 0.1 M formic acid.

As with the inositol phosphate separations, the elution conditions must be individually verified by stepwise elution of 1- to 2-ml fractions and by running labeled standards. [^{3}H] Glycerophosphoinositol standards can be prepared by mild alkaline hydrolysis of their corresponding phosphoinositides.

Scintillation Counting

For all of the methods detailed above, the detection of inositol phosphates or glycerophosphoinositols relies on the determination of the radioactivity associated with [³H]inositol. This is achieved by liquid scintillation counting in which an organic solvent containing a fluor (scintillant) is added to the final sample. Radioactivity present in the sample causes excitation of the fluor and subsequent emission of light that can be detected by a photomultiplier present in a scintillation counter. There are a number of points that must be considered when choosing an appropriate scintillation cocktail. The first concerns the problem of "quenching" which occurs when there is interference of the energy transfer between radioisotope, fluor, or photomultiplier. This can occur as a result of interference with energy transfer from the sample to the fluors by chemicals present in the sample (e.g., chloroform) or by optical quenching (e.g., due to an opaque final solution) interfering with the detection by the photomultiplier. Correction for quenching must be made and counts per minute (cpm) converted to disintegrations per minute (dpm) by external or internal standardization. The second problem occurs when chemical reactions in the sample-scintillant mixture excite the fluors to give a false reading (chemiluminescence). Many counters now have a system for detection and correction for chemiluminescence.

We have used a number of commercially available scintillants to count [³H]inositol phosphate fractions collected following anion-exchange chromatography. Fractions (1 to 1.5 ml) containing up to 1 M formate can be counted as a clear single phase in 12 ml of Biofluor Du Pont-New England Nuclear or similar emulsifier-containing scintillant (e.g., Readisolv, Beckman) at counter temperatures below 10°C with an efficiency of *ca.* 40%. Higher fraction volumes (2.5 to 5 ml) containing up to 1 M HCl or 2 M formic acid can be counted in a gel phase below 10°C in many of these cocktails at an efficiency of *ca.* 25% in most modern counters. We have routinely used Optiphase X (LKB). (*Note:* It is important that the samples be cooled immediately on mixing the sample and scintillant into a gel since the aqueous and organic phases will separate on standing at room temperature.)

EXAMPLES

Comparison of Extraction Techniques

Figure 3 shows the data from an experiment designed to compare the various extraction procedures for [³H]inositol phosphates in slices of guinea pig cerebellum. Slices were prepared and preincubated with [³H]inositol as described under "Procedures." The accumulation of [³H]inositol phosphates was then measured after a 45-min incubation in the presence (*open bars*) or absence (*stippled bars*) of 1 mM histamine. Incubations were terminated by one of four methods described under "Procedures." (Fig. 3). Values are mean $+/-$ SE of five replicate determinations. [³H]Inositol phosphates were separated as described under "Procedures," and the data shown represent the radioactivity in the first 5 ml (which accounted for *ca.* 90% of the radioactivity) of each inositol phosphate fraction eluted from the columns.

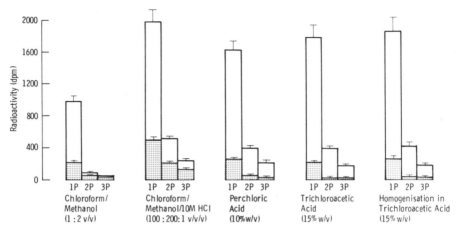

FIG. 3. Comparison of extraction techniques for [³H]inositol phosphates. Reproduced with permission from Donaldson J, Hill SJ. *Eur J. Pharmacol* 1986; 124: 255-265.

Separation of Inositol Phosphates

Figure 4 shows the effect of the muscarinic receptor agonist carbachol on the stimulation of [³H]inositol phosphate accumulation in slices of mouse cerebral cortex. The data were collected from experiments in which 25 μl of packed slices were incubated for 45 min with 1.5 μCi of [³H]inositol before addition of carbachol for 10 min. Five samples were combined for each separation. Figure 4A shows the separation of the [³H]inositol phosphates on Dowex 1 columns, and Fig. 4B, the separation on HPLC. The *broken line* in Fig. 4B indicates the concentration of ammonium formate in the eluting buffer during the run. The separations of [³H]Ins-1,4,5-P₃ and [³H]Ins-1,3,4-P₃ are clearly shown in Fig. 4B but not in Fig. 4A. However, many Dowex 1 column separations can be run concurrently, whereas only one HPLC separation, taking over 60 min in total, can be run at a time.

Pharmacological Studies of Total Inositol Phosphate Accumulation

Figure 5 illustrates the modulation by adenosine of histamine H_1-receptor function in guinea pig and mouse cerebral cortical slices observed by measuring total [³H]inositol phosphate accumulation. Guinea pig slices (50 μl) or mouse slices (25 μl) were incubated with increasing concentrations of histamine in the presence and absence of adenosine (300 μM) for 45 min. Values represent mean +/− SE of five replicate determinations. It can be seen that adenosine increases the response to histamine in the guinea pig and reduces the response to histamine in the mouse.

DISCUSSION AND APPLICATIONS

The phosphoinositide cycle is a series of biochemical events whose complexity appears to be growing at an alarming rate as an increasing number of workers focus

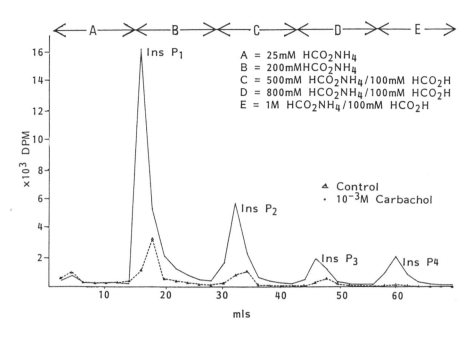

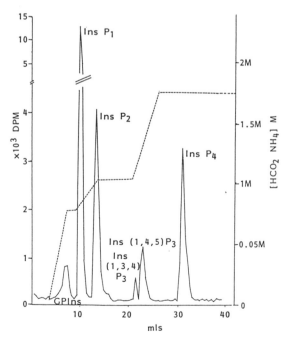

FIG. 4. Separation of inositol phosphates.

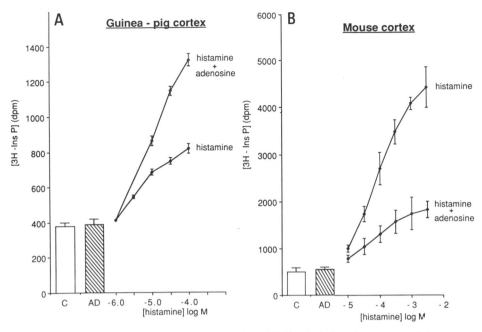

FIG. 5. Modulation of histamine-stimulated total [³H]inositol phosphate accumulations.

their attention upon it. This complexity can inhibit potential investigators from entering the field, but interested research workers should not be discouraged since there is a vast amount of information that can be gleaned by using simple technology to address simple and clearly formulated questions.

For instance, the following type of question could be posed: What is the effect of intervention X (could be a drug or tissue treatment, for example) on the activity of muscarinic receptors in the rat cerebral cortex? By measuring total [³H]inositol phosphate accumulation in response to, e.g., carbachol in lithium-treated brain slices prelabeled with [³H]inositol for 45 min, the simple answer (activity is increased/decreased/unchanged) could be produced. At this stage, the investigator might wish to ask more mechanistic questions about how the effect is produced, i.e., does it alter receptor number? (Follow up with ligand-binding studies.) Does it alter phosphoinositide synthesis? (Measure separate phosphoinositides by deacylation and separation of glyceroinositol.) Does it affect inositol phosphate kinases or phosphates? (Measure individual inositol phosphates and their isomers after HPLC separation.) Thus, the techniques to be used can be tailored to suit the complexity of the question that is posed, and there would, for instance, be no point in wasting time and resources on the separation of individual inositol phosphates in addressing the simple question originally posed: Is receptor activity affected?

Functional questions concerning *in vitro* drug efficacies and affinities for certain receptors can also be asked by employing the simple total phosphates assay. For instance, the partial agonist properties of certain agents can be investigated, and the receptor reserves in tissues can be determined by employing irreversible antagonists and parallel ligand-binding studies. It should be noted that there are often discrepancies in the apparent affinities of antagonists calculated from their antagonism of agonist-stimulated inositol phosphate production and those values determined from ligand-binding studies, and it is probable that the former values are the more physiologically relevant.

From a practical point of view, there are certain critical points in the assays to which special attention should be paid. (*a*) Radiolytic decomposition products of [³H]inositol can produce unacceptably high basal levels, and the label should be routinely purified on a daily basis as described under "Supplies." (*b*) In brain slice experiments, settling of the slices in the incubation vessels reduces responsiveness, and efforts should be made to keep them in suspension by gentle agitation throughout the experiment. (*c*) Retention times on the HPLC columns can vary quite widely due to temperature changes and other factors, and it is good practice to monitor the separation of ATP and GTP photometrically on the first run of the day.

Acknowledgment

The work performed in the authors' laboratories was supported by The Wellcome Trust and the Science and Engineering Research Council.

REFERENCES

1. Batty IR, Nahorski SR, Irvine RF. *Biochem J* 1985;232: 211–215.
2. Dean NM, Moyer JD *Biochem J* 1987; 242:361–366
3. Downes CP, Mussat MC, Michell RH. *Biochem J* 1982;203:169–177.
4. Downes CP, Hawkins PT, Irvine RF. *Biochem J* 1986; 238:501–506.

BIBLIOGRAPHY

Batty I, Nahorski SR. *Biochem J* 1987;247:797–800
Berridge MJ. *Biochem J* 1984;220:345–360
Berridge MJ, Downes CP, Hanley MR. *Biochem J* 1982;206:587–595.
Brown E, Kendall DA, Nahorski SR *J Neurochem* 1984;42:1379–1387.
Donaldson J, Hill SJ. *Eur J Pharmacol* 1986;124:255–265.
Downes CP, Wusteman MM. *Biochem J* 1983;216:633–640
Drummond AH. *Trends Pharmacol Sci* 1987;8:129–33.
Fisher SK, Agranoff BW. *J Neurochem* 1987;48:999–1017.
Hawkins PT, Stephens L, Downes CP. *Biochem J* 1986;238:507–516.
Hill SJ, Kendall DA. *Br J Pharmacol* 1987;91:661–669.
Irvine RF, Hemington H, Dawson RMC. *Biochem J* 1977;164:177–180.
Jolles J, et al. *Biochem J* 1981;194:283–291.
Kendall DA, Hill SJ. *J Neurochem* 1988;50:497–502
Kendall DA, Nahorski SR. *J Neurochem* 1984;42:1388–1394.
Kendall DA, Brown E, Nahorski SR *Eur J Pharmacol*, 1985;114:41–52.
Nahorski SR, Kendall DA, Batty I. *Biochem Pharmacol* 1986;35:2447–2453.
Wells MA, Dittmer JC. *Biochemistry* 1965;4:2459–2467.

Methods in Neurotransmitter Receptor Analysis,
edited by Henry I. Yamamura, et al.
Raven Press, Ltd., New York © 1990.

4

Analysis of Neurotransmitter Receptor-Coupled Cyclic Nucleotide Systems

Cyclic Adenosine 3':5'-Monophosphate and Adenylate Cyclase

*Samuel J. Strada, **Ronald S. Duman, and ‡S. J. Enna

*Department of Pharmacology, University of South Alabama College of Medicine,
Mobile, Alabama 36688;
**Department of Psychiatry, Yale University School of Medicine,
New Haven, Connecticut 06510; and
‡Nova Pharmaceutical Corporation, Baltimore, Maryland 21224

Adenylate Cyclase

Analysis of the activity of adenylate cyclase is a useful procedure for studying receptor function since it is one of the few enzymes that responds *in vitro* to hormonal signals. Signal transduction can be demonstrated at the subcellular level (i.e., in plasma membranes) indicating that, under these conditions, the receptors are "coupled" to adenylate cyclase. In this context, coupling refers to the process wherein the enzyme is activated as a consequence of a ligand-receptor interaction. Enzyme activity may be either activated or inhibited by receptor agonists, depending upon whether the receptor is coupled in a positive or negative manner to adenylate cyclase. Thus, a family of related guanine nucleotide-binding proteins (G-proteins) are involved in the coupling of the receptor to the enzyme. Some receptors (i.e., β-adrenergic) are coupled with a stimulatory G-protein (G_s), whereas others are coupled to the enzyme by way of an inhibitory G-protein (G_i).

Early studies of adenylate cyclase focused on measurements of overall enzyme activity in crude homogenates or subcellular fractions of tissue. However, recent advances have led to the identification and quantification of the individual components involved in the receptor-linked adenylate cyclase system. Since much of what has been gained from these approaches has been applied to the analyses of neurotransmitter-coupled systems, these techniques will be emphasized in this review. However, it is important to recognize that other components of the cyclic nucleotide cascade (i.e., cyclic nucleotide phosphodiesterases, protein kinases, and protein phosphatases) can be modified by neurotransmitters independent of the adenylate cyclase system. The precise definition of the influence of neurotransmitters on intracellular activity will only be obtained when it is possible to extrapolate data from cell-free systems to intact cells and tissues.

In Vivo Analysis of Cyclic Adenosine 5'-Monophosphate (AMP)

The level of cyclic AMP measured in tissues reflects a balance between the synthesis and degradation of the nucleotide. However, technical problems are encountered in determining the cyclic AMP content *in vivo*. For example, it is difficult in the whole animal to fix tissues rapidly so that an "instantaneous" cyclic AMP response to a drug or other condition can be assessed. Since cyclic AMP is chemically stable, some ingenious methods have been developed to inactivate the enzymes responsible for its synthesis and degradation, including rapid cooling (dropping the brain or "blowing the brain" into liquid nitrogen, freezing tissue *in situ* with a cryoprobe) or heating (microwave irradiation). Although these techniques are designed to prevent postexperimental changes, they all involve a finite delay in their ability to inactivate these enzymes, and most are associated with stress. The effectiveness of the procedure is dependent on the species, age of the animal, and the tissue being examined. In fact, postdecapitation changes in rat cerebellar cyclic AMP content are quite marked and are subject to modulation. Even if these methods of inactivation were perfected, problems of cellular heterogeneity would continue to confound the interpretation of them.

In Vitro Analysis of Cyclic AMP

The *in vitro* systems most widely used to analyze the effects of neurotransmitters on the cyclic nucleotide system are brain slices and cultured cells. Although data from brain slices are complicated by cellular heterogeneity, this approach allows a more direct analysis of changes in cyclic AMP content or turnover than can be achieved *in vivo*. The cyclic nucleotide content of brain slices can be measured either by radioimmunoassay or competitive binding assays. Alternatively, neurotransmitter or drug regulation of cyclic AMP production can be determined using a technique whereby the cyclic AMP pool is prelabeled with radioactive precursors (prelabeling techniques).

In addition to steady state concentrations, the rates of accumulation or degradation of cyclic AMP can be determined under appropriate conditions. In the presence of an inhibitor of phosphodiesterase (the enzyme that degrades cyclic AMP), the rate of accumulation of labeled cyclic nucleotide is directly proportional to adenylate cyclase activity. The rate of degradation may be monitored by following the disappearance of cyclic AMP when activation is reversed by the addition of an antagonist for the receptor mediating the stimulation of this enzyme.

Regulation of cyclic AMP production in brain tissue has also been examined by superfusing slices using an oxygenated chamber designed to circulate and collect the incubation buffer. A fraction of the intracellular cyclic AMP is released, with levels of the nucleotide in the effluent representing changes in production. The superfusion system allows for the incubation of the same batch of brain slices with different neurotransmitters or drugs, making it useful for studying relatively small brain regions.

Changes in cyclic nucleotides can be studied in both tissue slices and cell cultures using immunocytochemical techniques. These procedures employ fluorescent-tagged antibodies to cyclic AMP, with the nucleotides localized in sections of frozen tissue or fixed cells. Methods of tissue preparation and fixation allow for the analysis of only that portion of cyclic AMP bound to macromolecules. Thus, unlike other methods of analysis (radioimmunoassay, a binding technique, or by prelabeling), immunocytochemistry does not measure the total cyclic AMP levels.

Several factors are known to influence the responsiveness of the cyclic nucleotide system in brain slices. These include the age, sex, and species of animal, as well as environmental, dietary, and endocrine status.

The cyclic AMP levels in homogeneous cell cultures are known to be influenced by a variety of neurotransmitter substances. Such cultures are amenable to analysis of either cyclic nucleotide content and/or rates of accumulation using the prelabeling technique. With this approach, problems of cellular heterogeneity are circumvented, and chronic studies are simplified since the exact concentration and time of drug exposure can be controlled with precision. However, as in brain slices, a host of factors influences cyclic nucleotide responses in cell cultures, including the cell density, stage of the cell cycle, incubation medium, attachment to the substratum, and even the method used to harvest the cells. With cultured cells, changes in cyclic nucleotide content can be correlated with morphological parameters (neurite extension, sprouting) or biochemical events (induction of tyrosine hydroxylase). With brain slices, electrophysiological activity can be correlated with nucleotide levels. The effects of forskolin or cholera toxin, agents known to influence the intracellular synthesis of cyclic AMP, can be tested with either brain slices or cell cultures. Moreover, the specificity of a cyclic nucleotide response can be studied by analyzing the response to 8-bromo-cyclic AMP or other penetrable cyclic nucleotide derivatives. In addition, the involvement of cyclic AMP protein kinase can be examined in these systems following inhibition of the phosphorylating enzyme.

BASIC PRINCIPLES

Measurement of Adenylate Cyclase Activity

Analysis of receptor-coupled adenylate cyclase in cell-free systems is widely used because it allows the conditions for receptor regulation of enzyme activity to be precisely defined. In this way, it is possible to examine the contribution of each individual component (i.e., receptor recognition site, G-protein) in the regulation of enzyme activity. However, neurotransmitter receptor responses are reduced during homogenization of brain tissue in comparison with responses observed in brain slices.

Radioisotopic procedures are commonly used for measurement of adenylate cyclase activity. For these assays, radiolabeled adenosine 5'-triphosphate (ATP) is the substrate, and the product of the reaction, radiolabeled cyclic AMP, is isolated from unreacted substrate and metabolites. When this procedure was first introduced, [^{14}C]ATP was used as the substrate, and ion-exchange chromatography, paper chromatography, or precipitation with zinc sulfate and barium hydroxide was used to isolate the ^{14}C-cyclic AMP. Currently, [α-^{32}P]ATP is used since it can be labeled to much higher specific activity, and a dual-column separation technique combining Dowex ion-exchange chromatography and alumina oxide absorption is utilized for isolating radiolabeled cyclic AMP. This procedure offers many advantages over other techniques, including a greater degree of sensitivity. The main disadvantage of this approach is the expense of the radionucleotide. However, methods to synthesize the substrate at a considerably reduced cost have been devised.

The original discovery by Rodbell and coworkers of the obligatory role of guanine nucleotides in hormonal regulation of adenylate cyclase and hormone receptor interactions revealed the need to have guanosine 5'-triphosphate (GTP) or a non-hydrolyzable analogue such as guanyl-5'-yl imidophosphate [Gpp(NH)p] present to obtain hormonal stimulation. Half-maximal effects of guanine nucleotides are observed between 0.1 and 0.5 μM and saturating effects between 1 and 10 μM. The action of the guanine nucleotide may not be observed if the reagents are contaminated or if guanine nucleotides are introduced inadvertently into the assay with the particulate fraction. Successive washing of particulate fractions is needed to obtain membrane preparations devoid of nucleotide contamination.

Although receptor stimulation of adenylate cyclase is apparent in most brain regions, receptor inhibition of cyclic AMP production is readily apparent only in the neostriatum, where enzyme activity is approximately tenfold higher than in other brain areas. However, the ability of neurotransmitters to decrease adenylate cyclase is detectable in other brain regions if the enzyme is activated by forskolin or calmodulin. In addition, neurotransmitter receptor inhibition of cyclic AMP production is more apparent when the concentration of magnesium is less than 2 mM, since higher concentrations of this divalent cation, which regulates G-proteins and complexes with ATP to form the enzyme substrate, cause a stimulation of the enzyme which is not readily inhibited.

Assays for Discrete Components of the Adenylate Cyclase System

Hormonally sensitive adenylate cyclase consists of at least three components: (*a*) the receptor for the hormone or neurotransmitter; (*b*) the catalytic moiety of adenylate cyclase; and (*c*) regulatory component(s) that bind guanine nucleotides and are the sites of action for cholera toxin and pertussis toxin. The G_s confers guanine nucleotide and fluoride sensitivity to the catalytic component and can be extracted from brain tissue and analyzed by reconstitution with S49 Cyc⁻ membranes. This variant of S49 mouse lymphoma cells has receptors and the catalytic component but is deficient in the regulatory component.

The molecular characteristics of G-proteins have been studied extensively, first with the use of cholera- and pertussis toxin-catalyzed adenosine 5'-diphosphate (ADP)-ribosylation of G_s and G_i, respectively. Pertussis toxin also causes the ribosylation of another G-protein, G_o. Toxin-catalyzed ADP-ribosylation of G-proteins in the presence of radiolabeled nicotinamide-adenine dinucleotide (NAD) results in the covalent labeling of the G-proteins. Subsequent polyacrylamide gel electrophoresis and autoradiography of the samples yields the molecular characteristics and amounts of G_s and G_i.

Analysis of Cyclic AMP Accumulation by Prelabeling Techniques

Intracellular pools of adenine nucleotide (AXP), the precursor for ATP, are prelabeled to a steady state level with [³H]adenine. The accumulation of radiolabel into cyclic AMP is used to assess the effects of neurotransmitter, drugs, or other treatments on the accumulation of cyclic AMP.

Analysis of Cyclic AMP Content by Radioimmunoassay or Protein Kinase Activity Ratios

The accumulation of cyclic AMP in brain slices can be analyzed by measuring the endogenous content of the cyclic nucleotide by radioimmunoassay or other competitive binding assay techniques. In the latter case, the endogenous cyclic AMP is quantified by measuring its ability to displace iodinated cyclic AMP from tissue-binding sites.

The state of protein kinase activation in intact tissue can be used to measure the ability of neurotransmitters to alter intracellular levels of cyclic AMP. Two cyclic AMP-dependent protein kinase isozymes have been identified in various mammalian tissues and have been designated type I and type II based on their elution on DEAE-cellulose by salt gradients. Type II is the dominant species (70 to 80%) in mammalian brain. Putative neurotransmitters (adenosine), receptor-dependent (isoproterenol), and receptor-independent (forskolin) activators of adenylate cyclase are used to examine whether the elevation of cyclic AMP produced by these agents is accompanied by alterations in the activation of protein kinase in brain slices and cell-free particulate preparations.

Measurement of Cyclic AMP Turnover

Any of the above methods can be used to examine the effect of drugs and other treatments on cyclic AMP turnover. However, the prelabeling technique is the simplest and most reproducible. Once cyclic AMP levels have reached a steady state in response to an agonist, the decay constant may be determined provided that synthesis is inhibited and the basal rate is minor compared with the rate of degradation. Depending upon the agonist used to induce cyclic AMP accumulation, an appropriate antagonist is added at a concentration sufficient to inhibit agonist activity. The half-time for the decline can be assessed in relative terms by plotting the level of cyclic AMP (percent conversion, cyclic AMP content, or protein kinase activity ratio) at time zero as 100% (time when antagonist is added once maximum stimulation is obtained) against time. However, the rate of degradation of cyclic AMP in cells is not a simple unitary process and can be influenced by a number of factors including receptor desensitization. Despite these complications, it has been shown that the decay constant is the negative slope of the straight line obtained by plotting the natural log of the response (percent conversion-basal) versus time or ln $[C_t - C_\alpha]$ as a function of time. The slope of the line $= K_{dy}$. This first-order decay constant is an estimate of the fractional turnover constant.

SUPPLIES

Adenylate Cyclase Assay

1. $[\alpha\text{-}^{32}P]ATP$.
2. Cyclic $[^3H]AMP$ purchased commercially and purified periodically by Dowex 1-X8 ion-exchange chromatography.
3. Dowex 50-X4 AG 50W-X4, 200 to 400 mesh (H^+ form) purchased from Bio-Rad or Aldrich.
4. Aluminum oxide (neutral, Brockman activity grade I).
5. Glass columns, diameter 6×15 cm, with a no.18-16 gauge hole at the bottom and a 2.5-$\times$ 5-cm cup at the top. Kontes or Bio-Rad plastic disposable columns can be used instead, or 15 cm Pasteur pipettes fitted with plastic funnels.
6. Racks to hold columns and vials; they can be designed and made with Merck Plexiglass or purchased from Kontes.
7. Scintillation fluid with high capacity for H_2O (e.g., Aquasol, Du Pont-New England Nuclear; or Budget-Solve RPI).

Reconstitution Assays

1. Cell culture for S49 Cyc⁻ cells or source of cell membranes.
2. Other supplies for analysis of G_s reconstitution are the same as described above for above adenylate cyclase.

Ribosylation Assays

1. Pertussis toxin or cholera toxin.
2. Benzamidine.

3. Dithiothreitol (DTT).
4. Soybean trypsin inhibitor.
5. Isoniazide.
6. 3-Acetylpyridine adenine nucleotide.
7. GTP or Gpp(NH)p.
8. Triton X-100.
9. [^{32}P]NAD.
10. Sodium dodecyl sulfate (SDS).
11. *N*-Ethylmaleimide.
12. β- Mercaptoethanol.
13. SDS-polyacrylamide gels.
14. Acrylamide.
15. Bisacrylamide.

Prelabeling Procedure

1. O_2/CO_2 (95%/5%) oxygenation system for buffer and slices.
2. [^{3}H]Adenine.
3. Cyclic [^{14}C]AMP.

Cyclic AMP Assays

Protein Kinase

1. Phosphodiesterase (PDE) inhibitor.
2. Mixed histone or histone HF2B.
3. [γ-^{32}P]ATP.
4. Whatman P-81 phosphocellulose paper.
5. Phosphoric acid.

Radioimmunoassay

1. Phenol red.
2. Pasteur pipettes.
3. Methanol.
4. Rotary evaporator.
5. Dioxane.
6. Triethylamine.
7. Cyclic ^{125}I-AMP-tyrosine methyl ester.
8. Anti-cyclic AMP antibody.
9. Carrier protein.
10. Ethanol.

PROCEDURES

Measurement of Adenylate Cyclase Activity

1. Brain homogenate or subcellular fraction (e.g., synaptic membranes) are incubated in appropriate medium using $[\alpha\text{-}^{32}P]ATP$ as substrate.
2. Tissue preparation.
   a. Freshly dissected cerebral cortex or other brain region is homogenized gently (Teflon on glass) in 10 volumes of 0.32 M sucrose, 0.05 M [tris(hydroxymethyl)aminoethane] (Tris)-Cl (pH 7.6 at 4°C), 2 mM [ethyleneglycol-*bis*(aminoethylether)tetraacetate] (EGTA) and 1 mM DTT.
   b. Homogenate is centrifuged at $1,000 \times g$ for 10 min at 4°C and the resultant supernatant at $13,000 \times g$ for 20 min at 4°C to obtain a P_2 pellet.
3. Resuspend P_2 in 40 volumes of buffer without sucrose and centrifuge at 50,000 $\times g$ for 10 min at 4°C.
4. Resuspend the pellet as above and centrifuge twice more to obtain the final pellet (washed P_2 fraction). *Note:* Although repeated washing is required to remove endogenous GTP from membranes, the extra resuspensions and centrifugations also disrupt the coupling between receptors and G-proteins. Depending on the adenylate cyclase component of interest (receptor coupling or G-protein stimulation), these manipulations can be modified accordingly.
5. Resuspend the washed P_2 fraction in 8 volumes of 20 mM *N*-2-hydroxyethyl-piperazine-*N*'-2'-ethanesulfonic acid (HEPES), 2 mM $MgCl_2$, and 1 mM EGTA and divide into 0.5-ml portions.
6. These samples can be frozen on dry ice and acetone and stored at $-70°C$ until assayed.
7. For assay, frozen samples are thawed at 30°C and gently resuspended.
8. The incubation medium consists of 0.5 mM ATP, 2 mM $MgCl_2$, 1.0 mM EGTA, 0.1 mg/ml bovine serum albumin (BSA) (fraction V), 5.0 mM potassium phosphoenolpyruvate, pyruvate kinase (0.5 mg/ml), 80 mM HEPES (pH 8.0), 0.1 mM methylisobutylxanthine or other PDE inhibitor. These components of the reaction are combined into a "reaction mixture" at five times the final concentration and added to the incubation as a single aliquot. For example, a sample incubation volume of 100 µl would contain 20 µl of reaction mix (five times final concentration), 25 µl of assay buffer (which contains Tris buffer, four times final concentration), 25 µl of membrane suspension containing 10 to 100 µg of protein, and a 30-µl sample of drug or water (generally added in 10-µl aliquots).

   Any agents that are going to be present throughout the assay, such as GTP, can also be added as part of the reaction mix.
9. Add Gpp(NH)p, NaF, forskolin, or receptor agonist (in the presence of GTP, 10 µM) to the incubation medium and initiate reaction by adding 1 µCi of $[\alpha\text{-}^{32}P]ATP$ (included in the reaction mix) into each reaction tube, and incubate the samples for 20 min at 30°C (in cell-free systems, the catalytic unit is unsta-

ble at higher temperatures). Linearity of the assay is established by time course experiments. Blanks consist of buffer minus tissue or a preparation of tissue that has been heat inactivated.

10. Terminate the reaction by the addition of 800 µl of stopping solution containing 10 mM [^{3}H] cyclic AMP (approximately 10,000 cpm) to measure recovery, 40 mM unlabeled ATP, and 1% SDS followed by boiling of each assay tube for 3 to 4 min (boiling is optional).

11. [^{32}P] cyclic AMP and [^{3}H] cyclic AMP are separated from [α-^{32}P]ATP and its ^{32}P-metabolites using the combined Dowex 50 and aluminum oxide chromatography procedure described below under "Analysis of Cyclic AMP Accumulation by Prelabeling."

Example

Assay conditions: [ATP], 0.50 mM or 50,000 pmol/100 µl (incubation volume); time, 10 min; protein, 0.05 mg; [α-^{32}P]ATP, 1.5×10^6 dpm; [^{3}H] cyclic AMP, 10,000 dpm (added to sample after reaction stopped to measure recovery from column chromatography). GTPγS, guanosine 5'-3-O-(thio)triphosphate.

	Results from Double-column chromatography		Corrected for recovery
Assay Condition	[^{32}P]cAMP formed	[^{3}H]cAMP recovered	[^{32}P]cAMP
	(dpm)	*(dpm)*	*pmol/mg/min*
Blank (no protein)	40	6,567	
Basal	1,665	6,174	175
GTPγS (10 µM)	11,655	6,389	1,212
Forskolin (10 µM)	14,870	6,785	1,458

Results are expressed as [^{32}P] cyclic AMP formed in pmol/mg/min calculated as follows.

$$\frac{\text{pmol ATP (50,000)} \times \text{dpm [}^3\text{H]cAMP (10,000)}}{\text{dpm [}^{32}\text{P]ATP } (1.5 \times 10^6) \times 10 \text{ min} \times 0.05 \text{ mg protein}}$$

This factor is a constant (k) and is the same for each sample within a single experiment (equal to 667 for these conditions). This constant is used to calculate pmol cyclic [^{32}P]cAMP formed.

$$\text{Basal} = k \times \frac{\text{dpm [}^{32}\text{P]cAMP-blank}}{\text{dpm [}^3\text{H]cAMP}} = \frac{1,665 - 40 \times 667}{6,174} = 175 \text{ [}^{32}\text{P]cAMP pmol/mg/min}$$

Reconstitution of Adenylate Cyclase Components

1. Resuspend the particulate fraction (washed P_2) in 5 volumes of buffer containing 0.05 M Tris-Cl (pH 7.6), 2 mM EGTA, and 1 mM DTT (TED buffer) with 2% cholate.
2. Stir the suspension on ice for 60 min, and then centrifuge for 1 hr at $50,000 \times g$.
3. The supernatant (cholate extract) may be frozen on dry ice and acetone and stored at $-70°C$ until assayed.
4. To reconstitute, thaw the extract at 30°C and dilute to 2.6 mg/protein/ml with TED containing 1% cholate.
5. Incubate the samples for 15 min at 30°C to inactivate residual catalytic activity.
6. Dilute the samples with an equal volume of 0.1% Lubrol and 0.1 M NaCl in TED buffer.
7. The reconstitution of brain extracts with Cyc⁻ membranes involves a three-stage procedure.
   a. Incubate portions of the extract on ice with the Cyc⁻ membranes for 15 min in a volume of 40 μl. *Note:* Lubrol and cholate concentrations are 0.019 and 0.19%, respectively.
   b. Add Gpp(NH)p (100 μM), NaF (10 mM) or isoproterenol (10 μM) in a volume of 20 μl, and incubate the mixture for 15 min at 30°C. *Note:* When isoproterenol is used, the magnesium concentration is raised to 10 mM during this incubation period.
   c. Initiate the reaction by the addition of [^{32}P]ATP (in reaction mix), and incubate the samples for 20 min. The final concentrations of Mg^{2+} is 10 mM. The reaction is terminated by the addition of 1% SDS and isolation and measurement of [^{32}P] cyclic AMP produced in the assay.

Example

Cerebral cortex G_s was extracted with 1% cholate and 15 μg of extract protein was reconstituted with 25 μg of S49 Cyc⁻ membranes.

Results were calculated as described for the adenylate cyclase and are expressed as [^{32}P] cyclic AMP formed (pmol/mg/min).

	Cyc⁻	Cyc⁻ plus G_s extract
GTP (100 μM)	10	12
Gpp (NH)p (50 μM)	11	75
Isoproterenol (10 μM) + GTP (100 μM)	11	48

ADP-Ribosylation of G-Proteins

1. Tissue Preparation.
   a. For ADP-ribosylation experiments, the tissue is homogenized (10 mg, wet weight/ml) in buffer containing 50 mM Tris-HCl (pH 7.6), 5% sucrose, 6 mM $MgCl_2$, 1 mM EDTA, 3 mM benzamidine, 1 mM DTT, and 1.25 μg/ml soybean trypsin inhibitor.
   b. Homogenates of brain samples are centrifuged at $10,000 \times g$ at 5°C in a microfuge for 10 min.
   c. Pellets are resuspended (by homogenization or sonication) in the original volume of ice-cold buffer containing 100 mM Tris (pH 8), 10 mM thymidine, 10 mM isoniazide, 1 mM 3-acetylpyridine adenine dinucleotide, 5 mM $MgCl_2$, 2.8 mM DTT, 2.4 mM benzamidine, 0.8 mM ethylenediaminetetraacetate (EDTA), 2.5 mM ATP, 2 mM GTP, 4% sucrose, 0.8 μg/ml soybean trypsin inhibitor, and 0.5% Triton X-100. *Note:* The inclusion of Triton X-100 is necessary to obtain consistent levels of ADP-ribosylation of G-proteins in the brain stem nuclei, whereas it is necessary when studying other brain regions. The use of 100 μM Gpp(NH)p during ribosylation enhances incorporation by cholera toxin.
2. Toxins are activated by incubation in 20 mM DTT at room temperature for 1 hr: 50 μg of pertussis toxin in 50 μl or 250 μg cholera toxin in 250 μl; 20 mM DTT.
3. Portions (25 to 50 μg of protein) of the resuspended pellets (extracts) are subjected to ADP-ribosylation in duplicate in 1.5-ml microcentrifuge tubes for 1 hr at room temperature under the following conditions.
   a. For pertussis toxin experiments, 80-μl portions of the extract are incubated with 1 μg of purified pertussis toxin (List Biochemical Laboratories, Campbell, CA) and 10 μM [^{32}P]NAD (30 Ci/mmol) in a final volume of 100 μl.
   b. For cholera toxin experiments, 80-μl portions of the extract are incubated with 10 μg of purified cholera toxin α-subunit (List Biochemical Laboratories) and 20 μM [^{32}P]NAD (30 Ci/mmol) in a final volume of 110 μl.
   c. Reactions were terminated by the addition of 0.75 ml of ice-cold homogenization buffer, and the samples were centrifuged at $10,000 \times g$ for 10 min.
4. Sample Preparation.
   a. The pellets are resuspended by vortexing in 30 μl of a solution containing 40 mM Tris (pH 6.8), 1 mM DTT, and 2% SDS.
   b. The samples are incubated in a 75°C water bath for 5 min, after which 20 μl of 100 mM *N*-ethylmaleimide is added, and the mixtures are incubated for an additional 15 min at room temperature.
   c. A solution (50 μl) containing 40 mM Tris (pH 6.8), 2% SDS, and 50% glycerol/6% β-mercaptoethanol is then added and the mixture boiled for 2 min.
   d. The samples are then subjected to one-dimensional SDS-polyacrylamide gel

electrophoresis with 9% acrylamide/0.25% bisacrylamide in the resolving gels.

e. Resultant gels are dried and autoradiographed. Individual G-protein bands are excised from dried gels, and the amount of radioactivity is quantified by liquid scintillation spectrometry. Each step in this procedure is required to obtain sharp bands and consistent resolution of G_i and G_o in the final SDS gels. Under these assay conditions, ADP-ribosylation levels of G-proteins are linear over a fivefold range of tissue concentration and are 80% of maximal ADP-ribosylation levels obtained with much longer incubation times and higher concentrations of toxin and NAD.

Analysis of Cyclic AMP Accumulation by Prelabeling

Tissue Slice Preparation

1. Dissect the desired brain area over ice and mount it on a chopping block.
2. Chop the tissue in two directions with McIlwain chopper (Brinkmann Instruments) set at 350 μm (rotate the chopping block 90° for the second direction).
3. Place the slices into beaker with oxygenated buffer (approximately 10 ml/100 mg of tissue, wet weight).
4. Decant and add fresh buffer. Incubate for 15 min at 37°C while aerating with O_2/CO_2 (95%/5%). Aeration can be accomplished by gently bubbling O_2/CO_2 through the buffer to avoid foaming.

Prelabeling Preincubation Period

1. Decant and add fresh buffer.
2. Add [³H]adenine (14 to 20 Ci/mmol), approximately 30 μCi/100 mg tissue and incubate 45 min at 37°C while aerating.
3. Decant the buffer with [³H]adenine into a radioactive waste container and wash the slices twice with fresh buffer to remove nonincorporated adenine.
4. Collect the slices in a conical centrifuge tube (packed slices).

Cyclic AMP Accumulation-Drug Incubation Period

1. Place 50-μl portions of packed slices into minivials containing 440 μl of buffer (final volume for the assay is 500 μl; 50-μl slices, 440 μl of buffer, and 10 μl of experimental agent).
2. Aerate the vials and cap them; incubate for 5 to 10 min at 37°C in a shaking water bath with or without a PDE inhibitor.
3. Add drugs, aerate, and cap, and incubate for 10 min at 37°C in shaking water bath.

4. Stop the reaction with 580 μl of ice-cold 10% trichloroacetic acid (TCA). This stops the flux of radioactivity from prelabeled ATP pools into cyclic AMP pools and fixes the protein.

Sample Preparation

1. Disrupt the slices for 10 to 15 sec using a Polytron (Brinkmann Instruments) or tissue mixer.
2. Centrifuge at $10,000 \times g$ for 10 min.
3. Transfer 1.05 ml of supernatant to 12- $\times$ 75-mm glass test tubes.
4. Transfer 50 μl of 1.05-ml sample to minivials, add fluor, and count (for calculation of total [^{3}H]AXP pools).
5. Add 50 μl (*ca.* 10,000 cpm) of [^{14}C] cyclic AMP (recovery marker) to 1-ml samples and vortex.

Analysis: Double-column Method to Isolate Cyclic AMP

1. Add a 1-ml sample of the TCA extract with recovery marker to regenerated 1.5-ml Dowex columns (see below for regeneration procedure).
2. After the sample has run onto the resin, sequentially add 1 ml and then 1.5 ml of distilled water. Discard the initial eluate. The second eluate containing ATP and ADP can be collected or discarded. *Note:* New Dowex and alumina columns should be calibrated with radiolabeled cyclic AMP to determine the elution profile for the cyclic nucleotide.
3. Place Dowex columns over the alumina columns and add 4 ml of distilled water. This eluate containing the labeled cyclic AMP is allowed to flow directly into a fresh alumina column.
4. Remove the Dowex columns and add 1.5 ml of 0.1 M imidazole-HCl (pH, 7.5) to the alumina columns.
5. Place the alumina columns over the rack with 20-ml scintillation vials and add 3 ml of 0.1 M imidazole-HCl, eluting the labeled cyclic AMP fraction directly into scintillation vials.
6. Add 10 ml of fluor and determine the radioactivity by liquid scintillation counting using a dual-label (^{3}H/^{14}C) program (for adenylate cyclase, use a ^{3}H/^{32}P program).

Recovery

1. Recovery of ATP and ADP in the Dowex eluate is practically 100%.
2. Recovery of cyclic AMP in the final alumina eluate is 60 to 75%.

Calculations

Results are expressed as the percent of the total tritium pool represented by [^{3}H] cyclic AMP (percent conversion) and are calculated as follows.

1. Calculate the total [^{3}H]AXP from the 50-μl aliquot taken from the 1.05-ml supernatant (total [^{3}H]AXP in 1-ml sample is $20 \times$ cpm in a 50-μl aliquot).
2. Calculate the recovery of cyclic AMP from each column from the amount of [^{14}C] cyclic AMP recovered divided by [^{14}C] cyclic AMP standard.

3. Percent Conversion $= \dfrac{[^3\text{H}] \text{ cyclic AMP} \times 100}{[^3\text{H}]\text{AXP}}$

Preparation of Dowex 50 Columns

These columns are prepared by transferring 3 ml of a 50% suspension of Bio-Rad AG 50W-4X, 200 to 400 mesh (H$^+$ form) into columns containing a glass wool plug at the bottom, after which the column is subjected to three regeneration cycles before use. Each regeneration cycle consists of the successive washing of the resin columns with 20 ml of water, 20 ml of 2 N NaOH, 20 ml of water, 20 ml of 2 N HCl, followed by three additional washes with 20 ml of water. After each usage, the columns are activated by a single regeneration cycle. An abbreviated regeneration procedure (described below) can be used when the columns are utilized for the prelabeling procedure.

Preparation of Aluminum Oxide Columns

These columns are prepared by adding 1.2 g of dry aluminum oxide into plugged columns that have been filled with water to allow for an even flow of alumina. The material is stirred if necessary to eliminate air bubbles. After packing, the columns should not be allowed to dry and are stored under water when not in use. On the day of assay, the columns are removed from the water and washed once with 10 ml of 0.1 M imidazole-HCl (pH 7.5).

Column Regeneration

Dowex

1. Rinse the columns with distilled water.
2. Add 15 ml of 1 N HCl.
3. Rinse the columns two additional times with distilled water.

Alumina

1. Rinse the columns twice with distilled water.
2. Prior to use, add 15 ml of 0.1 M imidazole-HCl.
3. Following assay, store columns in water to prevent drying.

Buffer Composition: Modified Krebs-Ringer Bicarbonate with Glucose (pH 7.4)

The buffer contains (mmol/liter): NaCl, 118; KCl 5; $CaCl_2$, 1.3; $MgSO_4$, 1.2; KH_2PO_4, 1.2; $NaHCO_3$, 25. A mixture of 95% O_2 and 5% CO_2 is bubbled through the solution for at least 20 min prior to analysis. Mix NaCl, KCl, and $CaCl_2$ first, and then add $MgSO_4$, $NaHCO_3$, and glucose to the solution.

Assay condition	[^{3}H]cAMP	[^{14}C]cAMP[a]	[^{3}H]cAMP − 10% Spillover[b]	[^{3}H]cAMP adj. rec.[c]	[^{3}H]AXP	conversion[d]
	dpm	*dpm% recovery*			*dpm*	*%*
Basal	1,341	3,506/58%	991	1,708	1,029,770	0.16
Isopro. (10 μM)	5,525	3,436/57%	5,181	9,089	1,018,781	0.89
Forskolin (10 μM)	30,383	3,614/60%	30,022	50,037	1,050,789	4.76

[a]To measure recovery, 6,000 dpm [^{14}C]cAMP added to assay.
[b]To account for the "spillover" of ^{14}C into the ^{3}H channel, calculate the percent spillover from samples containing [^{14}C]cAMP only. This percent of the [^{14}C]cAMP for each sample must be subtracted from the [^{3}H]cAMP for each sample.
[c]The [^{3}H]cAMP is adjusted for the recovery: $991 \div 0.58 = 1708$.
[d]% Conversion $= 100 \times \dfrac{[^3H]cAMP\ (1708)}{[^3H]AXP\ (1,029,770)} = 0.16$

Measurement of Cyclic AMP by Protein Kinase Activity Ratio

1. Tissue slices are prepared and incubated as previously described.
2. The incubations are terminated by immersing the slices in liquid nitrogen.
3. For determining the cyclic AMP-dependent protein kinase activity ratio, approximately 20 mg of the frozen tissue is rapidly homogenized (use ground glass homogenizers) in 1 ml of 5 mM potassium phosphate buffer (pH 6.8) containing 320 mM NaCl, 5 mM EDTA, and a PDE inhibitor.
4. The homogenate is centrifuged at $12,000 \times g$ for 15 min.
5. The supernatant fraction is immediately assayed for cyclic AMP-dependent protein kinase activity using mixed histone or histone HF2B as a substrate.
6. The reaction mixture (100 μl) consists of the following: 10 μl of 100 μM cyclic AMP or water; 20 μl of HF2B (5 mg/ml); 25 μl of supernatant; and 50 μl of the

assay solution which contains (mM): KH_2PO_4, 10; KH_2HPO_4, 10; Mg^{2+} acetate, 24; ATP, 0.2 to 0.4; and 10^6 cpm of [γ-^{32}P]ATP (300 cpm/pmol).

7. Assays are initiated by the addition of tissue extract and conducted at 30°C for 5 to 10 min. *Note:* It is critical to establish linearity with respect to the duration of the incubation and amount of supernatant added for each system.

8. Reactions are terminated by pipetting 75 μl of the reaction mixture onto 1- × 2.5 × 2.5 cm squares of Whatman P-81 phosphocellulose paper which have been numbered with a lead pencil.

9. The squares are immersed immediately into a beaker (~200 ml) of 75 mM phosphoric acid and swirled gently for approximately 2 min.

10. The phosphoric acid is decanted and the squares washed twice more in 75 mM phosphoric acid.

11. Following the third wash, the squares are dried with a blow dryer, placed in 20-ml scintillation vials containing 8 ml of Budget-Solve (xylene-based scintillation fluid), and analyzed by liquid scintillation spectrometry.

Calculations

Protein kinase activity, measured by ^{32}P incorporation into histone, is expressed as the protein kinase activity ratio, i.e., the ratio of kinase activity in the absence of exogenous cyclic AMP to that in the presence of a maximally stimulating concentration of cyclic AMP (10 to 20 μM).

Measurement of Cyclic AMP Content by Radioimmunoassay

Isolation of Cyclic AMP

1. Homogenize the tissue slices or cells (use Polytron) in 1 to 2 ml of 50% methanol/0.04 N HCl.

2. Centrifuge the homogenate at $3,000 \times g$ for 15 min.

3. Neutralize the supernatant with 20 μl of 2 M Tris-Cl (pH 8.0) using phenol red as an indicator.

Purification of Cyclic AMP

1. Place a 0.5-ml Dowex 1 X8 slurry (1:4) into stuffed Pasteur pipettes or other columns.

2. Wash the column with 2.0 ml of distilled water.

3. Apply neutralized sample to the Dowex column.

4. Wash the column with 2.0 ml of distilled water.

5. Wash the column with 2.0 ml of 0.001 N HCl/50% methanol.

6. Wash the column with 0.4 ml of 0.01 N HCl/50% methanol.

7. Collect 1.0 ml of the 0.01 N HCl/50% methanol eluate in 12- × 75-mm disposable test tubes.
8. Evaporate the samples to dryness in rotary evaporator.

Sample Acetylation

1. Reconstitute the tissue samples such that each 80 µl contains approximately 0.01 to 0.098 pmol of cyclic AMP. (Dilute them in distilled water if necessary.)
2. Dilute standard concentrations of cyclic AMP and store them frozen.
3. To an 80-µl tissue sample or standard, add 10 µl of a dioxane/triethylamine/acetic anhydride (7:2:1) mixture.
4. Vortex and let it stand for 10 min.
5. To neutralize acetylation, add 10 µl of a solution containing 2 M Tris and 1 mg/ml BSA (pH 8.0).

Radioimmunoassay

1. Submerge the tubes containing acetylated standards or tissue samples (100 µl, total volume) in an ice-water bath.
2. Add 50 µl of ^{125}I-cyclic AMP-tyrosine methyl ester (20,000 to 30,000 cpm/50 µl).
3. Add 50 µl of anti-cyclic AMP antibody. The antibody dilution is predetermined such that it will bind about one-third of the added radioactive cyclic AMP in the absence of any unlabeled ligand (bound over free ratio of approximately 0.5).
4. Mix it well and let it stand overnight.
5. Add 100-µl portion of 20% dialyzed pig plasma (or other carrier protein) and 1.5 ml of 100% ice-cold ethanol (kept in salted ice bath during use) simultaneously to each sample to precipitate the antibody-ligand complex.
6. Mix thoroughly and let it stand for 30 min at 4°C.
7. Centrifuge at $3,000 \times g$ for 30 min (4°C).
8. Decant the supernatant and drain the tubes onto Kimwipe absorbant paper.
9. Count the radioactivity in pellet on a γ-scintillation counter.

Preparation of Standards

The concentrations of the cyclic AMP standards should range from 2.5 to 1200 fmol/80 µl. The standards are prepared from a stock solution of cyclic AMP dissolved in water, with the concentration verified spectrophotometrically (molar extinction coefficient, 14.65 at 259 mm) and stored frozen in aliquots at $-20°C$ until used.

Analysis of Standard Curve

The amount of cyclic AMP in the tissue samples is determined by computerized dose interpretation from the standard curve using a standardized radioimmunoassay program.

The standard curve is determined by assaying, in duplicate, each of the cyclic AMP standards. Blanks contain all reagents but no antibody.

DISCUSSION

Assessment of Adenylate Cyclase

The units of Adenylate cyclase activity are expressed as pmol of cyclic AMP formed/min/mg of protein. Both homogenates and particulate preparations contain cyclic nucleotide phosphodiesterases of much higher specific activity than the [^{32}P] cyclic AMP generated in the assay. To prevent hydrolysis of the radiolabeled cyclic nucleotide, saturating amounts of unlabeled cyclic AMP are included in the assay mixture. The coaddition of PDE inhibitor, such as 1-methyl-3-isobutylxanthine (MIX) or 4-(3-butoxy-4-methoxybenzyl)-2-imidazolidinone (RO 20-1724) is required if high concentrations (>1 mM) of cyclic AMP are unable to inhibit degradation of the labeled product completely. The effects of these inhibitors themselves must be determined since under certain circumstances, PDE inhibitors (especially the methylxanthines) may interfere with the assay.

Since brain homogenates and particulate fractions contain ATPases and other terminal phosphatases, it is necessary to maintain constant levels of substrate (Mg-ATP). Since the substrate for the Adenylate cyclase reaction is [^{32}P]ATP labeled in the α-position, it is possible to regenerate the substrate degraded by phosphatases without altering the specific activity of the ATP. Regeneration systems consisting of phosphoenolpyruvate and pyruvate kinase or myokinase and creatine phosphokinase circumvent the problem.

Magnesium ions are required in the assay since Mg-ATP rather than ATP is the substrate for the enzyme. Further Mg^{2+} ions in excess over ATP and EDTA are required to obtain expression of activity since Mg^{2+} is an activator of the enzyme. Maximum stimulating activities are generally seen in the range of 5 to 15 mM Mg^{2+}, whereas receptor inhibition of Adenylate cyclase is optimal at 1 to 2 mM Mg^{2+}. Since $MgCl_2$ is highly hygroscopic, magnesium acetate-Tris acetate buffers can be used if it is not possible to store $MgCl_2$ under anhydrous conditions.

The Tris salts of EDTA and EGTA (1 mM) are generally used in the assay. Their inclusion permits linear cyclic AMP accumulation over extended (10-to 90-min) periods of time. However, in some adenylate cyclase systems, e.g., with brain adenylate cyclase, trace amounts of calcium activate calmodulin, which stimulates adenylate cyclase activity three- to fivefold above basal. The degree of calcium/calmodulin-stimulated adenylate cyclase activity is dependent on the washing of tissue and the level of calcium, either endogenous or added to the assay.

The level of adenylate cyclase activity in brain is generally five- to tenfold higher than that of peripheral tissues. As discussed above, adenylate cyclase activity requires GTP and Mg^{2+}. In addition to these important regulatory molecules, there are a variety of other factors that influence cyclic AMP production in brain. The presence of monovalent cations, different buffers, and method of tissue preparation may alter the adenylate cyclase response. The sensitivity of this second messenger system to a variety of factors requires that the conditions of the assay be precisely defined to ensure consistent data.

The alumina oxide columns can be used between 20 and 50 times depending on the amount of radioactive ATP in each assay. With the "wet procedure," the columns are washed with 25 ml of water immediately after use and are kept under water to avoid drying. The columns are never stirred since this increases the blank, especially after several uses as the column becomes progressively saturated with labeled materials.

Alumina oxide purchased from Sigma (neutral grade) can be stored in columns in a dry state ensuring much faster flow rates during separations if used in the prelabeling procedure.

Assessment of G_s Activity by Reconstitution Assays

Adenylate cyclase activity is expressed as pmol of [^{32}P] cyclic AMP formed/20 min, and the data are plotted as a function of extract protein present in the reconstitution assay. This procedure is simply a bioassay for reconstituted activity of the regulatory component. The level of extract required for half-maximal expression of reconstituted activity is determined from the concentration-response curve, which represents relative units of reconstituted activity. However, as with any bioassay, a number of factors influence the results. Thus, when making comparisons among animals or between treatment groups, it is important to employ a standardized and reproducible procedure. Optimal conditions for solubilization and reconstitution need to be established for each membrane system.

The choice of detergent for solubilization is predicted by the behavior of the detergent in subsequent reconstitution procedures. For example, the addition of a small amount of Lubrol-PX (0.019%) yields four- to fivefold more isoproterenol or fluoride stimulation in the reconstituted Cyc$^-$ membrane with cholate extracts of cerebral cortex. Also, the reconstitution of transmitter-receptor-activated Adenylate cyclase in Cyc$^-$ membrane is dependent upon the use of saturating concentrations of extract protein. For example, 2 μg of extracted protein yields less than a twofold and 16 μg, greater than fourfold isoproterenol stimulation when incubated with 25 μg of Cyc$^-$ membranes.

The thermolability of both the catalytic and regulatory components depends upon the detergents used for solubilization. An inactivation profile for catalytic activity must be determined whenever the detergent or its concentration is altered or if the particulate preparation is modified. For instance, whereas both the catalytic and regulatory components are more labile in cholate solutions, cholate is often the preferred detergent for extraction since it permits stable reconstitution as well as reconstitution of hormonal or transmitter receptor-activated Adenylate cyclase in the Cyc − membranes. Addition of KCl (100 to 500 mM) can be used to increase the yield of extractable proteins from membrane fractions.

Linear velocity measurements are made with fixed-time incubations if the reconstitution is allowed to proceed for a period sufficient to eliminate any lag and for the enzyme to reach steady state (velocity no longer changes with time). A simple method to accomplish this is to incubate the reaction mixture in the presence of all additives except the radiolabeled ATP. The [α-^{32}P]ATP is then added and the reaction allowed to proceed for another 10 to 20 min before assaying the amount of [^{32}P] cyclic AMP.

It is advisable to purify commercial supplies of cholic acid prior to use by recrystallization from ethanol. This is accomplished by adding cholic acid to boiling absolute ethanol (ratio of 1:1) and stirring until the acid is in solution. Any residue should be removed by filtration through Whatman no. 2 filter paper. The filtrate is poured into 200 ml of ice-cold distilled water to precipitate the cholic acid. This suspension is kept at 0 to 4°C for at least 4 hr prior to removing the supernatant by either centrifugation or aspiration. The precipitate is redissolved in the original volume of boiling alcohol and the above procedure repeated. Following three cycles of successive recrystallizations, the cholic acid is dried in an oven at 50°C.

ADP-Ribosylation of G-Proteins

The pertussis- and cholera toxin-catalyzed ADP-ribosylation procedures have been important tools for analyzing the molecular and functional characteristics of G-proteins. Cholera- and pertussis toxin-mediated ADP-ribosylation has been used to demonstrate the regional distribution of G-proteins in brain and the influence of chronic morphine treatment on G-proteins. However, factors such as the functional state of G-proteins and soluble constituents that influence the ribosylation reaction may confound the interpretation of these data. An absolute change in the level of G-proteins can be verified by using specific antibodies for Western blot analysis of the various G-proteins.

Assay of Cyclic AMP Content

The type of homogenization, ionic strength, and composition of the incubation medium are known to alter basal protein kinase activity ratios. Therefore, these conditions must be optimized for each tissue being investigated and whenever alterations are made in the procedure. Blanks consist of boiled supernatant or reagent blanks alone. The values obtained are generally 0.03 to 0.05% of the total radioactivity and should not exceed 0.1%. Endogenous protein kinase other than the cyclic AMP-dependent form can phosphorylate exogenous histone substrates. Thus, a heat-stable inhibitor of protein kinase should be added to a set of tubes to determine what portion of the incorporation is cyclic AMP dependent. If the basal protein kinase activity ratio is high (>0.5) before activating the cyclase, it will be difficult to demonstrate dose-response relationships and small changes in the intracellular levels of cyclic AMP since the maximum change in ratio is only twofold.

The most widely used procedure for measuring cyclic AMP is radioimmunoassay. The antibodies for cyclic AMP and the iodinated antigen are commercially available (Du Pont-New England Nuclear). The results are expressed as pmol of cyclic AMP/mg of tissue protein. The acid precipitate is dissolved in 1 N NaOH and protein content determined in individual samples by standard assay techniques. This will minimize variation among slices divided into individual samples.

In addition to cost, there are other drawbacks to this procedure. Although basal levels of cyclic AMP can be determined, the procedure is less sensitive to changes in cyclic AMP content than is the prelabeling technique. This is due to the fact that a large portion of the endogenous store of cyclic AMP does not change in response to a receptor-cyclase interaction and the possibility that different nucleotide pools have differences in turnover rate.

Both of these procedures can be used to assess changes in cyclic AMP turnover. However, the most commonly used for this purpose is the prelabeling technique. Following incubation of slices for 45 to 60 min with [^{3}H]adenine to label endogenous nucleotide pools, the slices are washed and incubated with a saturating concentration of agonist until a steady state level of cyclic AMP is attained (percent conversion no longer changes over time).

A 50-μl suspension of slices is rapidly transferred into fresh buffer containing 200 μM propranolol or 0.55 units of adenosine deaminase when isoproterenol or adenosine is used as agonist, respectively. Various inhibitors of cyclic nucleotide PDE can be tested to assess their effects on degradation in intact tissue. The incubation is allowed to proceed until cyclic AMP levels return to basal. The reaction is terminated by the addition of an equal volume of 10% TCA at various times (1 to 20 min). Following homogenization, the samples are centrifuged and the extracted cyclic AMP isolated by the Dowex 50/alumina column method.

For turnover studies, it is necessary to conduct the postincubation period long enough to return to the basal state. If the decay plot deviates from linearity, it is not a first-order process and will require more extensive analysis.

BIBLIOGRAPHY

Superfusion of Brain Slices

Schoffelmeer ANM, Hogenboom F, Mulder AH. *Arch Pharmacol* 1987;335:278–284.

ADP-Ribosylation

Bokoch GM, Katada T, Northup JK, Hewlett EL, Gilman AG. *J Biol Chem* 1983;258:2072–2075.
Cassel D, Pfeuffer T. *Proc Natl Acad Sci USA* 1978;75:2669–2673.
Duman RS, Enna SJ. *Brain Res* 1986;384:391–394.
Katada T, Ui M. *Proc Natl Acad Sci USA* 1982;79:3129–3133.

Nestler EJ, Tallman JF. *Mol Pharmacol* 1988;33:127–132.
Sternweis PC, Robishaw JD. *J Biol Chem* 1984;259:13806–13813.
Tamir A, Gill DM. *J Neurochem* 1988;50:1791–1797.

Adenylate Cyclase and G-Proteins

Asano T, Semba R, Ogasawara N, Kato K. *J Neurochem* 1987;48:1617–1623.
Gilman AG. *Cell* 1984;36:577–579.
Gierschik P, Milligan G, Peres M, Goldsmith P, Codina J, Klee W, Spiegel A. *Proc Natl Acad Sci USA* 1986;83:2258–2262.
Hatta S, Marcus MM, Rasenick MM. *Proc Natl Acad Sci USA* 1986;83:5439–5443.
Howlett, AC, Sternweiss PC, Macik BA, VanArsdale DM, Gilman AG. *J Biol Chem* 1979;254:2287–2295.
Krishna G, Weiss B, Brodie BB. *J Pharmacol Exp Ther* 1968;163:379–385.
Neer EJ, Salter RS. *J Biol Chem* 1979;256:2287–2295.
Perez-Reyes E, Cooper DMF. *Mol Pharmacol* 1987;32:212–216.
Rasenick MM, Stein PJ, Bitensky MW. *Nature* 1981;294:560–562.
Rodbell M, Birnbaumer L, Pohl SL, Krans HMJ. *J Biol Chem* 1971;246:1877–1882.
Rosenberg GB, Storm DR. *J Biol Chem* 1987;262:7623–7628.
Ross EM, Gilman A. *Proc Natl Acad Sci USA* 1977;74:3715–3719.
Ross, EM, Howlett AC, Ferguson KM, Gilman AG. *J Biol Chem* 1978;253:6401–6412.
Salomon Y. *Adv Cyclic Nucleotide Res* 1979;10:35–55.
Salomon Y, Londos C, Rodbell M. *Anal. Biochem* 1974;58:541–548.
Stryer L, Bourne HR. *Annu Rev Cell Biol* 1986;2:391–419.
Worley PF, Baraban JM, Van Dop C, Neer EJ, Snyder SH. *Proc Natl Acad Sci USA* 1986;83:4561–4565.
Worley PF, Baraban JM, DeSouza EB, Snyder SH. *Proc Natl Acad Sci USA* 1986;83:4053–4057.

Receptor-Mediated Inhibition of Adenylate Cyclase

Fredholm BB, Lindgren E, Lindstrom K. *Br J Pharmacol* 1985;86:509–513.
Devivo M, Maayani S. *J Pharmacol Exp Ther* 1986;238:248–253.
Ahlijanian MK, Halford MK, Cooper DMF. *J Neurochem* 1987;49:1308–1315.
Ahlijanian MK, Cooper DMF. *Mol Pharmacol* 1987;32:127–132.
Neer EJ, Lok JM, Wolf LG. *J Biol Chem* 1984;259:14222–14229.
Rasenick MM, O'Callahan CM, Moore CA, Kaplan RS. In: De Brabander M, De Mey, J, eds., *Microtubles and microtuble inhibitors*. New York: Elsevier Science Publishing Co, 1985.

Cyclic AMP and Protein Kinase

Daly JW. *Cyclic nucleotides in the nervous system*. New York: Plenum Publishing Corp, 1977.
Davis CW. *Life Sci* 1985;37:85–94.
Shimizu H, Daly JW, Creveling CR. *J Neurochem* 1969;16:1609–1619.

Effects of Drugs and Other Treatments on Adenylate Cyclase System

Daly JW, Padgett W, Creveling CR, Cantaeuzene D, Kirk KL. *J Neurosci* 1981;1:49–59.
Donaldson J, Brown AM, Hill SJ. *Biochem. Pharmacol* 1988;37:715–723.
Duman RS, Enna SJ. *Neuropharmacology* 1987;26:981–986.
Duman RS, Strada SJ, Enna SJ. *J Pharmacol Exp Ther* 1986;234:409–414.
Duman RS, Strada SJ, Enna SJ. *Brain Res* 1989;477:166–171.
Duman RS, Tallman JF, Nestler EJ. *J Pharmacol Exp Ther* 1988;246:1033–1039.
Nestler EJ, Erdos JJ, Terwilliger RZ, Duman RS, Tallman JF. *Brain Res* 1989;476:230–239.
Perkins JP, Moore MM. *J Pharmacol Exp Ther* 1973;185:371–378.
Schwabe U, Daly JW. *J Pharmacol Exp Ther* 1977;202:134–143.
Stone EA, Platt JE, Herrera AS, Kirk KL. *J Pharmacol Exp Ther* 1986;237:702–707.

Methods in Neurotransmitter Receptor Analysis,
edited by Henry I. Yamamura, et al.
Raven Press, Ltd., New York © 1990.

5

Receptor Solubilization, Characterization, and Isolation

Morley D. Hollenberg

*Endocrine Research Group, Department of Pharmacology and Therapeutics and
Department of Medicine, University of Calgary, Faculty of Medicine,
Calgary, Alberta, T2N 1N4 Canada*

Perhaps faster than the information can be assimilated, the detailed amino acid sequences of a variety of neurotransmitter receptors are now appearing in the literature. Although the complete sequence information has come from the analysis of cloned receptor cDNA, in all instances, the studies have also relied heavily on partial amino acid sequence data that have been obtained from purified receptor preparations. The hallmark for such studies can be seen in work with the nicotinic receptor for acetylcholine (1, 2). Not only has the complex oligomeric structure of this ligand-regulated ion channel been determined, but the amino acid sequences of the four distinct receptor polypeptide sequences have been deduced from the cloned cDNAs. This work represents a remarkable chapter that began at the turn of the century with Langley's interest in the mechanism whereby nicotine affects striated muscle (3). Progress of the kind illustrated by work with the nicotinic receptor has been made possible by the development of a number of biochemical approaches for dealing with membrane-localized receptors. In summary, the key methodologies for receptor characterization comprise: (*a*) preparation of suitable radioligand probes; (*b*) selection of a suitable detergent for solubilization of the receptor from a rich membrane source; (*c*) development of a rapid, reliable method for detecting the soluble receptor; (*d*) use of appropriate lectin and other selective ligand affinity chromatography columns for receptor isolation; (*e*) cross-link labeling of receptors either with photoprobes or with chemical cross-linking reagents; (*f*) analysis of cross-link-labeled receptor preparations by biochemical approaches (e.g., chromatographic, electrophoretic, proteolytic mapping); (*g*) preparation and use of anti-receptor antibodies; and (*h*) microsequence analysis and cDNA probe synthesis, followed by receptor cloning and sequencing. A number of review articles, including those resulting from our own work, have described in general many of the methods used for receptor solubilization and isolation (4–7). It will be the aim of this chapter to provide sufficient details for the methods routinely used so that the interested reader could (*a*) reproduce the work reported previously in the literature and (b) adapt the procedures for use with an as yet uncharacterized receptor system. At the outset, it must be emphasized strongly that each receptor system presents its own challenges and idiosyncracies, such that no single method of approach will be applicable for all receptors that one may encounter. However, in principle, all receptor isolation studies reported so far have faced analogous challenges; and essentially the same directions with common goals have been followed by all studies. Thus, for this chapter, I have chosen to draw on my past experience with the receptors for insulin, insulin-like growth factor I [IGF-I or basic-somatomedin (BSM)] and epidermal growth factor-urogastrone (EGF-URO). Although these polypeptides do not, of themselves, function as neurotransmitters, the approaches developed for the solubilization and purification of their receptors can be seen as a model for the purification of receptors for neurotransmitters (both peptide and nonpeptide alike). The specific examples that have been selected for the chapter are those that have been essentially student tested in my laboratory and that might serve as a basis for a "hands-on" graduate course in receptor isolation and characterization.

GENERAL CONSIDERATIONS

Before proceeding with the purification of a putative receptor molecule, it is useful to consider a number of questions.

1. Does the radiolabeled ligand probe possess a radiochemical specific activity sufficient for the ligand-specific detection of the receptor upon solubilization? For instance, polypeptides used generally for receptor probes as ^{125}I-labeled species usually possess specific activities of 600 to 1,200 µCi/nmol (1 Ci $= 2.70 \times 10^{10}$ becquerels). Thus, there is usually no problem in detecting the receptor, upon solubilization, even when samples become diluted during the various steps of purification. However, difficulties may be encountered with ^{3}H-labeled ligand probes, which are often available only with specific activities of 2 to 6 µCi/nmol. Another property of the radiolabeled probe which merits attention relates to its stability and behavior (e.g., adsorption to gel chromatography matrices) in the various systems (e.g., high pressure liquid chromatography (HPLC), ultracentrifugation) that may be used for receptor purification.

2. Are sufficient receptor-specific competitive ligands available to ensure that the solubilized binding protein, upon isolation, displays the ligand specificity expected of the receptor being studied? It is easily overlooked that, upon solubilization, membranes may release nonreceptor constituents that can bind ligands with high affinity but without the kind of specificity that is exhibited by the true receptor.

3. Does the starting material (e.g., isolated membrane preparation) possess a sufficient abundance of receptor to make its isolation feasible? By their nature, receptors represent a vanishingly small fraction of the proteins present in the membrane, and on average, membrane preparations containing 10 to 20 pmol

of receptor protein/mg of membrane protein can be considered as "rich" sources of receptor. Very often, receptor abundance in membrane preparations is far below this value, thereby increasing the difficulty of the task of receptor isolation.

4. Is the affinity of the radiolabeled ligand probe sufficient to permit the detection of the receptor, should the process of solubilization lead to a reduction in ligand affinity? For binding constants that are in the range of 10^9 or greater, a reduction in affinity of up to an order of magnitude need not present a problem. However, affinities in the 10^7 to 10^6 M^{-1} range would present problems because of the rapid ligand dissociation rates that would be encountered, rendering problematic the measurements of binding to the solubilized receptor.

5. Can receptor binding be specifically and rapidly measured for the solubilized receptor species? Indeed, the development of a convenient reliable assay for the solubilized receptor (to be discussed below) represents the key to any planned purification protocol. Unfortunately, upon release from the membrane environment, some receptors simply to not bind a ligand efficiently.

MATERIALS

Although it is assumed that general laboratory reagents, equipment, and supplies (e.g., analytical grade chemicals; β- or γ-counters; centrifuges and rotors; chromatography and electrophoresis equipment, micropipettes) will be available, there are a number of specialized reagents and pieces of equipment which are required of a laboratory involved in receptor studies.

Source of Radiolabel and Labeling Facility

For those without the luxury of purchasing prelabeled ligand probes, it is essential to equip the laboratory for synthetic purposes and to secure a reliable source of radioisotope (usually, ^{3}H or ^{125}I). In practice, the procedures to be outlined below require 1 to 2 mCi of carrier-free ^{125}I, obtained from the supplier as soon as possible after the production date. Suitable dedicated laboratory space and disposable micropipettes required for the safe handling of the isotope are essential.

Tissue Homogenizer

In searching for a suitable tissue source for a receptor of interest, it may be necessary to prepare membranes from a variety of organs from a number of species. In such a search, and for the procedures to be outlined below, an efficient rotary knife tissue homogenizer (of the Polytron-type) that can process large amounts of material is essential.

Filter Manifold and/or Microcentrifuge

The heart of a receptor isolation procedure is the binding assay. As will be outlined below, this assay may require the trapping and washing of a precipitated ligand-receptor complex on a filter or the collection of a bead-bound or membrane-bound receptor complex by centrifugation. For these procedures, which may involve the processing of up to 100 samples in a single assay, it is highly desirable to use a multiwell manifold-type filter machine or, alternatively, a multisample microcentrifuge (e.g., of the Beckman or Eppendorf type). Whether the assay to be employed uses membrane filters (e.g., Millipore E-series or Whatman glass fiber-type) or centrifuge tubes (e.g., 1-ml or 0.5-ml Polythene microcentrifuge tubes), it is essential to make sure that nonspecific binding of the radiolabeled probe either to the filter or to the tube does not complicate the measurements of receptor binding. To eliminate nonspecific bindng from this source, it may be necessary to evaluate tubes and/or filters of different chemical composition from a variety of suppliers.

Source of Membranes

As alluded to above, receptor isolation procedures require a readily available source of membranes that possess a comparatively high abundance of the receptor of interest (e.g., 10 to 20 pmol of receptor/mg of membrane protein). For neurotransmitter receptors, the cerebral cortex has often been a focus of interest because of the obvious localization of neurotransmitter receptors of many types in the central nervous system. However, the brain need not be the best tissue to use in terms of receptor abundance. For instance, the α_1-adrenergic receptor, although clearly present in many brain regions at a level of 80 to 200 fmol/mg of protein, is present in liver tissue at much higher levels (400 to 1200 fmol/mg of protein). The human placenta, which will be used as a tisssue source for the examples to be described below, is not only an excellent source of receptor for insulin, EGF-URO and other growth factors, but also may be a suitable source of receptors for neurotransmitters (e.g., the β-adrenergic receptor). For some receptor studies, it is possible to use fresh-frozen tissue; for studies in which a receptor property apart from ligand recognition may be of interest (e.g., ligand-regulated tyrosine kinase activity), the use of freshly obtained tissue is preferable. In the examples to follow, either rat liver or human placental tissue will be used as a source of receptor. For the study of receptors for insulin and EGF-URO, the procedures to be described will work equally well. It is only because of my laboratory's familiarity with the procedures to be described that rat liver and human placenta have been singled out as tissue sources to be used as an example. In principle, analogous procedures should work for the isolation of other receptors (including those for neurotransmitters) from these two tissue sources; and it should be possible to adapt the described procedures for use with other tissues.

METHODS

The following methods were developed to study the receptors for insulin, IGF-I, and EGF-URO. In many ways, methods worked out first for the insulin receptor have served as a paradigm for work with many other receptors in terms of the solubilization, gel filtration, and affinity chromatography procedures. Some of the challenges presented by the difficulties of detecting the solubilized EGF-URO receptor led to the cross-link-labeling and lectin immobilization assays that have proved of use for a variety of receptor systems. Taken together, the methods to be described should prove of use for the study of new receptor systems displaying sufficiently high ligand affinities to permit the measurement of binding upon receptor solubilization.

Preparation of Radioligand Probe

For peptide ligands, it is frequently possible to introduce carrier-free ^{125}I at tyrosine residues using a modification of the chloramine-T-metabisulfite procedure originally described by Greenwood and coworkers (7a) and outlined in the following paragraph. On average, the procedure described results in the introduction of one atom of iodine/peptide molecule. Higher degrees of substitution with ^{125}I may interfere with the binding properties of insulin or EGF-URO. Radiolabeled insulin or EGF-URO prepared in the manner described can be used for binding studies without further purification. For other peptides, it is essential to demonstrate that neither the oxidation/reduction conditions nor the introduction of the iodine atom alters the biological activity of the parent compound. Should the peptide lack an accessible tyrosine residue (sulfhydryls or histidine residues may also become substituted with ^{125}I) or should the iodination procedure destroy the peptide's biological activity, alternative methods of labeling (e.g., use of a ^{125}I-labeled N-succinimidyl ester reagent, developed by Bolton and Hunter, that can be coupled to the primary amino group of the peptide or to the ε-amino group of lysine) must be sought.

Other methods of preparing radioactively labeled ligands do not yield the very high specific activities obtained with carrier-free ^{125}I or ^{131}I. Among the more useful alternatives are tritium exchange, especially with the use of microwave discharge activation of tritium gas; chemical modification of sulfhydryl groups with radioactive organomercurials or analogous metals; substitution of free amino groups with $[^3H]$acetyl moieties by using $[^3H]$acetic anhydride (available commercially at 8 Ci/mmol); reaction of primary amino groups with tritiated methyl ester of acetamide to give acetamido derivatives; oxidation (reversible) of terminal galactose residues followed by reduction with NaB^3H_4; dehalogenation of an iodinated derivative by substitution of tritium for iodine and by the specific substitution of tritiated pyridoxal groups. In the past, the incorporation of $[^{35}S]$sulfate (into insulin) has also been used. References for the details of these alternative procedures, which are beyond the scope of this chapter, are to be found elsewhere (6). The routine method for peptide iodination is summarized in the following paragraph.

Stock peptides (about 1 mg/ml) are routinely dissolved in 50 mM sodium bicarbonate. The precise concentration of peptide can be measured spectrophotometrically using measurements at 215 and 225 nm for samples diluted in phosphate buffer, according to the formula

$$(E_{215} - E_{225}) \times 155 = \mu g/ml$$

Carrier-free Na^{125}I (or ^{131}I) (1 to 3 mCi in a volume of 5 to 10 µl) is added to 100 µl of 0.25 M sodium phosphate buffer, pH 7.5 (4.15 g of Na$_2$HPO$_4$ + 0.51 g of NaH$_2$PO$_4$·H$_2$O/100 ml), and polypeptide (5 µl of a 1 mg/ml solution in 0.05 M NaHCO$_3$) is then added with a glass capillary so as to avoid bubbling the solution. Immediately, 20 µl of a freshly prepared solution of chloramine-T (0.5 mg/ml in distilled H$_2$O) is added with gentle agitation, and the oxidation reaction is allowed to proceed for 20 to 30 sec; then sodium metabisulfite (20 µl of 1 mg/ml in distilled H$_2$O) is added, and the consequent reduction step is allowed to proceed for a period of 10 to 15 sec. The reaction mixture is then diluted with 200 µl of 0.1 M sodium phosphate buffer, pH 7.5, containing 0.1% (w/v) crystalline bovine serum albumin. An aliquot (10 µl) is quickly withdrawn so as to quantitate by crystal scintillation counting the amount of radioactive iodine present in the reaction medium. The remaining solution is transferred either to a preequilibrated (albumin-containing phosphate buffer) 10-ml column (disposable 10-ml pipette, 18×0.9 cm) of Sephadex G-10 or to a heavy walled 12-ml conical centrifuge tube containing a talc pellet (25 mg, Gold Leaf Pharmaceutical Co.), which is then crushed and triturated with a Pasteur pipette so as to adsorb the iodinated peptide. The small amount of solution remaining in the reaction vessel (12- × 75-mm glass test tube) is diluted with approximately 0.5 ml of albumin-containing buffer and saved for the measurement of the percentage of ^{131}I or ^{125}I incorporated into peptide. The gel filtration column is eluted with the 0.1% albumin-containing 0.1 M phosphate buffer at a flow rate of about 0.5 ml/min; the radiolabeled peptide, collected in 0.5-ml fractions from the column, is usually recovered in fractions 4 to 8. In order to recover the peptide from talc, the talc-adsorbed peptide is suspended in about 10 ml of albumin-containing buffer and pelleted by centrifugation; the pellet is washed four more times in this manner. The labeled polypeptide is then eluted from the final pellet by suspension in 2 to 3 ml of a solution comprised of 3 ml of 1 N HCl, 2.5 ml of H$_2$O, and 0.5 ml of 20% crystalline albumin (either in H$_2$O or in Krebs-Ringer-bicarbonate buffer, pH 7.4). The suspension is clarified by centrifugation (3,000 rpm, 40 min), and the ^{125}I-labeled peptide is transferred to a tared vial and the exact volume determined by weight. Several drops of 0.25 M phosphate buffer, pH 7.4, are added, and the solution is adjusted to near neutrality (pH 4 to 7, indicator paper) by the dropwise addition of 1 N NaOH up to an amount just under half the original volume measured as described above. Should the solution inadvertently become alkaline, a drop of 1 N HCl is added, and the pH is then readjusted to near neutrality. Although the gel filtration method of recovery is by far the most convenient and is suitable for preparing radiolabeled EGF-URO, the talc-adsorption procedure can prove to be an advantage for certain peptides (like insulin) in that the intact radiolabeled peptide can be purified from "damaged" peptide reaction productions that do not adsorb well to the talc. An aliquot (20 μl) of the solution of radiolabeled peptide is withdrawn to measure the precipitability of the preparation by trichloroacetic acid (TCA) and the specific radioactivity of the peptide. As an alternative to the two procedures outlined above, the entire reaction mixture can be purified by HPLC. Although this procedure is not necessary for work with radiolabeled insulin and EGF-URO, the separation of mono- and diiodo derivatives of certain peptides may be essential for the reliable estimate of binding to solubilized receptors.

The incorporation of ^{125}I is estimated in the following manner. An aliquot, e.g., 50 μl, of the residual diluted reaction mixture is mixed into 1.0 ml of 0.1 M phosphate buffer, pH 7.5, containing 1% (w/v) bovine serum albumin. An equal aliquot (50 μl) is withdrawn for measurement of radioactivity. TCA [0.5 ml of a 10% (w/v) solution in H_2O] is then added, and the precipitate is chilled in ice and then sedimented in a clinical centrifuge. An aliquot of the supernatant (50 μl) is withdrawn, and the radioactivity is measured. It is assumed that the radioactivity remaining in the supernatant represents nonincorporated ^{125}I. The fraction (f) of ^{125}I incorporated into the peptide is given by the formula

$$f = (RA\ initial\ -\ 1.5\ RA\ final)/RA\ initial$$

where RA initial and RA final refer to the radioactivity in aliquots before and after the addition of TCA, respectively. If in the initial reaction mixture containing 5 μg of peptide there were C μCi present, the specific activity (SA) of the preparation is given by the equation

$$SA\ = (fC/5)\ \mu Ci/\mu g \qquad [1]$$

In a procedure identical to the one described in the preceding paragraph, the fraction of ^{125}I-labeled peptide precipitated by TCA is determined for an aliquot of the purified iodopeptide solution. In practice, 90 to 99% of the radioactivity is precipitated for a preparation of ^{125}I-peptide that is fully biologically active and yields good binding data. The number of radioactive iodine molecules, on average, that are incorporated can be calculated using a value of 1.62×10^7 mCi/milliatom for ^{131}I and 2.8×10^6 mCi/milliatom for ^{125}I.

The use of the lactoperoxidase technique also yields highly radioactive ^{125}I-substituted peptides. However, this method employs H_2O_2 in the reaction to generate free iodine and thus does not avoid exposure of the peptide to a strong oxidizing agent. The enzymatic procedure thus does not offer a fundamentally distinct chemical iodination procedure. Nonetheless, the enzymatic method has been found to yield ^{125}I-labeled derivatives of some polypeptides better suited to receptor studies than derivatives prepared by the chloramine-T method.

Preparation of Membranes

Either rat liver or human placental tissue can be used. Freshly isolated tissue (fresh-frozen tissue that is thawed before processing can also be used, but optimal results are obtained with fresh tissue) is rinsed free from blood with 25 mM [tris(hydroxymethyl)aminomethane] (Tris)-HCl-buffered (pH 7.4) 0.25 M ice-cold sucrose and is minced at 4°C in Tris-buffered isotonic sucrose solution containing 200 mg of phenylmethylsulfonyl fluoride [dissolved in 10 ml of dimethyl sulfoxide (DMSO)/liter and 1 mM iodoacetate. The inclusion of iodoacetate is optional; this agent appears to preserve the tyrosine kinase activity of the insulin and EGF-URO receptors. The sensitivity of the sulfhydryl-containing receptors to this reagent should be evaluated prior to proceeding with solubilization and isolation protocols. The tissue is diluted to 10 volumes (w/v) with the buffered sucrose solution and homogenized at 0°C with a rotary knife homogenizer (Brinkmann Instruments Polytron, setting 7, 90 sec). The homogenate is then filtered through two layers of cheesecloth and centrifuged at $10,000 \times g$ for 30 min at 4°C to remove debris. The supernatant solution is then made up to 0.1 M in NaCl and 0.2 mM $MgSO_4$ by the addition of concentrated solutions of these salts and then recentrifuged at $48,000 \times g$ for 40 min at 4°C. The resulting pellet is washed once by resuspension in 50 mM Tris-HCl, pH 7.6, and membranes are harvested by centrifugation ($48,000 \times g$ for 30 min at 4°C). The resulting pellet (0.15 g from 300 g, wet weight, of tissue) is resuspended (1 ml of buffer for each 10 g of tissue processed) in 50 mM Tris-HCl buffer to yield a suspension (2 to 8 mg/ml of protein) that can be stored frozen ($\leq -20°C$) as 1-ml aliquots for further use.

Membrane Solubilization and Measurement of Binding to Solubilized Receptors

Selection of a Detergent and General Approaches to Measuring Binding

Many detergents are now available to solubilize membrane proteins for further characterization (8,9). The key preliminary experiments comprise (*a*) the selection of a detergent that will solubilize the receptor in an active form from its membrane source; and (*b*) the design of a suitable assay to measure the binding of ligand to the soluble receptor. It is important to keep in mind that the "activity" of the receptor may comprise not only its ability to bind a ligand with high affinity and specificity but also its ability to function in a reconstitution system (e.g., as a ligand-regulated tyrosine kinase, as an ionophore, or as a regulator of adenylate cyclase in a liposome reconstitution system). Thus, the ability to remove the detergent by dilution, by adsorption to polystyrene beads (e.g., Bio-Beads SM-2 or XAD-2 Amberlite), or by dialysis may be an important factor in the choice for receptor solubilization. Thus, it is important to know the critical micelle concentration (CMC) for a selected detergent as well as the micelle size. The CMC represents the highest concentration of detergent at which monomers remain in solution; above this concentration, micelles of varying size [e.g., M_r 1,000 to 2,000 for octylpoly (oxyethylene); M_r 60,000 to 90,000 for Lubrol PX] can form so as to retard or prevent removal by dialysis. In practice, detergents such as Triton X-100 (CMC 0.1 to 0.4 mM) Lubrol PX (CMC≅.1 mM), octyl glucoside (CMC, 10 to 24 mM), digitonin (CMC≅0.25 mM), and cholate (CMC = 2 to 10 mM) have been used successfully. In our own work, it has proved important, when studying receptor kinase activity, to remove sulfhydryl-oxidizing contaminants from commercially available detergents by borohydride reduction and silicic acid chromatography, as described in detail elsewhere (10). These contaminants, if present, do not appear to affect receptor binding.

Initial experiments are usually performed to determine the optimum detergent concentration for receptor solubilization and for measuring binding. Even if binding cannot be monitored efficiently in the protein extract, it is possible to detect extraction of the receptor from the membranes by repeating the membrane-binding assay on washed membranes before and after detergent treatment. Often, the concentration of detergent required to release the receptor from the membrane [e.g., 1% (v/v) Triton X-100 for the insulin receptor] may be above the concentration at which binding can be measured; to measure binding, it is necessary to dilute the detergent concentration to below 0.1% (v/v). For peptide receptors, it has proven fruitful to measure binding to the solubilized receptor by two main approaches: (a) by gel filtration, whereby the receptor-bound ligand is eluted in a volume smaller than that at which free ligand appears, and (b) by precipitation of the ligand-receptor complex [e.g., with polyethylene glycol (PEG) or ammonium sulfate] under conditions in which the free ligand remains in solution. Both of these approaches for detecting the insulin receptor are illustrated in a following section. In the event that binding cannot be measured in the presence of detergent, it may be possible to immobilize the receptor on a solid matrix so as to wash away the detergent prior to the measurement of ligand binding. The lectin immobilization assay using this approach will be described below.

Membrane Solubilization

Both liver and placental membranes, suspended in 50 mM sodium phosphate buffer (pH 7.5) at a concentration of about 2 mg/ml of protein, are extracted for 12 h at 4°C with 2% (v/v) Triton X-100. Shorter extraction periods can be used with a somewhat reduced yield of receptor. Insoluble material is removed by centrifugation ($48,000 \times g$ for 60 min at 4°C). The extract can either be used directly for binding and gel filtration experiments, or the insulin receptor can be precipitated with ammonium sulfate [15% (w/v) fraction, collected by centrifugation] redissolved (0.8 mg/ml of protein) in phosphate buffer containing 0.1% (w/v) Triton X-100, and dialyzed at 4°C against detergent-containing buffer (4 hr against 1 liter of buffer) to remove excess salt. The receptor-containing extract can be stored at 4°C for further use.

Gel Filtration Method

Two aliquots (0.1 to 0.5 ml) of soluble receptor are equilibrated with radiolabeled ligand usually for about 1 hr at 24°C (e.g., for insulin) or up to 17 hr at 4°C (e.g., IGF-I) in the absence of or, after preequilibration (10 to 20 min) with a 100- to 1,000-fold excess of unlabeled ligand. After equilibration, both aliquots are applied to gel filtration columns (e.g., 90×1.5 cm of Sepharose 6B) and are eluted with detergent-containing buffers. Radioactivity in the eluted fractions is monitored. The elution volume of the receptor corresponds to a peak for which the radioactivity is reduced in the sample pretreated with an excess of unlabeled ligand (see Fig. 1). This approach provides not only a means of detecting the soluble receptor but also provides information about the hydrodynamic properties of the receptor (apparent Stokes radius).

PEG Method

This method, adapted from immunoassay procedures, has been used successfully for a variety of receptors, including the one for insulin (11). In brief, a concentration of PEG is sought which is sufficient to precipitate the ligand-receptor complex, leaving the labeled ligand in solution. The appropriate PEG concentration is arrived at by trial and error. The procedure for the insulin or IGF-I receptor follows.

For measurement of insulin binding, 5 to 50 µl of detergent-extracted receptor is added to 0.2 ml of Krebs-Ringer bicarbonate buffer, 0.1% (w/v) albumin, pH 7.4, containing ^{125}I-insulin with (control tubes only) or without 25 to 50 µg of native insulin/ml. Phosphate buffer (0.1 M, pH 7.4) may also be used for the binding assay provided the pH is maintained between 7.0 and 7.4; buffers containing Tris-HCl, however, appear to interfere with the PEG precipitation. Equilibration of binding is achieved in about 20 to 50 min at 24°C, at which time 0.5 ml of ice-cold 0.1 M sodium phosphate buffer (pH 7.4) containing 0.1% bovine γ-globulin (a carrier for precipitation) is added, and the tubes are placed in ice. Cold 25% (w/v) PEG (0.5 ml) is added [final concentration, 10% w/v], and the tubes are thoroughly mixed and placed in ice for 10 to 15 min. The suspension is then filtered under reduced pressure on cellulose acetate (Millipore EG or EH) filters, and the collected precipitate is washed with 3 ml of 8% (w/v) PEG in 0.1 M phosphate buffer (pH 7.4) before measurement of trapped radioactivity by crystal scintillation counting. In some instances, it may be possible to collect and wash the ligand-receptor precipitate by centrifugation with a microcentrifuge. As for the measurements of binding with cells and membranes, the specific binding is determined by subtracting from the total radioactivity bound that which remains bound in the presence of a high concentration (25 to 50 µg/ml) of native insulin. Under the above conditions, less than 0.5% of the total free ^{125}I-insulin is precipitated or adsorbed nonspecifically, and nearly quantitative precipitation of the insulin-receptor complex occurs.

Concentrations of PEG less than 8% (w/v) incompletely precipitate the complex;

concentrations higher than 12% significantly precipitate free insulin. The presence of γ-globulin is essential as a carrier for the precipitation reaction, but concentrations above 0.1% (w/v) cause precipitation of free insulin. If the pH of the buffer containing the γ-globulin is above 8 or below 7, the complex is less effectively precipitated; phosphate buffers (0.1 M, pH 7.4) can be used effectively in the incubation medium. A final concentration of Triton X-100 in the assay mixture in excess of 0.2% (v/v) results in decreased insulin binding. The membrane extracts are therefore diluted before assay so that the final concentration of Triton X-100 is usually less than 0.1% and always less than 0.2% (v/v). For the estimation of rate data (association/dissociation), it is assumed that the addition of the cold PEG-γ-globulin solutions stop the binding reaction at the timed intervals. It is expected that for each hormone studied, different conditions will be necessary to precipitate the maximum amount of hormone-receptor complex, leaving most of the free ligand in solution. The procedure that has been used for the insulin receptor may serve as a prototype for other studies. In principal, any analogous method for selective precipitation of hormone-receptor complexes (ammonium sulfate or other salting-out agent; TCA; change in pH) should provide a means of assaying soluble receptor, provided the complex is not dissociated by the precipitating agent. For example, salt fractionation has been used to examine the properties of soluble cholinergic receptor proteins. The analysis of soluble receptors for other ligands by a precipitation technique should similarly be possible. In principle, any procedure like precipitation which leads to a rapid separation of receptor bound from free ligand should work. For instance, in some cases, the selective adsorption of the receptor-ligand complex to a filter (e.g., ion-exchange disc or glass fiber) may serve as an alternative to precipitation. It is apparent that if the half-life of the receptor-ligand complex is not sufficiently prolonged at low temperatures (4°C), the dilution of the sample (about five-fold in the procedure described above) and the time allowed for precipitation may shift the binding equilibrium appreciably; appropriate corrections of the data will then be necessary. The use of the gel filtration and PEG methods together has led to the detection of soluble receptor forms that might have gone undetected had either assay been used in isolation (e.g., see Fig. 2).

Lectin Immobilization Assay

It can often happen (as with the EGF-URO receptor) that the soluble receptor may not be readily detected by either of the above methods. In such instances, it has proven useful to aggregate the soluble receptor with an insoluble or soluble lectin [concanavalin A (ConA), wheat germ agglutinin (WGA)] prior to the ligand-binding assay. For the immobilization assay, the receptor is absorbed from solution on beads of lectin-agarose, and the binding assay is done on the bead-bound receptor.

We have observed that the most readily available and useful lectin for the assay is ConA. However, other lectins (e.g., WGA) appear to work equally well, and in principle, it should be possible to optimize any assay of interest by an appropriate choice of lectin. ConA-Sepharose 4B-CL (approximately 2 mg of ConA/ml) is used in 50-µl aliquots for the adsorption of replicate samples of soluble membrane protein (approximately 100 µg of protein) in 12- × 75-mm glass tubes (15 min at 24°C; final reaction volume, approximately 300 µl). A variety of detergents (Triton X-100; Ammonyx-L0; Lubrol PX) do not interfere significantly with the adsorption of protein. The bead-bound protein is then washed by dilution with 5 ml of ice-cold buffer, immediately harvested by centrifugation (2 min at 1,000 rpm), and is then incubated with radiolabeled ligand either with or without an excess (usually 10- to 100-fold) of unlabeled ligand. After equilibration (usually 1 hr at 24°C), the samples are again washed by suspension in 5 ml of ice-cold buffer and harvested by centrifugation (2 min at 2,000 rpm) for measurement of bead-bound radioactivity upon removal of the supernatant solution by aspiration. As in other studies, the "specific" ligand binding is calculated by subtracting from the total radioactivity bound in the absence of unlabeled ligand, the amount of radioactivity bound in the presence of about a 100-fold excess of unlabeled ligand.

The method offers the advantages that the receptor can conveniently be transferred via the beads to a buffer optimized for the measurement of ligand binding and that dilute receptor samples (e.g., column effluent fractions) can be concentrated on the beads for the study of ligand binding.

As a useful variant of this approach, the soluble receptor is first equilibrated with soluble ConA. The binding of ligand is then measured by the PEG method, using the usual procedure. The addition of the soluble lectin facilitates the precipitation of the ligand-receptor complex and evidently does not interfere appreciably with the binding of ligand to the soluble receptor.

The binding of radiolabeled EGF-URO to its soluble receptor by the PEG method is estimated after a 45-min equilibration at 25°C in the presence of 100 µg of ConA, 0.1% bovine serum albumin, and 0.2% Triton X-100 in 0.5 ml of 20 mM N-2-hydroxyethylpiperazine-N'-2-ethanesulfonic acid (HEPES), pH 7.5, buffer. The ^{125}I-EGF-URO-receptor complex is precipitated by the addition of 1 ml of 20 mM HEPES buffer, pH 7.5, containing 0.1% bovine γ-globulin and 1 ml of 21.3% (w/v) PEG 6000 in buffer. The resulting precipitate is collected by centrifugation for the measurement of precipitated radioactivity. Nonspecific binding is determined in replicate tubes containing 1 µg/ml unlabeled EGF-URO.

Alternative Methods for Measuring Binding

Although the above methods have proven sufficient for measuring the binding of insulin, IGF-I, and EGF-URO to their receptors, other approaches may be necessary for other receptors. These approaches include equilibrium dialysis (adsorption of the radioligand probe to the membrane may be a problem); ion-exchange separation of receptor-bound from free ligand; fluorescent probe analysis (the fluorescence of either the receptor or a fluorescent probe may change, upon formation of the ligand-receptor complex); and differential adsorption of the free ligand (e.g., charcoal or talc may sequester the radiolabeled ligand, leaving the receptor-bound probe in solution). For literature pertaining to these alternative methods, the reader is referred elsewhere (6).

Use of Chemical Cross-linking Reagents

Even if it proves impossible to detect ligand binding after receptor solubilization, a great deal of information can be obtained about the physical properties of the soluble receptor through the use of a cross-link labeling approach. The radiolabeled ligand probe can be covalently attached to the receptor by one of several methods. The simplest method employs a bifunctional amino-specific cross-linking reagent like disuccinimidyl suberate (DSS) which can link an amino group of the receptor to a nearby amino group on the radiolabeled ligand. This approach, used principally for peptides, takes advantage of the high affinity and specificity of ligand binding and uses the principle of binding site protection (with an excess of unlabeled ligand) to establish the identity of the specifically cross-link-labeled protein, representing the putative receptor. Alternatively, specific photoreactive reagents can be synthesized (12, 13) in which the radioligand receptor probe is attached to a photoactivatable azido group. Upon binding, the ligand-receptor complex is exposed to intense light to activate the photoprobe, which then forms a covalent bond with the receptor. As a variant of this procedure, it has been discovered that photolysis itself may activate a radiolabeled ligand probe (e.g., fluorinated derivatives of benzodiazepines), so as to form a reactive species that can bind covalently to the receptor. In principle, the cross-link-labeling procedures can employ either cleavable (e.g., by disulfide reduction) or noncleavable reagents. Once labeled covalently in a ligand-specific manner, the receptor can be solubilized both for analysis by many of the procedures to be described below (gel filtration, sedimentation velocity, proteolytic mapping) and for subsequent receptor isolation by a variety of approaches.

Chemical Cross-linking with a Bifunctional Reagent

The most commonly used bifunctional cross-linking reagent used for peptide receptors has been DSS. One-milliliter aliquots of the particulate membrane preparation [2 to 4 mg of membrane protein/ml in 50 mM Tris-HCl buffer, pH 7.4, containing 0.1% (w/v) bovine serum albumin] are equilibrated (5 to 17 h at 4°C; 60 min at 22°C) with ^{125}I-labeled peptide (insulin, IGF-I, or EGF-URO; 0.5 to 1 nM) either with or without an excess (e.g., 100 nM) of unlabeled peptide. It is convenient to perform all of the procedure in 5-ml polyallomer ultracentrifuge tubes (Beckman). After equilibration, the chilled reaction mixture is diluted with 4 ml of ice-cold phosphate buffer, pH 7.4, and the membranes are harvested at 4°C by centrifugation for 20 min at 15,000 rpm using a swing-out rotor (Beckman SW 50.1) The supernatant solutions are discarded, and the pellets are taken up and resuspended in 1 ml of albumin-free phosphate buffer using Teflon resin pestles in 10-ml Potter-Elvehjem tissue grinders. Cross-link labeling with DSS is achieved by adding 10 μl of a freshly prepared solution of DSS (100 mM in DMSO) to the resuspended washed membranes. The cross-linking reaction is allowed to proceed for 15 min on ice and is then quenched by the addition of 4 ml of 50 mM Tris-HCl, pH 7.4. The cross-link-labeled membranes are again sedimented by centrifugation, and the pellets are resuspended as described above, with the exception that after centrifugation, the resuspension buffer is 1 ml of 10 mM Tris-HCl, pH 7.4. Aliquots of these cross-link-labeled membranes can be either solubilized with Triton X-100 [2% (v/v)] for analysis (e.g., see Fig. 3) on gel filtration columns (1.5- × 85-cm Sepharose 6B or Sephacryl S-200) or solubilized with electrophoresis sample buffer for analysis by sodium dodecyl sulfate polyacrylamide gel electrophoresis (SDS-PAGE) employing autoradiographic detection of the labeled receptor.

Chemical Cross-linking with a Photoprobe

The succiminide ester reagent, possessing a photoactivatable azido group, N-succinimidyl-6-(4'-azido-2-nitrophenylamino)hexanoate (SANAH, Pierce Chemical Co., Rockford, IL), has proven useful for the preparation of radiolabeled peptide photoaffinity probes. In principle, this reagent can be coupled, via a peptide amino group, to any radiolabeled peptide receptor probe so as to generate a photoprobe. The procedure used to prepare a photoprobe of EGF-URO is as follows. The peptide is first labeled with ^{125}I using the insoluble oxidizing agent, Iodogen (Pierce). In brief, 10 to 20 μg of EGF-URO is mixed with 100 μl of 0.1 M sodium phosphate buffer, pH 7.5, in acid-washed borosilicate glass tubes precoated with 40 μg of Iodogen. To coat the tubes, Iodogen is dissolved (2 mg/ml) in chloroform, and 20 μl of the solution is added to the tubes. The tubes are shaken using a Vortex mixer, and the chloroform is evaporated using a gentle stream of nitrogen. The iodination reaction is initiated by the addition of 0.5 to 1.0 mCi of ^{125}I (Amersham Corp., Arlington Heights, IL, IMS-300) to the EGF-containing phosphate buffer. After 15 sec, the reaction mixture is removed from the Iodogen tube and filtered through a glass wool-plugged Pasteur pipette into an aluminum foil-covered 5-ml specimen vial. Aliquots of the reaction mixture are then removed for the determination of peptide-incorporated counts by TCA precipitation. The volume of the reaction mixture is made up to 2 ml with 0.1 M sodium phosphate buffer, pH 7.5, and the solution is gently stirred using a Teflon-coated stir bar and magnetic stirrer. The photoaffinity-labeling reagent, SANAH is dissolved (1 mg/ml) in DMSO in a light-protected screw-top 2-ml specimen vial. Freshly prepared SANAH solution (200 μl) is added to the iodinated EGF-URO reaction mixture (2 ml). Coupling of SANAH to ^{125}I-EGF-URO is allowed to proceed at room temperature for 30 min, and the reaction is quenched by the addition of 0.5 ml of 0.5 M lysine HCl. The SANAH-^{125}I-EGF can be stored at 4°C until used for photoaffinity labeling. If not used immediately, the reagent should usually be used within 24 to 48 hr of its production. The reaction mixture can be used without further purification.

To photoaffinity label the EGF-URO receptor in placenta membranes, 100 μl of SANAH-^{125}I-EGF reaction mixture is mixed with 1 ml of membranes (2 to 4 mg/ml of membrane protein) in 50 mM Tris-HCl, pH 7.4, containing 0.1 M NaCl. Binding of SANAH-^{125}I-EGF is allowed to proceed to equilibrium in the dark, at room temperature, for 60 min. The binding and subsequent steps are conveniently carried out in a 5-ml polyallomer centrifuge tube (Beckman). After bindng, the membranes are diluted to 5 ml with ice-cold binding buffer and are sedimented by centrifugation at 15,000 rpm for 20 min (4°C) using a Beckman SW -50.1 rotor. The resulting supernatant solution can be discarded and the pellet resuspended in 1 ml of binding buffer using a Potter-Elvehjem tissue grinder as described above. The pellet resuspension step is performed under dim lighting conditions with the tissue grinder immersed in ice. After resuspension, the membranes are transferred back into a 5-ml polyallomer centrifuge tube that is placed in ice. To cross-link bound SANAH-^{125}I-EGF to the receptor, the membranes are exposed for 10 min to the light from two 200-W incandescent light bulbs placed 10 cm from the mouth of the centrifuge tubes. A shallow Pyrex baking pan or Petri dish filled with 3 to 5 cm of water and placed between the lights and the membranes is sufficient to prevent melting of the ice and excessive warming of the sample. After exposure to light, the volume of the mixture is increased to 5 ml with ice-cold 10 mM Tris-HCl buffer, and the membranes are again sedimented by centrifugation as described above. The resulting pellet is either resuspended in 1 ml of 10 mM Tris-HCl buffer for solubilization with Triton X-100 or dissolved directly in SDS sample buffer prior to SDS-PAGE analysis. Using the conditions described above, it can be shown that the cross-linking of SANAH-^{125}I-EGF to the receptor requires the light activation step. However, in intact cell preparations, specific cross-linking of an iodopeptide (insulin or EGF-URO) to a membrane receptor can occur via an as yet unidentified reaction simply by the incubation of the cell preparation at room temperature for 1 hr with nanomolar concentrations of iodopeptide.

Biochemical Analysis of Soluble Receptors

When a method for detecting the soluble receptor has been developed and when procedures for cross-link labeling the receptor are available, a variety of analytical procedures can be used to characterize the receptor. In principle, one might prefer to use methods that do not expose the receptor itself to a bifunctional cross-linking reagent, so as to opt for using a photoprobe for cross-link labeling. However, in practice, the results obtained with the receptors for insulin and EGF-URO have been equivalent using either photoprobes or bifunctional cross-link-labeling reagents. *A priori*, any of the conventional methods of protein analysis (gel filtration, SDS-PAGE, ultracentrifugation, and proteolytic domain analysis) can be considered for studying receptor properties.

Gel Filtration

Chromatography of crude soluble receptor preparations on columns of Sepharose 6B can yield estimate of the apparent Stokes radius of the receptor by two methods. Using *method 1*, two aliquots (0.5 ml) of the soluble membrane extract (liver or placenta; 0.4 mg of protein) are preequilibrated (1 hr at 22°) with ^{125}I-labeled peptide (e.g., ^{125}I-insulin; 0.9 nM) either with or without an excess of unlabeled peptide (e.g., 1 μM insulin). In separate runs on the identical column, both samples are applied at 4°C to a column (1.5 × 85 cm) of non–cross-linked Sepharose 6B preequilibrated with 50 mM Tris-HCl buffer, pH 7.4, containing 0.1% (v/v) Triton X-100. The column is precalibrated with the molecular size markers thyroglobulin, apoferritin, γ-globulin, and albumin. The sample is eluted at a flow rate of 15 ml/hr and 1.8-ml fractions are collected. Radioactivity in the fractions eluted from the column is monitored by crystal scintillation counting. The presence of receptor is indicated by a reduction in radioactivity in fractions in which unlabeled insulin is present, compared with the identical fractions in which unlabeled insulin is absent from the initial binding reaction. In *method 2*, only one aliquot of solubilized receptor is applied to the column. Eluted fractions are then monitored for ligand-binding activity using an assay like the PEG method described above. In practice, for analysis of the insulin receptor, aliquots (50 to 100 μl) of each column fraction are used for the assay described under "PEG Method" (above).

Analysis of Receptors by Sedimentation Velocity

The hydrodynamic data obtained from gel filtration experiments can be greatly amplified by studies of the sedimentation velocity of receptors in sucrose gradients. In practice, the receptor can be detected either by the assay of fractions from the gradient using the PEG method or by monitoring the sedimentation of the radioactive ligand, which is assumed to be bound to the receptor. In the latter kind of experiment, two receptor aliquots are analyzed. Prior to sedimentation analysis, each aliquot is equilibrated with radioligand either with or without an excess (100- to 1,000-fold) of unlabeled ligand. As with the gel filtration experiments outlined above, the peak of radioactivity which is reduced in the presence of excess unlabeled ligand is assumed to represent the receptor.

In both the gel filtration and sedimentation velocity experiments, the properties of the receptor (Stokes radius; Svedberg constant) are determined with respect to the properties of well-studied proteins like thyroglobulin, myosin, and ovalbumin, which are used to construct calibration curves. Both the Stokes radius and sedimentation constant of the receptor are determined from the calibration curves. Further, using gradients made with either H_2O or D_2O, it is possible to estimate the partial specific volume (v̄) of the detergent-receptor complex (see ref. 40 and "Sucrose Gradient Centrifugation"). The hydrodynamic parameters can be used to calculate the apparent molecular weight of the soluble detergent-receptor complex, according to the formula

$$\frac{6\pi N\eta}{1 - \bar{v}p} R_S S_{20,w}$$

where R_S is Stoke's radius; N is Avogadro's number; η is the viscosity of water at 20°C; and p is the density of water at 20°C. The molecular weight of the receptor determined in this way can be corrected for the amounts of bound detergent. It is most instructive to compare the molecular weight of the receptor observed in detergent solutions with the data obtained by cross-link labeling and gel electrophoresis analysis.

Sucrose gradient centrifugation of a solubilized receptor preparation is done as follows.

A 4.5-ml linear gradient of sucrose [5 to 20% (w/v)] is prepared from concentrated solutions of sucrose in buffer (0.1 M sodium phosphate, pH 7.4) containing 0.1% bovine serum albumin (BSA) (w/v) and 0.2% (v/v) Triton X-100. The solubilized membrane extract (300 μl), with or without prior dialysis against the above buffer, is layered onto the top of the sucrose gradients. These are then centrifuged at 100,000 × g for 16 hr at 4°C (Beckman SW 50.1 rotor). Fractions (0.2 ml each) are collected by flotation with 70% (w/v) sucrose injected by piercing the bottom of the tubes (1.0 × 5.0 cm); ligand-binding activity is measured for 50-μl aliquots by the PEG method. Reference proteins used to calibrate the gradients are ^{14}C-methylated myosin and [14C]ovalbumin (obtained from Amersham Corp.) and a ^{14}C-acetyl derivative of γ-globulin prepared in the laboratory with [14C]acetic anhydride. The sedimentation verlocity of ^{125}I-labeled ligand (e.g., insulin) is also measured. If it is not possible to use the PEG or another method to detect the receptor after centrifugation, two aliquots (300 μl) of soluble receptor are equilibrated with ^{125}I-labeled ligand (60 min at 22°C; 16 hr at 4°C), one without and the other with an excess of unlabeled ligand. Both aliquots are layered onto two identical gradients and centrifuged as outlined above. Radioactivity in the fractions (0.2 ml) collected from the gradient by flotation is monitored by crystal scintillation counting. This method is analogous to the gel filtration method 1 outlined above.

Analysis of Receptors by PAGE

One of the most useful approaches for receptor analysis has employed PAGE of the cross-link-labeled receptor, followed by autoradiographic detection of the receptor. Done in the presence and absence of reducing agents, this approach can yield information about receptor subunit composition. In addition, analysis of the receptor in this manner both before and after treatment with proteases and glycosidases can provide information about receptor domain structure and about the degree of receptor glycosylation. Although the majority of studies of this kind have been done using autoradiographic detection of the cross-link-labeled receptor, the non–cross-link-labeled receptor can also be localized after separation by electrophoretic transfer from the gel to diazopaper. Once bonded to the paper, the receptor can be detected using a "ligand-blotting" technique to be referred to below (14, 15). In principle, the unlabeled receptor can also be analyzed by isoelectric focusing experiments done in solutions of ampholytes. After equilibrium, the fractions collected from the isofocusing apparatus may be analyzed by the PEG procedure, provided that the interference of the ampholytes can be eliminated.

Electrophoretic analysis of cross-link-labeled receptor can be done routinely using SDS-PAGE performed in slab gels (either 5% or 4 to 10% gradient gels can be used) according to methods originally developed by Laemmli (16) and O'Farrell (17). Experiments are usually done both in the presence and absence of a reducing agent [50 mM dithiothreitol or 5% (v/v) β-mercapthoethanol]. Washed cross-link-labeled membranes are solubilized directly in SDS-containing sample buffer by heating for 5 min at 100°C. Aliquots (50 μl) are transferred to the gel sample lanes and subjected to electrophoresis with cooling (4°C) at constant current (17 mA/0.75-mm × 11-cm gel) for approximately 4 hr. Gels are then fixed and stained in methanol/acetic acid/water [5:10:30 (v/v)] containing 0.1% (w/v) Coomassie Brilliant Blue. After destaining, gels are dried under vacuum onto filter paper. A fluorescent pen (e.g., Ultemit, Du Pont-New England Nuclear) is then used to identify the positions of proteins used for gel calibration. For this purpose, the following proteins of nominal molecular mass (kDa) have proven useful (18): thyroglobulin (669 and 330); ferritin (440); catalase (232 and 60); lactate dehydrogenase (140); and albumin (67). Alternatively, erythrocyte membrane proteins (19) can be used as markers. The fixed dried gel is then exposed (for 4 days to 2 weeks) at $-70°C$ to x-ray film (e.g., Kodak, X-Omat R) using an intensifying screen (Du Pont, Cronex). The apparent molecular mass of the receptor-ligand complex can then be determined from the calibrated autoradiogram according to the plot of relative distance of migration versus log molecular mass. Should the receptor prove to be a ligand-regulated tyrosine kinase, like those for insulin, IGF-I, and EGF-URO, the molecular mass of the receptor phosphorylated in the presence of $AT^{32}P$ can also be determined by the autoradiographic procedure outlined above.

Analysis of Receptor Domains by Proteolytic Mapping

Proteolytic domain analysis can be done without the need for obtaining pure receptor, provided the receptor can be covalently labeled either with a receptor-specific ligand, as outlined above, or with a radiolabeled probe (e.g., ^{32}P) that requires for its insertion the presence of a receptor-specific ligand. For instance, ligand-stimulated receptor autophosphorylation in the presence of $AT^{32}P$ provides one avenue for this approach. However, the binding of ligand to a receptor may expose other reactive sites (e.g., sulfhydryls) that may be amenable to radiolabeling. Aliquots of specifically radiolabeled receptor-bearing membranes (e.g., 50 μl of a suspension) can be subjected to proteolysis by a variety of enzymes [e.g., 10 μl of 1-tosylamido-2-phenylethyl chloromethyl ketone (TPCK)-treated trypsin (0.25 mg/ml) or 10 μl of chymotrypsin (1 mg/ml)] for 15 min at room temperature. Proteolysis is terminated by heating samples for 10 min in a boiling water bath after the addition of 60 μl of twofold-concentrated SDS sample buffer and 10 μl of β-mercaptoethanol. Alternatively, 50 μl of cross-link-labeled particulate membranes is dissolved in 50 μl of twofold-concentrated SDS sample buffer and heated for 2 min in a boiling water bath. The samples are transferred to a 37°C water bath and incubated for 30 min with 10 μl of TPCK-treated trypsin (2.5 mg/ml) or 10 μl of chymotrypsin (1.0 mg/ml). Proteolysis is terminated by the addition of 10 μl of β-mercaptoethanol and heating the samples in a boiling water bath for 8 min. After analysis by SDS-PAGE, the peptides are visualized by autoradiography. When particulate membranes are subjected to proteolysis, only those receptor domains that are external to the lipid bilayer should be accessible to cleavage by the enzymes. Conversely, peptide maps that are observed when SDS-solubilized receptors are subjected to proteolysis reflect receptor domains that are internal to the membrane-lipid bilayer. For the above procedures, it may be preferable to excise a radiolabeled receptor protein, detected as outlined under "Analysis of Receptors by PAGE," and subject the labeled receptor to proteolytic domain analysis by the in- or out-of-gel method developed by Cleveland and coworkers (20).

Receptor Isolation

One of the major goals of work with receptors is to isolate amounts of sufficient purity and quantity that will permit the analysis of receptor amino acid sequence and the study of reconstituted receptor systems. To this end, a variety of approaches has been developed, using both conventional biochemical procedures (e.g., salting-out, gel-permeation and ion-exchange chromatography) and adaptations of affinity chromatographic techniques. For instance, ammonium sulfate precipitation and chromatographic separations, using columns of DEAE- and carboxymethyl-cellulose, have played an important role in isolation procedures for the insulin and EGF-URO receptors (21–23). In addition, lectin-agarose affinity chromatography, employing a variety of immobilized lectins (most comonly, ConA and WGA) has proved to be a useful preliminary purification step in which the membrane glycoprotein fraction, containing many pharmacological receptors, is freed from other nonglycosylated membrane proteins. Other nonspecific methods that can be employed for receptor isolation include the use of Sepharose derivatized with cibacron blue (this dye can form a specific complex with proteins having a "dinucleotide" fold) and solid matrices derivatized with anti-phosphotyrosine antibodies. The above mentioned nonspecific methods of protein separation can be combined with specific ligand affinity columns to achieve the final purification of a receptor. Only the use of these receptor-specific affinity columns will be described in detail in the sections that follow.

Ligand-specific Affinity Chromatography

Affinity chromatography using receptor-specific immobilized ligands, like insulin, has played a key role in the isolation of many receptors. In principle, any ligand with a free amino group can be coupled to cyanogen bromide-activated beaded agarose. The agarose can either be used for coupling ligands directly to the activated matrix, or the support can be derivatized with a reactive "spacer arm" to which a receptor-specific ligand can be subsequently coupled. Many derivatized solid matrices can now be purchased commercially (e.g., Bio-Rad or Pierce). In practice, the most useful procedures in my laboratory have proven to be the simplified method for cyanogen bromide activation of agarose, developed by March et al. (24) and the reaction of ligands via a primary amino group with a succinimide ester-derivatized agarose support; Affi-Gel 15 (Bio-Rad) has been particularly useful for preparing insulin-agarose derivatives.

The cyanogen bromide activation procedure developed by March et al. (24) is as follows.

One volume of a slurry of washed agarose beads (Sepharose 4B, Pharmacia LKB Biotechnology Inc.) consisting of equal volumes of gel and water, is added to 1 volume of 2 M sodium carbonate and mixed by stirring slowly. The rate of stirring is increased, and 0.05 volume of an acetonitrile solution of cyanogen bromide (2 g of cyanogen bromide/ml of acetonitrile) is added all at once. The cyanogen bromide solution is prepared by adding 50 ml of dry redistilled acetonitrile to a 100-g bottle of cyanogen bromide and is stored at $-20°C$ when not in use. The amount of cyanogen bromide solution used can be varied to achieve the degree of activation desired. The slurry is stirred vigorously for 1 to 2 min after which the slurry is poured onto a course sintered-glass funnel, washed with 5 to 10 volumes each of 0.1 M sodium bicarbonate, pH 9.5, water, and the buffer that is to be used in the subsequent coupling reaction. When activation is performed at 4°C, the beads may become sticky and tend to clump during the first wash. For this reason, the beads should not be filtered to a compact cake during washing. After the final wash, the beads are filtered to compactness to facilitate transfer of the gel to the coupling solution. The cake is resuspended promptly after transfer to ensure uniform dispersion of the beads. For coupling to the amino ligand, the activated agarose is transferred to a plastic bottle containing the ligand (e.g., 1 to 50 mg/ml) dissolved in 1 volume of 0.2 M sodium bicarbonate, pH 9.5. The coupling reaction is allowed to proceed for 20 hr at 4°C. At 20 hr, the gel is washed free from unreacted ligand, and unreacted groups on the agarose gel are masked by resuspending the gel in 0.5 M glycine for at least 4 hr at 24°C. Other nonnucleophilic buffers may be used in place of sodium bicarbonate in the coupling step. For use as an affinity column, it is essential that the agarose derivative be thoroughly washed (see below for insulin-agarose) to remove all traces of free ligand from the matrix.

Using a commercially available coupling matrix (Affi-Gel 15), efficient insulin-agarose derivatives can be prepared essentially as heralded by the work of Cuatrecasas (22). Coupling can be performed in 0.1 M sodium phosphate buffer, pH

7.4, containing 6 M freshly deionized urea and insulin at a final concentration of 1 mg/ml. One volume of settled gel and 2 volumes of insulin-containing buffer are mixed to initiate the coupling reaction, which is allowed to proceed for 1 hr at 4°C. The gel is then washed free of insulin and resuspended in 0.5 M glycine to block unreacted gel sites; after 24 hr at 4°C the gel is rinsed free of glycine with six washes of 50 mM Tris-HCl, pH 7.4, and preconditioned for chromatography by the following sequence of washes, done in a 25-ml bed volume column (2.7×5.3 cm): (*a*) 50 mM Tris-HCl, pH 7.4; (*b*) 50 mM Tris-HCl, pH 7.4, containing 1 M NaCl; (*c*) 0.1 M sodium phosphate buffer, pH 7.4, containing 6 M urea. The column is then washed extensively and equilibrated with 50 mM Tris-HCl buffer, pH 7.4, containing 0.1% Triton X-100 and 0.1 mM phenylmethylsulfonyl fluoride (PMSF) prior to sample application. On average, this procedure yields a coupling of about 150 µg of insulin/ml of packed gel.

Although most problems associated with the use of affinity matrices (leakage of the ligand from the support or requirement for a specific spacer arm) can usually be overcome, it is frequently the success of the column in adsorbing the receptor with high affinity which presents the major difficulty in obtaining good yields of active receptor from the affinity column. In practice, good recovery of the insulin receptor has been achieved by eluting the washed affinity column either with 50 mM sodium acetate buffer, pH 5, containing 1 M NaCl and 0.1% (v/v) Triton X-100 or with 50 mM sodium acetate buffer, pH 6, containing 4 M urea and 0.1% Triton X-100. The receptor-containing fractions are eluted into equal volumes of a neutralizing buffer (e.g., 0.5 M Tris-HCl, pH 7.4, containing 0.1% Triton X-100) so as to dilute the urea and return the pH toward neutrality. To recover material from antibody-Sepharose derivatives, elution at alkaline pH may be necessary. In essence, the affinity chromatography approach, first developed for purifying enzymes and then adapted for purification of the insulin receptor, has proven to be of enormous value in the isolation of many other receptors.

Immunoaffinity Chromatography

This approach was developed (25) because of the difficulty encountered in adsorbing the human placental receptor for EGF-URO to columns of EGF-URO-agarose. The principle of the approach comprises first cross-link-labeling the receptor with a specific ligand and then using an antiligand antibody coupled to agarose to isolate the ligand-receptor complex. In practice, cross-link-labeled receptor, prepared by the photoaffinity-labeling method described above, is solubilized in detergent (e.g., 0.5% Nonidet P-40 or Triton X-100), and the receptor-containing glycoprotein fraction is recovered by purifying aliquots on small columns (0.3 ml) of WGA-agarose (4 mg of WGA/ml of beads, prepared by the cyanogen bromide activation procedure described above). The affinity-labeled receptor is eluted from the WGA-agarose column with 0.2 M *N*-acetylglucosamine and applied in the same buffer (50 mM Tris-HCl, pH 7.6, containing 0.2 M NaCl and 0.1% detergent) to a column

(0.3 ml) of anti–EGF-URO-antibody-agarose. The antibody-agarose column is also prepared by the cyanogen bromide activation procedure, using the immunoglobulin fraction from a rabbit antiserum developed against pure mouse EGF-URO. The receptor adsorbed to the washed antibody-agarose column can be recovered by elution with 10% (v/v) formic acid. A variant of this procedure employs a protein A-agarose column to adsorb the antibody-bound ligand-receptor complex. Five-milliliter aliquots of the solubilized cross-link-labeled membranes, or the pooled fractions from the WGA-agarose column, are incubated for 24 hr at 4°C with anti-ligand antiserum (10 μl of a high-titer serum). Ten milligrams (dry weight) of washed protein A-agarose (Pharmacia) is then added, and incubation is continued with gentle stirring for 1 hr at room temperature. The mixture is them passed through glass wool-plugged Pasteur pipettes, and the trapped bead-bound antibody-receptor complex can then be washed and eluted for further analysis. In principle, the same procedure can be used for receptor isolation, should antireceptor antibodies be available. The advantage of the immunoaffinity approach is that analytical amounts of receptor can be efficiently recovered for further analysis (proteolytic mapping). A variant of the procedures described above was developed to isolate the insulin receptor (26). The disadvantage of the approach is that the receptor can only be recovered as a complex with the ligand such that further studies of receptor function may not prove possible. In addition, the approach is not easily scaled up for the isolation of large amounts of receptor entirely free from other contaminating proteins (e.g., immunoglobulin or Staphylococcus aureus protein A) that may leak from the solid support.

Receptor Sequencing and Reconstitution

The procedures outlined above will yield a great deal of information about the receptor and will provide a means for isolating reasonable amounts of receptor for further study. Two major directions that are of interest will be the determination of receptor sequence and the reconstitution of the receptor into a functional system. Although the detailed methodologies of the procedures are beyond the scope of this chapter, a brief overview will be provided.

Central to the reconstitution and amino acid sequence studies will be the transfer of the receptor into a suitable detergent. The use of lectin affinity columns to which the receptor can be adsorbed for elution into a suitable buffer provides a very useful means of switching the receptor from one solution to another. For analytical purposes, the removal of the last vestiges of lectin may represent the only minor difficulty with this approach. Once isolated, conventional methods of protein microsequencing can be applied, so as to obtain sufficiently unique sequences that can be used as a basis for preparing suitable oligonucleotide probes. Alternatively, the isolated receptor can be used for the preparation of both polyclonal and monoclonal antibodies. Monoclonal antibodies provide the advantage that completely pure receptor need not be used for antibody production. Indeed, very useful monoclonal antireceptor antibodies have been obtained using crude membrane preparations. The screening of an appropriate cDNA library can be achieved either with the use of such suitable oligonucleotide probes as was done for the insulin and somatomedin (IGF-I) receptors (27–29), or alternatively, a protein expression system can be used in conjunction with an antibody screen, employing antireceptor antibodies. Both of these approaches have their merits and pitfalls. Ultimately, however, the proof that the cDNA that has been sequenced does indeed represent the receptor will require both a match of the cDNA sequence with the partial amino acid sequence obtained by microsequencing and a reconstitution experiment wherein some function of the receptor (e.g., ligand binding or ligand-regulated ion flux) can be measured.

Receptor reconstitution experiments can be done both with isolated receptor and with recombinant receptor using either liposomes or crude membrane acceptor systems, as summarized elsewhere (30). Alternatively, if receptor mRNA is available, receptor expression can be observed in *Xenopus* oocytes, wherein the properties of a fully functional receptor can be measured as has been done for the nicotinic acetylcholine receptor (31). Transfection experiments, in which receptor cDNA is introduced into a mammalian cell like Chinese hamster ovary cells can also be used to evaluate not only the function of the cloned receptor gene but also the function of receptor genes subjected to site-directed mutagenesis. As summarized elsewhere (32), this approach has been used for a variety of receptors including the one for insulin (33, 34).

ILLUSTRATIVE EXAMPLES OF RECEPTOR CHARACTERIZATION AND PURIFICATION

The followng examples illustrate the use of the methods described above to characterize the receptors for insulin, IGF-I [also called BSM or somatomedin C (SM-C)], and EGF-URO. Although the illustrations are drawn from work in my own laboratory, the results typify observations that have been made for many other receptor systems. In essence, the approach stems primarily from the hallmark studies of the insulin receptor done by Cuatrecasas in the early 1970s (11, 21, 22). The interested reader is strongly encouraged to consult these early studies of the insulin receptor, which have set the stage for most of the work that has been done to date.

Ligand-binding Assay for Crude and Purified Soluble Insulin Receptor

Figure 1 illustrates the use of the PEG-binding assay (see "PEG Method") to characterize the receptor for insulin either before (Fig. 1A) or after (Fig. 1B) purification by insulin-agarose affinity chromatography (35). In Fig. 1A, aliquots of a solubilized placenta membrane preparation (65 µg of protein, solubilized with 0.2% Ammonyx-LO), fractionated by ammonium sulfate, were assayed for ^{125}I-insulin binding by the PEG method. The binding at increasing concentrations of ^{125}I-insulin was corrected for the nonspecific binding (about 25% of total binding) observed in

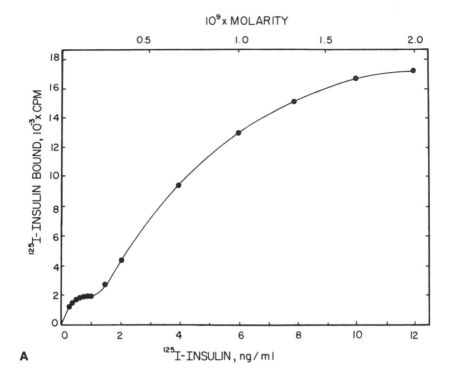

A

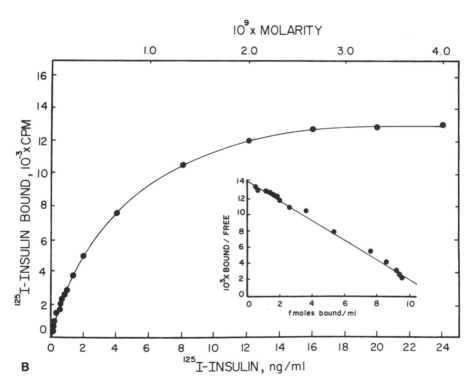

B

the presence of an excess of unlabeled insulin. The soluble receptor preparation analyzed in Fig 1A was purified by insulin-agarose affinity chromatography (see below and also under "Ligand-specific Affinity Chromatography"), and the binding of ^{125}I-insulin to the purified receptor (Fig. 1B) was measured as in Fig. 1A. The binding data were plotted according to Scatchard (ref. 36 and the *inset*, Fig. 1B). The two binding curves are shown (*a*) to illustrate the use of the PEG method for measuring a binding isotherm; and (*b*) to illustrate differences in receptor binding which may be observed before and after affinity chromatographic purification.

Measurement of Hydrodynamic Properties of the Soluble Receptor

Gel Filtration

Figures 2 and 3 illustrate the behavior of the receptors for IGF-I (Fig. 2, *somatomedin*, or *basic-SM*) and EGF-URO (Fig. 3) on gel filtration columns. The experiments show four different methods for detecting the receptor on the columns. In Fig, 2A, the crude soluble receptor has been preequilibrated with ^{125}I-somatomedin (IGF-I) both in the absence (*open circles*) and presence (*closed circles*) of excess unlabeled polypeptide. Both aliquots were then analyzed sequentially on the column (1.5 × 85 cm) of Sepharose 6B, and radioactivity in the fractions was measured. The reduction in radioactivity in the peak with $K_{AV} = 0.32$ (apparent Stokes radius, 7.2 nm) signals the position of the receptor. As an alternative, shown in Fig. 2B, unlabeled receptor was chromatographed on the same column, and aliquots from the eluted fractions were monitored for the binding of radiolabeled somatomedin (IGF-I) using the PEG assay (37).

The data obtained for the EGF-URO receptor (Fig. 3) illustrate two further ways the receptor can be visualized upon gel filtration (38). On the one hand, receptor cross-link-labeled with an EGF-URO photoprobe (see "Chemical Cross-linking with a Photoprobe") was solubilized, partially purified on a WGA-agarose column (see below), and was subjected to chromatography on a Sephacryl S-200 column (1.5 × 87 cm) in a 50 mM Tris-HCl buffer, pH 7.4, containing 0.15 M NaCl, 1 mM CaCl$_2$, 1 mM MnCl$_2$, and 0.1% (w/v) Ammonyx-LO. The elution of the specifically radiolabeled receptor was monitored by measuring radioactivity in the eluted fractions (*closed circles, righthand ordinate*, Fig. 3). On the other hand, an unlabeled receptor aliquot was subjected to chromatography on the same column, and aliquots (0.8 ml) of the effluent fractions were monitored for EGF-URO binding (*open circles, lefthand ordinate*, Fig. 3) using the lectin immobilization binding assay described (under the section with that title in the text). The receptor was

---

FIG. 1. Ligand-binding properties of the soluble insulin receptor before (**A**) and after (**B**) purification by insulin-agarose affinity chromatography. The crude (**A**, *upper*) and affinity-purified (**B**, *lower*) soluble receptor was analyzed for insulin binding by the PEG method, as described in the text. (from Maturo et al., ref. 35, with permission.)

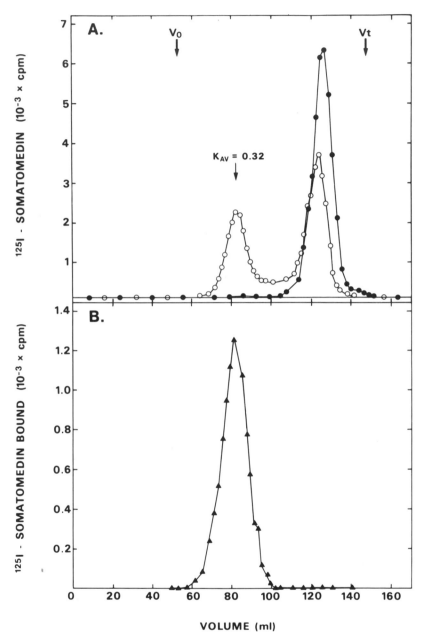

FIG. 2. Gel filtration of the receptor for IGF-I/basic-somatomedin. As outlined in the text, the receptor was detected either (**A,** *upper*) by preequilibration with ^{125}I-somatomedin (IGF-I) in the absence (○) or presence (●) of unlabeled peptide or (**B,** *lower*) using the PEG assay for aliquots of fractions eluted from the column. (From Bhaumick et al., ref. 37, with permission.)

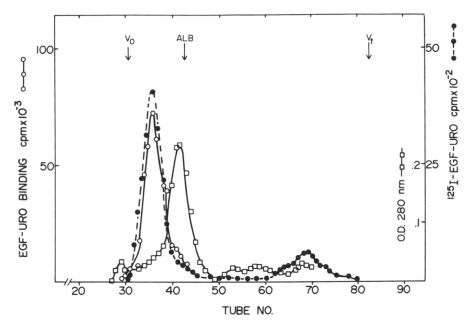

FIG. 3. Gel filtration of the receptor for EGF-URO. Either the cross-link-labeled receptor (●) or an unlabeled receptor preparation (○) was analyzed on the same column, as outlined in the text. The radioactivity profile (*righthand ordinate*) shows the position of the cross-link-labeled receptor; the lectin immobilization assay was used to detect the unlabeled receptor (*lefthand ordinate*). ALB = bovine serum albumin. (From Nexø et al., ref. 38, with permission.)

eluted well before the bulk of the membrane protein (OD, 280 nm; *open squares, righthand ordinate*, Fig. 3). Both methods of receptor detection indicated that under the conditions of chromatography, the apparent Stokes radius of the receptor was 5.1 nm.

Sucrose Gradient Centrifugation

In principle, the same four approaches illustrated above to detect the receptor for gel filtration experiments (i.e., displacement of radiolabeled ligand with the un-labeled ligand, the PEG assay, cross-link-labeling with a photoprobe, and the lectin immobilization assay) can be used to localize the receptor in sucrose gradients. In the example shown in Fig. 4 (39), the receptor for BSM (IGF-I) has been detected in using the PEG assay for aliquots (50 µl) of fractions (0.2 ml) collected from a linear sucrose gradient [5 to 20% (w/v) sucrose] that was centrifuged at $100,000 \times g$ for 16 hr at 4°C. In parallel gradient tubes (1.0×5.0 cm), rabiolabeled marker proteins (^{125}I-BSM; ^{14}C-labeled ovalbumin, myosin, and thyroglobulin) were layered onto the gradient; radioactivity in the eluted fractions from these calibration gradients

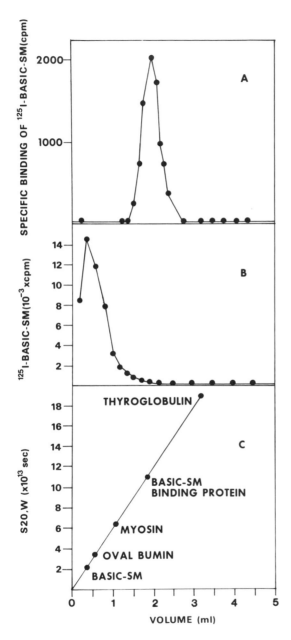

FIG. 4. Sucrose gradient centrifugation of the IGF-I (*basic-SM*) receptor. The sedimentation of the receptor (*upper*) detected in gradient fractions by the PEG assay was compared (*lower*) with the sedimentation of marker proteins, as outlined in the text. (From Bhaumick et al., ref. 39, with permission.)

was measured to construct the calibration curve shown in the *lower panel*. As outlined under "Gel Filtration," the sedimentation coefficient (S = 11.0) estimated from this experiment was combined with the estimate of the Stokes radius ($R_S = 7.2$ nm), determined from the data in Fig. 2 and the receptor's partial specific volume ($\bar{v} = 0.777$; ref. 40), to calculate a molecular mass of 402 kDa for the receptor-detergent complex, according to the formula, molecular mass = R_SS $[6\pi N\eta/(1-\bar{v}p)]$. In theory, these parameters should be corrected to values that obtain at 20°C. The calculated value for the molecular mass compares favorably with the value that would be expected from the heterodimer $\alpha_2\beta_2$ (450,000), suggested for the receptor structure, wherein the α-subunit has a molecular mass of 135 kDa (see below), and the β-subunit has a molecular mass of 90 kDa.

Analysis by PAGE

Molecular Weight of Receptor Subunits

Electrophoretic analysis of the receptor in SDS-containing gels, both in the absence and presence of a reducing agent, yields important information about receptor subunit composition and about the molecular weights of receptor subunits. Most often, this analysis is used for cross-link-labeled receptor that can be visualized by autoradiography. Nonetheless, in principle, the analysis should be possible using other methods of receptor detection (14, 15), as mentioned under "Analysis of Receptors by PAGE." Using the cross-link-labeling approach (DSS cross-linking with ^{125}I-insulin and ^{125}I-somatomedin), the receptors for insulin and somatomedin (IGF-I) are compared in Fig. 5. In the experiment shown, each receptor was cross-linked to the ^{125}I-labeled ligand at a ligand concentration (about 1 nM) that was entirely specific for each of the two receptors, which were both present in the same human placenta membrane preparation (39, 41). The major bands detected by autoradiography in Fig. 5 were eliminated in the presence of an excess of the appropriate unlabeled ligand (e.g., unlabeled insulin abolished the labeling of the insulin receptor but not the IGF-I receptor, and vice versa; not shown). In Fig. 5, major receptor bands are seen corresponding to molecular masses of 270 and 130 to 140 kDa. A minor band at about 100 kDa is observed for the insulin receptor. (*lane A*, Fig. 5). It is now suspected that the 270-kDa band may represent cross-link-labeled receptor subunits (e.g., α_2), wherein the cross-linking reagent has prevented the complete dissociation of the receptor polypeptide chains upon reduction (42). For both the insulin receptor and the somatomedin (IGF-I) receptor, the 140-kDa band represents the receptor α-subunit; and for the insulin receptor, the band at about 100 kDa represents the β-subunit. It is important to point out that the use of insulin receptor photoprobes instead of chemical cross-linking reagents has provided additional interesting information about the insulin receptor based on the approach illustrated in Fig. 5 (12).

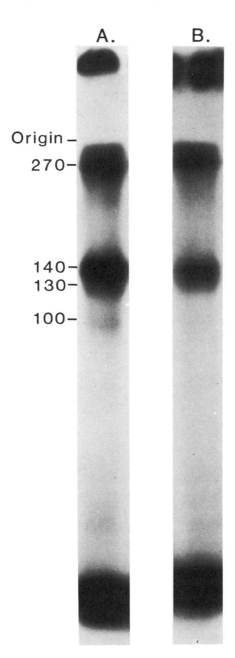

FIG. 5. Electrophoretic analysis of cross-link-labeled receptors for insulin (*lane A*) and IGF-I/basic somatomedin (*lane B*). Receptors were cross-link-labeled and analyzed by SDS-PAGE under reducing conditions as outlined in the text. The molecular weights of the radiolabeled receptor species, detected by autoradiography of fixed dried gels, were estimated relative to the mobilities in the same gel of marker proteins. (From Armstrong et al., ref. 41, with permission.)

Proteolytic Mapping

The use of the proteolytic mapping procedure (described under "Analysis of Receptor Domains by Proteolytic Mapping") to analyze the receptors for insulin and somatomedin (IGF-I) is illustrated in Fig. 6 (39). Receptors for both polypeptides were first specifically cross-link-labeled using DSS (see "Chemical Cross-linking with a Bifunctional Reagent") with either ^{125}I-insulin or ^{125}I-IGF-I, as shown in Fig. 5. The specifically labeled membranes were first solubilized in electrophoresis sample buffer containing SDS and were then treated for 30 min at 37°C with the indicated amounts of chymotrypsin in a final volume of 120 μl. The samples were then subjected to gradient slab gel electrophoresis followed by autoradiographic detection of the radiolabeled receptor fragments. In Fig. 6 it can be seen that chymotryptic digestion yielded some fragments of comparable molecular weight for both receptors, whereas some fragments were distinct for either the insulin receptor (*lanes A, C, E,* and *G*) or the somatomedin (BSM or IGF-I) receptor

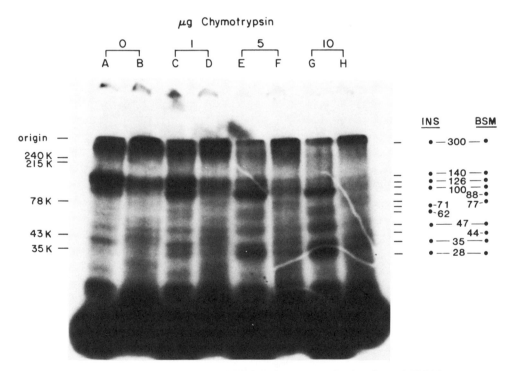

FIG. 6. Proteolytic mapping of cross-link-labeled receptors for insulin and IGF-I/basic-somatomedin. Receptors for either insulin (*INS; lanes A, C, E, G*) or IGF-I/basic-somatomedin (*BSM; lanes B, D, F, H*) were specifically cross-link-labeled, solubilized, and subjected to chymotryptic digestion followed by SDS-PAGE as outlined in the text. Proteolytic domains from the two receptors with similar and distinct molecular weights are denoted (●) on the *right*. (From Bhaumick et al., ref. 39, with permission.)

(*lanes B, D, F*, and *H*). The proteolytic map experiments are entirely in keeping with the closely related amino acid sequences that have been determined for the two receptors (27–29).

Receptor Isolation

Lectin-Agarose Affinity Chromatography

Affinity chromatography using columns of lectin-agarose, as illustrated in Fig. 7, is not only a most useful preliminary step for the recovery of solubilized receptors free from other nonglycosylated membrane proteins, but the procedure also provides a means for transferring the receptor from one detergent environment to another. In the experiment shown in Fig. 7, a 1% Lubrol PX extract of a human placental membrane preparation (500 mg of protein in 250 ml) was applied at room temperature to a WGA-Sepharose 4B column (1.5 × 11 cm, 3 mg of WGA/ml of beads; equilibrated with 25 mM Tris-HCl buffer, pH 7.6, containing 0.15 M NaCl and 0.1% Lubrol PX). After applying the sample, the column was washed with 190 ml of buffer. The adsorbed protein was then eluted by 0.2 M *N*-acetylglucosamine

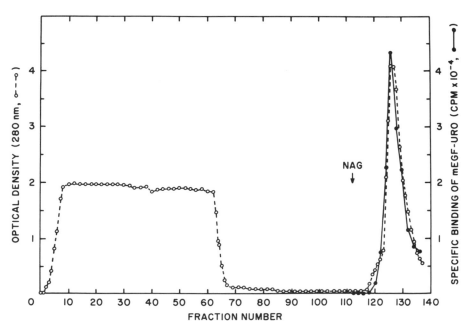

FIG. 7. Partial purification of the receptor for EGF-URO using lectin-agarose chromatography. Receptor solubilized in a large volume of detergent-containing buffer was applied to a column of WGA-Sepharose 4B. After the column was washed, the receptor was eluted (*arrow*) with 0.2 M *N*-acetylglucosamine (*NAG*). Receptor binding in the column effluent was monitored using the lectin immobilization assay. (Courtesy of RA Hock and MD Hollenberg, unpublished observations.)

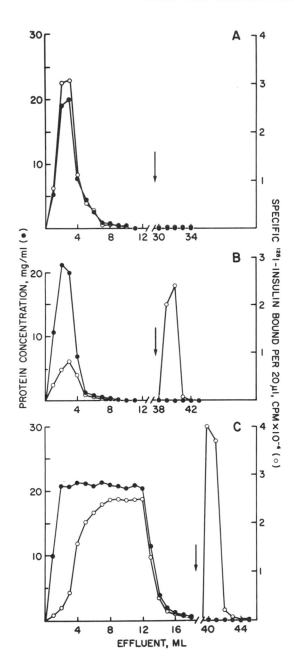

FIG. 8. Affinity chromatography of the insulin receptor. As outlined in the text, solubilized receptor from rat liver membranes was applied either to unsubstituted agarose or in increasing amounts (*B*, 2 ml; *C*, 12 ml) to columns of diaminodipropylamino - succinyl - *N* - phenylalanyl - insulin-agarose. Receptor was eluted in urea-containing acetate buffer, pH 6. Insulin binding in the column effluent was monitored with the PEG assay. (From Cuatrecasas, ref. 22, with permission.)

in the above buffer. Fractions of 4.5 ml were collected before elution with the sugar. When elution with the sugar was begun, the fraction volume was changed to 0.6 ml. Aliquots (50 μl) of the fractions were assayed for EGF-URO-binding activity by the lectin immobilization assay (see section with that title). The fraction eluted from the WGA column contains not only the EGF-URO receptor but also the insulin receptor, the somatomedin (IGF-I) receptor, and a variety of other glycosylated membrane receptors. This protein fraction can be used for further purification by the ligand-specific affinity chromatography approach to be described in the next section.

Insulin-Agarose Affinity Chromatography

This procedure, developed originally by Cuatrecasas (22) for purification of the insulin receptor has been successfully adapted to many other receptor systems using a variety of ligands coupled to agarose. The original procedure described by Cuatrecasas (22) is illustrated in Fig. 8. A 2% Triton X-100 extract of rat liver membranes dialyzed against Krebs-Ringer bicarbonate buffer, pH 7.4, containing 0.1% Triton was applied to columns (1.3 ml in Pasteur pipettes of either unsubstituted agarose (Fig. 8A) or to columns of diaminodipropylaminosuccinyl-*N*-phenylalanyl-insulin-agarose (Fig. 8, B and C). Either 2-ml (Fig. 8B) or 12-ml (Fig. 8C) aliquots of the membrane extract were applied to the small columns, which were washed with buffer until protein (*closed circles*) and insulin-binding activity (*open circles*) had returned to baseline. The columns were then eluted (*arrows*) with 50 mM sodium acetate buffer, pH 6.0, containing 4.5 M urea and 0.1% (v/v) Triton X-100. After application of the elution buffer to the column, the flow was stopped for 15 min to allow for desorption of the receptor before resumption of chromatography. The insulin-binding activity in fractions (1 ml) eluted from the columns was measured for 20-μl aliquots using the PEG method (see text). This isolation procedure was the key for the recovery of sufficient amounts of receptor to yield the microsequence data that led ultimately to the elucidation of the complete sequence of the insulin receptor (27, 28). It is to be hoped that this goal can be reached for other receptors by applying the general procedures outlined in this chapter.

Acknowledgments

The author is greatful for the long-term support of the Medical Research Council of Canada. Much of the work described in this chapter stems from innovative approaches originally developed by Dr. Pedro Cuatrecasas, to whom all of us involved in receptor isolation studies are greatly indebted.

REFERENCES

1. Conti-Tronconi BM, Raftery MA. *Ann Rev Biochem* 1982;51:491–530.
2. Noda M, Takahashi H, Tanabe T, et al. *Nature* 1982;299:793–797.
3. Langley JN. *Proc R Soc Lond* (*Biol*) 1906;78:170–194.
4. Armstrong GD, Hollenberg MD. In: Larner J, Pohl SL, eds. *Methods in diabetes research*, vol 1, *Laboratory methods*. New York: John Wiley & Sons, 1984;3–24.
5. Hollenberg MD, Cuatrecasas P. In: Busch H, ed. *Methods in cancer research*, vol 12. New York: Academic Press, 1976;317–366.

6. Cuatrecasas P. Hollenberg MD. *Adv Protein Chem* 1976;30:251–451.
7. Venter JC, Harrison LC, series eds. *Receptor biochemistry and methodology*, vols 1–6. New York: Alan Liss & Co., 1987.
7a. Greenwood FC, Hunter WM, Glover JS. *Biochem J* 1963;89:114–123.
8. Helenius A, Simons K. *Biochim Biophys Acta* 1975;415:29–79.
9. Tanford C, Reynolds JA. *Biochim Biophys Acta* 1976;457:133–170.
10. Chang H-W, Bock E. *Anal Biochem* 1980;104:112–117.
11. Cuatrecasas P. *Proc Natl Acad Sci USA* 1972;69:318–322.
12. Yip CC, Moule ML. *Diabetes* 1983;32:760–767.
13. Brandenburg D, Ambrosius D, Bala-Mohan S, et al. In: Goren HJ, Hollenberg MD, Roncari DAK, eds. *Insulin action and diabetes*. New York: Raven Press, 1988;13–27.
14. Fernandez-Pol JA. *FEBS Lett* 1982;143:86–92.
15. Daniel TO, Schneider WJ, Goldstein JL, et al. *J Biol Chem* 1983;258:4606–4611.
16. Laemmli UK. *Nature* 1970;227:680–685.
17. O'Farrell P. *J Biol Chem* 1975;250:4007–4021.
18. Goren HJ, Elliott C, Dudley RA. *J Cell Biochem* 1983;21:161–177.
19. Fairbanks G, Steck TL, Wallach DFH. *Biochemistry* 1971;10:2606–2617.
20. Cleveland DW, Fischer SG, Kirschner MW, et al. *J Biol Chem* 1977;252:1102–1106.
21. Cuatrecasas P. *J Biol Chem* 1972;247:1980–1991.
22. Cuatrecasas P. *Proc Natl Acad Sci USA* 1972;69:1277–1281.
23. Hock RA, Nexø E, Hollenberg MD. *J Biol Chem* 1980;255:10737–10743.
24. March SC, Parikh I, Cuatrecasas P. *Anal Biochem* 1974;60:149–152.
25. Hock RA, Nexø E, Hollenberg MD. *Nature* 1979;277:403–405.
26. Heinrich J, Pilch PF, Czech MP. *J Biol Chem* 1980;255:1732–1737.
27. Ebina Y, Ellis L, Jarnagin K, et al. *Cell* 1985;40:747–758.
28. Ullrich A, Bell JR, Chen EY, et al. *Nature* 1985;313:756–761.
29. Ullrich A, Gray A, Tam AW. *EMBO J* 1986;5:2503–2512.
30. Levitzki A. *Biochim Biophys Acta* 1985;822:127–153.
31. Mishina M, Tobimatsu T, Imoto K, et al. *Nature* 1985;313:364–369.
32. Hollenberg MD. *Trends Pharmacol Sci* 1987;8:197–199.
33. Ebina Y, Araki E, Taira M. *Proc Natl Acad Sci USA* 1987;84:704–708.
34. Chou CK, Dull TJ, Russell DS, et al. *J Biol Chem* 1987;262:1842–1847.
35. Maturo JM III, Shackelford WH, Hollenberg MD. *Life Sci* 1978;23:2063–2072.
36. Scatchard G. *Ann NY Acad Sci* 1949;51:660–672.
37. Bhaumick B., Bala RM, Hollenberg MD. *Proc Natl Acad Sci USA* 1981;78:4279–4283.
38. Nexø E, Hock RA, Hollenberg MD *J Biol Chem* 1979;254:8740–8743.
39. Bhaumick B, Armstrong GD, Hollenberg MD, et al. *Can J Biochem* 1982;60:923–932.
40. Siegel TW, Ganguly S, Jacobs S, et al. *J Biol Chem* 1981;256:9266–9273.
41. Armstrong GD, Hollenberg MD, Bhaumick B, et al. *J Cell Biochem* 1982;20:283–292.
42. Pilch PF, Czech MP. *J Biol Chem* 1980;255:1722–1731.

Methods in Neurotransmitter Receptor Analysis,
edited by Henry I. Yamamura, et al.
Raven Press, Ltd., New York © 1990.

6

Methods for Studying Receptors with Cultured Cells of Nervous Tissue Origin

Michael A. Pfenning and Elliott Richelson

*Departments of Psychiatry and Pharmacology, Mayo Foundation,
Rochester, Minnesota 55905*

Cultured cells have been very useful as model systems to study a variety of cellular processes relating to the function of the nervous system. Therefore, this chapter will present details of the techniques the reader will need to grow and propagate cultured cells, mainly established cells of nervous tissue origin, and to use them in *intact* form to study their receptors. Techniques for these receptor studies include direct measurement of receptor binding sites by radioligand-binding assays and measurement of receptor function from receptor-mediated synthesis of cyclic adenosine $3':5'$-monophosphate (AMP), cyclic guanosine $3':5'$-monophosphate (GMP), and inositol phosphates. These last compounds are products from the metabolism of polyphosphoinositides and, along with the cyclic nucleotides, may be second messengers, the first messenger being the neurotransmitter or neurohormone.

The protocols presented in this chapter make use of murine neuroblastoma clone N1E-115, since it is a widely studied clone with which we have the most experience. However, other intact cells may be substituted with little or no modification of most assay conditions.

Established (immortal) cells, that is, cells that divide indefinitely in culture, used in intact form offer distinct advantages over tissue or broken cell preparations. Thus, these cells can provide a readily accessible, homogeneous population of cells with neuronal properties. The nervous sytem is made up of so many different cell types, the normal neurons of which do not divide in culture. Hence, the availability of a homogeneous population of cells for research markedly simplifies experimentation and interpretation of results and contributes significantly to the reproducibility of experiments. However, care must be taken to ensure this reproducibility. In addition, since these cells can be studied in a precisely controlled environment, pharmacologists can enjoy studying the actions of drugs without concern in most circumstances for pharmacokinetic variables that can confound *in vivo* studies.

Another important advantage of the use of intact cultured cells is the ability to obtain results under identical or nearly identical conditions from direct binding assays of a receptor and from functional assays of that same receptor. This approach will assure that the data from radioligand-binding experiments relate to the reality of receptor function and not to an artifact of the binding technique. In addition, such experiments can yield interesting information about the relationship between response of a receptor and occupancy of that receptor by agonist, since there are many examples in which the magnitude of a particular biological response is not simply related to receptor occupancy.

The use of cultured cells has some disadvantages. In cases in which the cells being studied are derived from a tumor or are virally transformed, it is often necessary to demonstrate that the receptor or any other property being studied in the model system is similar to that found in normal tissue and is not altered as a consequence of the cellular transformation. Furthermore, although the environment can be precisely controlled, it is an artificial one nonetheless, and its global effect on cellular processes is unknown.

A final point to consider when using an intact cell system in performing binding studies is whether one measures true binding to a surface protein or uptake of the labeled material into the cell. Usually, transport into the cell can be obviated by the use of a hydrophilic ligand (for example, N-methylscopolamine instead of quinuclidinyl benzilate for studies of muscarinic receptors) or assay at 0°C. Reduction of temperature is also necessary when radioligands are peptides that can be rapidly degraded by enzymes on the surface of the cell.

Clone N1E-115, which is the focus of this chapter, was isolated from the uncloned murine neuroblastoma C-1300 cell line, which had been established in culture from the cells of a spontaneous tumor of a strain A/J mouse. This clone possesses a number of characteristics associated with adrenergic neurons, such as some of the enzymes needed for catecholamine synthesis (Table 1). Curiously, they lack L-aromatic amino acid decarboxylase. N1E-115 cells have electrically excitable membranes and display many of the morphological characteristics of neurons. Importantly, N1E-115 cells contain a variety of receptors that mediate the release of arachidonic acid and inositol phosphates, the synthesis of cyclic AMP and cyclic GMP, the inhibition of cyclic AMP, and the regulation of their electrical potential (Table 2). Because of these properties, this clone has become the most widely studied murine neuroblastoma clone, serving as an invaluable model system for the neurobiologist and neuropsychopharmacologist.

TABLE 1. *Properties of murine neuroblastoma clone N1E-115*

Biochemical	Electrophysiological
Transport system for L-tyrosine	Action potential mechanism
Tyrosine 3-monooxygenase	Anatomical
Dopamine β-hydroxylase	Neurons with microtubules and microfilaments
Monoamine oxidase	Synthesis of Polypeptides
Catechol methyltransferase	Methionine enkephalin
Acetylcholinesterase	VIP*

*Vasoactive intestinal peptide.

TABLE 2. *Receptors and their effects on cyclic nucleotides and inositol phosphates*[a]

| Receptor | Cyclic nucleotides | | Inositol phosphates |
	Cyclic AMP	Cyclic GMP	
Adenosine	+	0	?
Angiotensin	?	+	+
Bradykinin	?	+	+
Glucagon	+	0	?
Histamine H_1	0	+	+
Muscarinic M_1	0	+	+
Muscarinic M_2	−	0	0
Neurotensin	0	+	+
Opiate	−	0	0
Prostaglandin E_1	+	+	+
Secretin/VIP[b]	+	0	?
Somatostatin	−	0	?
Thrombin	?	+	+

[a]The symbols used are: +, stimulates; −, inhibits; 0, no change; ?, unknown effect.
[b]Vasoactive intestinal peptide.

CELL CULTURE

Principle

The culturing of cells is required for the propagation of an established cell line. It is important to maintain sterile technique, to be aware of any potential health hazards relative to the cell line, and to use consistent procedures in maintaining the cell line. Any changes in the conditions or techniques need to be examined for possible effects on the variables being measured.

The Cell Culture Laboratory

The proper use of cell cultures requires some specialized equipment. Usually, a separate room is set aside, which may be equipped with a sliding door to diminish the flow of air currents when opened and closed and with ultraviolet lights for sterility. Hoods of various types are employed for work in tissue culture. The least expensive are those that simply provide an air pocket, that is, an enclosure that is free from room air currents. Vertical laminar flow hoods confine aerosols generated during laboratory manipulation and offer greater protection from contamination for the worker and cultures. Horizontal laminar flow hoods have an open work area and, because they blow air in the face of the worker, offer less protection. An inverted phase-contrast microscope is essential to a tissue culture laboratory for observation of cells on monolayer surfaces. A CO_2 incubator with a method for humidifying the air is also required as most media for culture use a sodium bicarbonate-CO_2 buffering system requiring usually 5% CO_2/95% air or 10% CO_2/90% air. CO_2 incubators are available with or without water jackets. Those without water jackets are usually less expensive, and the advantages of a water jacket (e.g., less extreme fluctuations of temperature) may not be worth the extra cost.

Because the osmolality of solutions used in the cultivation of tissue is a variable that is very important and easily monitored, an osmometer is a necessary piece of equipment in the cell culture laboratory.

An ordinary light microscope and a hemocytometer are used for counting of cells. Viability of cells is determined with this equipment using dye (e.g., nigrosin) that is excluded by viable cells. Electronic cell counters are also available, although they are very expensive. A low-speed centrifuge capable of a force of 250 to $500 \times g$ for 15- and 50-ml tubes is necessary for isolation of cells. An automatic pipetter, although not essential, greatly enhances the efficiency of the pipetting chores required for feeding cells.

Consumables include 75 cm^2/250-ml tissue culture flasks; 15- and 50-ml sterile centrifuge tubes; and 5-, 10-, and 20-ml sterile glass or disposable plastic pipettes.

TABLE 3. *Solutions used in the culture and assay of intact cells*

I.	DMEM[a]

(0.03 μM D-biotin, 1.0 μM vitamin B_{12}, 1.0 μM DL-α-lipoic acid, 44 mM $NaHCO_3$)

Bubble in CO_2 for approximately 5 min to adjust pH
Establish an osmolality of 340 ± 5 mosM[b]
Filter sterilize[c]
Screen for mycoplasma and bacterial contamination[d]
Supplemented with 10% (v/v) calf serum[e] before use

II.	Modified Puck's D1 solution

(5.5 mM glucose, 5.4 mM KCl, 58.4 mM sucrose, 0.17 mM $Na_2HPO_47H_2O$, 138 mM NaCl, 0.22 mM KH_2PO_4)

pH Adjusted to 7.4 ± 0.05 with 0.1 N NaOH or 0.1 N HCl
Establish an osmolality of 340 ± 5 mosM[b]
Filter sterilize[f]

III.	PBS with glucose and sucrose (PBS-GS)

110 mM NaCl, 1.0 mM $MgCl_2$, 70 mM sucrose, 5.3 mM KCl, 1.8 mM $CaCl_2$, 2 mM Na_2HPO_4, 25 mM glucose)

pH Adjusted to 7.4 ± 0.05 with 0.1 N NaOH or 0.1 N HCl
Establish an osmolality of 340 ± 5 mosM[b]

[a] DMEM (no pyruvate) containing L-glutamine and 4,500 mg/liter glucose. The glucose is necessary for neuronal cell types as they require a high glucose concentration. This medium is available from GIBCO* and Mediatech.* (Asterisks refer to items appearing in the "Suppliers" section.)
[b] Osmolality is adjusted with either sucrose or H_2O to increase or decrease the osmolality, respectively.
[c] An acceptable filter apparatus would be model 316 (142 mm) from the Millipore Corp.* using prefilter; 1.2-, 0.45-, and 0.22-μM filters and driven under CO_2 pressure.
[d] Several techniques are available for mycoplasma screening: microbiological assay (ref. 33); fluorescent microscopy using Hoechst 33258 stain (ref. 34); or scanning electron microscopy (ref. 35).
[e] Either fetal or newborn bovine calf serum serves equally well as a supplement and both are available from a number of commercial sources including GIBCO* and Hyclone.*
[f] A 0.22-μM filter* under vacuum will suffice.

Growth Medium

It is essential that the medium in which the cells are cultured provide all essential components and cofactors necessary for normal growth, viability, and receptor function. The growth medium used for N1E-115 cells, Dulbecco's modified Eagle's medium (DMEM) with 10% (v/v) fetal calf serum (newborn calf serum may be substituted, but characteristics for certain receptors may be altered by this change), is a complete, although undefined medium because of the serum supplement (Table 3). Defined media have been formulated which do not require serum. Although these will sustain cell growth, viability, and functional integrity for some cell types (1), receptors that mediate cyclic GMP synthesis in clone N1E-115 cells function poorly, if at all, when these cells are grown under these conditions (2).

Streptomycin and penicillin are antibiotics that are frequently added to media. However, with the use of antibiotics it is possible to suppress a bacterial infection that becomes obvious several weeks later after drug-resistant strains have grown out. It is therefore wise to omit antibiotics from media so that infections may develop within days rather than weeks. Also since PPLO (pleuropneumonia-like organisms) may be coinfectors with bacterial cells but are not susceptible to penicillin or streptomycin, it is possible for the antibiotics in the media to take care of one but not the other infection. In this regard, it is important to test cultures periodically for infection with PPLO.

Culture

1. Grow cells in 75-cm^2 flasks in 20 ml of solution I in an atmosphere of 90% humidified air and 10% CO_2 at 37°C.
2. Feed cells daily after the 5th day from subculture by adding 10 ml of fresh solution I and then removing 10 ml. This method of replenishing one-third of the growth medium has proven successful and cost effective.
3. Do not subculture cells indefinitely. Cells used routinely in our assays are between passages 8 and 22. A passage is defined as the subculturing of a flask of cells which on average is performed every 10 to 14 dyas. Use only confluent flasks of cells in the experiments described here to ensure that all cells are in stationary phase when they are functionally similar between various studies (3, 4).

Subculture

1. Remove the growth medium and subculture cells by incubating them for 7 to 10 min in 10 ml of solution II at 37°C. The neuroblastoma cell requires divalent cations, especially Ca^{2+}, to adhere to the surface of the flask as a monolayer. Solution II lacks appreciable calcium.
2. Dislodge cells by gentle tapping on the sides of the flask.

3. Collect cells with the medium using a 10-ml sterile pipette and transfer them to a 15- or 50-ml sterile centrifuge tube.
4. Centrifuge suspended cells at $250 \times g$ for 1.5 min to pellet them.
5. Aspirate the medium with the use of a sterile Pasteur pipette, and resuspend the pelleted cells in 10 ml of fresh solution I (per 10 flasks of cells to be inoculated) by gentle trituration.
6. Seed 1-ml aliquots into 75-cm^2 flasks containing 20 ml of fresh solution I.

Note that from a confluent parent flask, approximately 5 million cells can be collected. This amount enables inoculation of each new flask with 500,000 cells when subculturing with a split ratio of 1:10.

Harvesting Cells for Assay

1. Harvest cells for use in experiments by the same procedure described above for subculturing. As an alternate means of harvesting the cells, scrape the surface of the flask with a sterile Teflon-coated scraper. The advantage of the former method is that it subjects the cells to much less physical duress, a point that is important when working with cells that are morphologically very differentiated (that is, have long cellular extensions). Scraping the cells, however, offers the advantage of speed. Cells could be removed by scraping in a matter of 15 to 30 sec and immediately centrifuged, whereas the treatment with solution II involves a lengthy incubation.
2. Pellet cells by centrifugation at $250 \times g$ for 1.5 min, aspirate the medium, and resuspend cells in 10 ml of solution III by *gentle* trituration.
3. Centrifuge the cells again, aspirate the medium, and resuspend the cellular pellet in a convenient volume of solution III. Typically, 2 ml of solution III is used for every two flasks of cells harvested.
4. Remove a small aliquot (e.g., 20 μl) for enumeration of cells with the use of a hemocytometer or electronic cell counter. As an alternate means of expressing the results of an assay, determine the amount of protein present in the aliquot.

Additional Comments

The entire process of harvesting cells for use in an experiment will take approximately 20 to 30 min using the incubation method. If on the other hand, the cells are procured by scraping them from the flasks, the process can be accomplished in as little as 3 to 5 min.

In the procedure described above, solution III in which the cells are resuspended is listed as a phosphate-buffered saline (PBS) (Table 3). Other buffers may be substituted. For example, an N-2-hydroxyethyl piperazine-N'-2'ethanesulfonic acid (HEPES) buffer (25 mM) may be used when either a stronger buffer or a buffer containing magnesium salts is needed.

Finally, we want to reemphasize that with the murine neuroblastoma clone N1E-115, we routinely culture only until passage 20 to 22. Recent findings in our laboratory (5, 6), which are analogous to findings obtained for other cultured cell lines, suggest that the properties of these cells change with prolonged culturing. Specifically in this clone, we have found a marked change in the proportion of the muscarinic receptor subtypes and a decrease in the total muscarinic receptor population with passage as measured by receptor binding and by biochemical assays of cyclic nucleotide synthesis and inositol phosphate formation.

RECEPTOR BINDING STUDIES

Principle

The reader is directed to Chapters 1, 3, and 7 in *Neurotransmitter Receptor Binding*, 2nd ed. (ref. 6a) for a more detailed description of many of the parameters under which receptor binding assays are performed. These include the requirements that the tissue concentration be within the linear range of binding; that optimal pH and temperature are used; that the radioactively labeled ligand be of high specific activity and high purity; and that the equilibrium conditions have been reached as described below. Failure to ensure that these conditions are met may invalidate any results obtained in your studies and lead to erroneous conclusions.

The principle of the assay is no different from that of a binding study involving membranal preparations. In the absence of a competitor and with a fixed concentration of receptor, the quantity of radioligand bound specifically to a given receptor is related to the concentration of the ligand and to its equilibrium dissociation constant. In general, conditions of this assay are similar for a variety of different receptors. However, changes in the protocol may be necessary, and precise assay conditions need be established for each receptor studied.

Supplies[1]

Reagents:
    Puck's modified D1 solution (see Table 3)
    PBS, solution III (see Table 3)
    Bovine serum albumin (BSA)
    Polyethylenimine
    [^{3}H]Neurotensin* (highest specific activity available) or other labeled ligand
    Neurotensin (or analogues) dilutions in solution III
Materials:

    Filters (glass fiber type GF/B*)
    Scintillation vials (7- or 20-ml capacity)
    Scintillation fluid for aqueous samples*
Equipment: Filtration device*

---

[1]See "Suppliers" section for a partial list of vendors for items marked with an asterisk throughout.

Procedure

The assay detailed here will be a competition study involving [³H]neurotensin and competing unlabeled neurotensin analogues binding to receptors on clone N1E-115 (7–12). We have selected this receptor as an example because it involves several additional steps and is likely one of the more difficult binding assays that we routinely perform. When relevant, we will attempt to clarify these differences. The reader is reminded to refer to Table 4 and the references contained therein for specific details regarding a particular receptor of interest.

1. Resuspend cells isolated as described above under "Harvesting Cells for Assay" after the final centrifugation in 2 ml of solution III containing 0.1% (w/v) BSA. The BSA is included in the assay for neurotensin receptor binding to reduce nonspecific binding and to inhibit proteases located on the surface of cellular membrane which are capable of nonspecifically degrading the neurotensin. The incubation is also done at 0 to 4°C to reduce further any possible degradation of ligands by proteases. The concentration of BSA cannot be significantly increased beyond that stated because it slows the filtration time when using a multiple filtration unit such as the cell harvester offered by Brandel.

2. Remove a small aliquot (e.g., 20 μl) for cell enumeration or for protein determination. If the amount of protein is to be measured, the aliquot must be removed prior to the resuspension in buffer containing BSA.

3. Dilute the cell suspension in solution III containing 0.1% BSA to provide between 300,000 and 400,000 cells/assay tube. Because of the density of neurotensin receptors, a minimum of 200,000 cells/tube is necessary to provide sufficient bound radioactivity to perform the data analysis. At the other extreme, the maximum number of cells/tube is approximately 400,000. Any significant increase over this cell number leads to clogging of the filtration apparatus.

4. Cool the cell suspension to 0 to 4°C in an ice bath prior to its distribution to 12- × 75-mm tubes. To prevent any deterioration of the viability of the intact cell suspension which might result from a prolonged equilibration period at 0 to 4°C, prepare the drug dilutions and assay tubes prior to harvesting the cells.

5. Add a 700-μl aliquot of cell suspension (300,000 to 400,000 cells) to 12- × 75-mm polypropylene tubes containing 100 μl of [³H]neurotensin (2 to 3 nM final concentration) and 100 μl of competing nonradioactive neurotensin, its analogues or fragments, in duplicate in a final volume of 1.0 ml. We use a filtration apparatus as described above which is capable of filtering 24 samples simultaneously in a matter of 30 to 60 sec including washes. Other models are available which will filter a smaller or larger number of samples. Therefore, when preparing tubes for an assay, we stagger the addition of the cells to each group of 24 tubes by approximately 3 min. Futhermore, we include in each run of 24 tubes, which routinely encompasses one competition curve, duplicate estimates of total binding in which no unlabeled competing peptide is added and an estimate of nonspecific binding in which excess unlabeled neurotensin (1 μM final concentration) is added.

6. Vortex the tubes gently, and incubate the cells for 20 min at 0 to 4°C. We have

found that equilibrium binding conditions are reached quite rapidly with this receptor. Thus, by 20 min, equilibrium has been achieved at this temperature. This is not the typical situation found with most other receptors on this clone (see Table 4), and the proper conditions must be determined for each receptor.

7. Terminate the assay after the 20-min incubation by rapidly filtering the samples through a type GF/B glass fiber filter that had previously been pretreated for approximately 30 to 60 min with 0.1% (w/v) polyethylenimine to reduce further nonspecific binding to the filters.

8. Rinse each tube with three 4-ml additions of ice-cold solution III, and apply each rinse to the filter.

9. Remove the filters, and place them in scintillation vials to which 7 ml of counting cocktail is added. Measure the amount of radioactivity after a minimum of 4 hr to allow for the solubilization of labeled material from the filters.

10. Analyze data. In our laboratory we routinely analyze data by the LIGAND program (13), which we have modified to give estimates of the Hill coefficient, a variable that provides information about whether the binding follows the law of mass action. We have found this program to be extremely efficient in analyzing data that correspond to one class of binding sites.

Other Comments

The choice of the concentration of labeled ligand used in this study was made after performing both saturation and tissue linearity studies with [^{3}H]neurotensin. If possible, attempt to use a concentration of labeled ligand which is less than 10 to 20% of its K_D. This is not always possible, but every effort should be made (including the choice of labeled ligand) to keep the concentration of labeled material well below its K_D yet still provide for adequate specific binding.

Peptides in general are very susceptible to proteolytic digestion as evidenced by the precautions taken in the above example (0 to 4°C assay temperature and inclusion of 0.1% BSA). Failure to prevent possible degradation can lead to the total loss of labeled ligand, in which case no specific binding will be evident, and to a complete loss of the unlabeled competing peptide, in which case no competition will be observed when the radioligand is resistant to degradation. The more common situation is that of partial degradation of the peptides which can lead to erroneous estimates of the binding parameters. In addition, it may lead to very high nonspecific binding that can further distort the analysis of the data. A second property of many peptides is that they adsorb to many materials, especially untreated glassware. This is the reason we have used polypropylene tubes. Alternately, one can experiment to determine whether polystyrene or silanized glassware will sufficiently reduce the peptide's binding to the surface of the tubes to warrant their use in the assay.

Finally, we want to emphasize that the dilutions used in the neurotensin binding assays for all analogues and fragments of the peptide are prepared immediately before use and are not stored for future use. Typically, we store only 10^{-2} or 10^{-3} M stock solutions of these peptides in very small aliquots (20 to 50 μl) at −70°C and discard any unused material after it has been thawed.

TABLE. 4. *Binding assays*

Receptor	Source	Parameters for labeled ligand			Estimate nonspecific	Incubation		Ref.
		Ligand	K_d^a	B_{max}^b		Time	Temperature	
						min	°C	
	Established cell lines							
Acetylcholine								
Nicotinic	BC3H-1 muscle	^{125}I-Bungarotoxin			100 µM Tubocurarine	60	23	36
	Neuroblastoma	[^{3}H] α-toxin		3.4×10^{7c}	Unlabeled toxin	20	23	37
Muscarinic	108CC15	[^{3}H]QNB	0.14		0.3 µM Atropine	60	37	38
	108CC15	[^{3}H]NMS	0.06	21	0.3 µM Atropine	30	37	38
	N1E-115	[^{3}H]QNB	0.4	25	1 mM Oxotremorine	60	24	39
	N1E-115	[^{3}H]Scopolamine		25	100 µM Scopolamine	60	24	39
β-Adrenergic	C6 glioma	[^{3}H]CGP-12177			2 µM Propranolol	60	37	40
Angiotensin	NG108-15	^{125}I-A$_{II}$	0.32	7.13	150 nM A$_{II}$	30	25	41
ANP	A10 muscle	^{125}I-ANP	0.157	115	1 µM ANP	30	37	42
Bradykinin	N1E-115	[^{3}H]Bradykinin	1.0^d	$160^{d,e}$	1 µM Bradykinin	90	25	43
Calcium channel	PC12	[^{3}H]PN200-110	0.04–0.6	$0.6–1.8^e$	1 µM Nifedipine	90	25	44
EGF	Fibroblast	^{125}I-EGF	0.2–0.4	$100,000^c$	20 µg EGF	60	37	45–47
Growth hormone	RIN-5AH	^{125}I-GH	0.2–0.4	$2,700^{c,d}$	100 µg/ml GH	60	37	48
	3T3 fibroblast	^{125}I-GH	0.13	$4,000^c$	10^4ng/ml GH	120	30	49
Insulin	Glial blastoma	^{125}I-Insulin			100 µg/ml Insulin	180	15	50
IFN	L1210	^{125}I-IFN	0.14	$5,000^c$	IFN (excess)	90	37	51
Neurotensin	N1E-115	[^{3}H]Neurotensin	10	215^e	1 µM Neurotensin	20	0	12
Opiate	NG108-15	[^{3}H]MEA	1.6		10 µM Naloxone		37	52–54
	N4TG1	[^{3}H]Enkephalin	1–2	30^e	1 µM Cold ligand	60	24	55–57
	N4TG1	[^{3}H]Naloxone			1 µM Naloxone	60	24	58
PDGF	3T3 fibroblast	^{125}I-PDGF	0.7	$400,000^c$	4 µg/ml PDGF	60	22	59
Prostaglandin	N1E-115	[^{3}H]PGE$_1$	10^d	$220^{d,e}$	1 µM PGE$_1$	90	15	60
Thrombin	N1E-115	^{125}I-Thrombin	1.11^d	$41.9^{d,e}$	10 units/ml Hirudin	15	37	61

Primary Cultures

Receptor	Source	Ligand	K_d	B_{max}	Displacer	Binding capacity		Ref.
Acetylcholine								
Nicotinic	Chick ganglia	^{125}I-Bungarotoxin	1.0	8.6[f]	10 µM Bungarotoxin	60		62
Muscarinic	Neurons/cortex	[^{3}H]QNB	0.17	250,000[c]	1 µM Atropine	30	37	63
	Avian retina	[^{3}H]NMS	0.6	33[g]	10 µM Atropine	15	37	64
β-Adrenergic	Chick glial	[^{3}H]DHA	0.04	3.3[e]	1–10 µM Alprenolol	30	37	65
Angiotensin	Rat neuron	^{125}I-A_{II}	1.0	6,000[c]	84 nM A_{II}	30	24	66
	Rat neuron	^{125}I-A_{II}	0.25–0.6	40–280	50–150 nM A_{II}	90	24	67
	Spinal neuron	[^{3}H] or ^{125}I-A_{II}	0.43[d]	8.3[d,e]	10 µM A_{II}	120	37	68
Benzodiazepine	Hippocampus	[^{3}H]Diazepam	4.8	960[f]	10 µM diazepam	30	4	69
	Spinal neuron	[^{3}H]Flunitrazepam	6.1	822	10 µM Clonazepam	30	24	70
	Astrocyte	[^{3}H]Flunitrazepam	7.0	6,033	50 µM Flunitrazepam			71
	Interneuron	[^{3}H]Flunitrazepam	11	450	1 µM Clonazepam		25	72
	Mouse glial	[^{3}H]Diazepam	25.3	7,575	100 nM R05-4864	60	4	73
GABA	Interneuron	[^{3}H]Muscimol	12.5	500	1 mM GABA	15	25	72
K$^+$ channel	Rat astrocyte	^{125}I-Apamin	0.09	3	50 nM Apamin	90	1	65
Neurotensin	Mouse neuron	^{125}I-Neurotensin	0.3	178	1 µM Neurotensin	45	37	74
Transferrin	Chick myotube	^{125}I-Transferrin	37	7,500[c]	1,000-Fold excess	90	4	75

The abbreviations used are: ANP, atrial natriuretic peptide; EGF, epidermal growth factor; IFN, interferon; PDGF, platelet-derived growth factor; GABA, γ-aminobutyric acid; QNB, quinuclidinyl benzilate; NMS, N-methylscopolamine; DHA, Dihydro-L-alprenolol; A_{II}, angiotensin II; CGP, (±)-4-(3-tert-butylamino-2-hydroxypropoxl) benzimidazole-2-on HCl; GH, growth hormone; MEA, Methionine enkephalinamide.

[a] K_d values are nanomolar unless otherwise indicated.
[b] Binding capacities are fmol/mg protein unless indicated.
[c] Sites/cell.
[d] High-affinity binding site only.
[e] Femtomoles 10^6 cells.
[f] Femtomoles 10^4 cells.
[g] Femtomoles/well or dish.

Application

Here is a representative example of data generated using the techniques described above. The conditions were: labeled ligand, [^{3}H]neurotensin; competing ligand, neurotensin; maximum cpm bound, 350; nonspecific cpm bound, 145; total cpm/tube, 125,600; efficiency of counting, 41.6%; labeled [^{3}H]neurotensin concentration/tube, 3.3×10^{-9} M; cells/tube, 400,000.

Tube no.	Average cpm/tube	Competing unlabeled neurotensin	Comment
		M	
1–2	334	4×10^{-10}	
3–4	334	8×10^{-10}	
5–6	319	2×10^{-9}	
7–8	306	4×10^{-9}	
9–10	288	6×10^{-9}	
11–12	262	8×10^{-9}	
13–14	214	2×10^{-8}	
15–16	186	4×10^{-8}	
17–18	165	8×10^{-8}	
19–20	154	1×10^{-7}	
21–22	350	0	Maximum binding
23–24	145	1×10^{-6}	Nonspecific

These data were entered in the LIGAND program, and the following results were obtained: K_D for neurotensin, 1.08×10^{-8} M; B_{max} for neurotensin, 2.43×10^{-11} M; Hill coefficient, 1.01.

Graphs were generated using the final parameter estimates given above and are shown in Fig. 1. These results suggest that neurotensin is binding to a single class of receptors based on the linearity of the Scatchard plot and on a Hill coefficient of approximately unity. The maximum number of binding sites determined from the x-intercept of the Scatchard plot can be converted to the number of receptor sites per cell or per specified unit of protein based on the enumeration of cells or protein determination performed earlier.

A second example (Fig. 2) depicts a more extensive study involving competition experiments at the neurotensin receptor with a series of neurotensin analogues and fragments.

MEASUREMENT OF CYCLIC GMP IN INTACT CELLS

Principle

Cyclic GMP is likely a second messenger (14, 15) of many different receptors (Table 5). Those receptors that mediate cyclic GMP in a calcium-dependent manner (16) do so only in intact cell preparations and therefore appear not to be directly coupled to soluble guanylate cyclase, the enzyme that synthesizes this cyclic nucle-

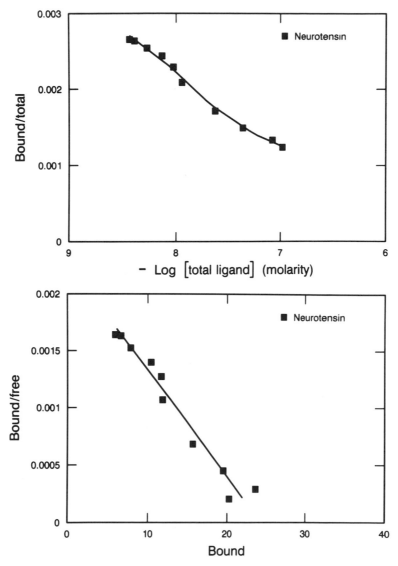

FIG. 1. Competition of [³H]neurotensin binding by increasing concentrations of unlabeled neurotensin. **A**, competition plot of data using final estimates from LIGAND program (13). **B**, Scatchard plot of data.

otide from guanosine 5′-triphosphate (GTP) (17–19). Atrial natriuretic peptide(s) stimulates a receptor that is directly coupled to the particulate form of the enzyme present in the membrane (20). The activation and competitive antagonism of receptors mediating cyclic GMP formation provide a physiological response, the data from which may be compared with radioligand-binding data. Clone N1E-115 cells contain a number of receptors that mediate the formation of this nucleotide in a robust fashion (Table 1) and thus serve as an excellent model system in which to study these receptors by measurement of this putative second messenger.

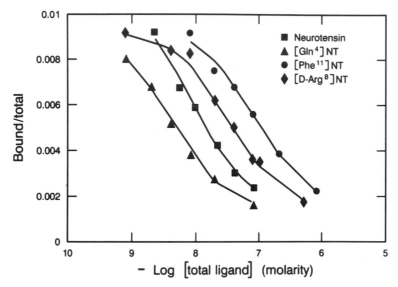

FIG. 2. Competition of [³H]neurotensin binding by increasing concentrations of unlabeled neurotensin or analogues. Data taken from Gilbert et al. (12).

This assay as well as those described below measuring cyclic AMP and inositol phosphates exploits one of the major advantages of using an intact cell preparation, namely, the ability to measure a product in radiolabeled form by feeding cells a radiolabeled precursor. However, this technique will measure only relative changes in the product of interest; absolute changes require the use of an assay that measures endogenous unlabeled compound. Radioimmunoassay is an example of such an assay.

Isolation of cyclic [³H]GMP from the cells prelabeled with [³H]guanine or [³H]guanosine that is incorporated into [³H]GTP is accomplished by cation-exchange column chromatography and a one-step precipitation-centrifugation procedure to purify the product further. The assay is very straightforward, relatively easy to perform, relatively sensitive, and convenient, since large numbers of samples can be processed in 1 day.

Supplies

Reagents:
Puck's modified D1 solution (see Table 3)
PBS, solution III (see Table 3)
[³H]Guanine sulfate or [³H]guanosine* (5 to 15 Ci/mmol) (Each radioactive precursor works equally well. However, [³H]guanosine is significantly less expensive than [³H]guanine.)

TABLE 5. *Cyclic nucleotide, inositol phosphate, and electrophysiological assays*

Receptor	Source[a]	AMP	GMP	IP	Electrochemical	Ref.
		Cyclic				
Acetylcholine						
Nicotinic	PC12				*	76, 77
	NX31				*	78
Muscarinic	N1E-115	*	*	*	*	17, 79 80, 81
	NG108-15	*				82
	108CC15	*				83
	108CC25	*				83
Adenosine	C6 glioma	*				84
	138MG glial	*				84
	N18	*				84
	41A3	*				84
	N1E-115	*				84, 85
Adrenergic						
α	NG108-15	*				86
	1' Cortical neuron	*				87
	TCX11,17				*	88
β	C6 glioma	*				89, 90
	C6TG1A glioma	*				91
	1' Fetal mouse neurons	*				87
Angiotensin	N1E-115		*	*		92
	Endothelial		*			93
ANP	A10 muscle cell		*			42
Bradykinin	N1E-115		*	*		43
	108CC15		*			94
	C6-4-2		*			94
	NG108-15		*	*	*	95
Dopamine	1' Retinal ganglia				*	96
DA$_1$	1' Striatal neurons	*				97
DA$_2$	1' Striatal neurons	*				97
GABA	1' Chick ganglia				*	98
Glucagon	108CC15	*				99
Histamine H$_1$	N1E-115		*	*	*	100–102
	Endothelial		*			93
Neurotensin	N1E-115		*	*		103–105
Opiate	N1E-115	*				106, 107
	N4TG1		*			108
	N18TG2	*				109, 110
	NG108-15	*			*	109, 111 112
Prostaglandin	N1E-115	*	*	*		85, 106 113, 114
	108CC15	*			*	83, 99 115
	108CC25	*				83
	NG108-15	*				82
	TCX11,17				*	115
Secretin/VIP	108CC15	*				99
Serotonin (5-HT$_1$)	1' Hippocampus neuron	*				116
	NG108-15				*	112, 117
Somatostatin	Neuroblastoma × glioma	*				118
Thrombin	N1E-115	*				119
	CCL39 fibroblast			*		120
Vasopressin (V$_{1a}$)	1' Aortic myocytes			*		121
VIP	1' Striatal neurons	*				97

[a]Established cell lines and primary cultures.

Cyclic [^{14}C] GMP* (1,200 to 1,400 dpm/100 μl in H_2O, 0.5 nCi)
Agonist and antagonist solutions in solution III
Trichloroacetic acid (TCA) [50% (w/v)]
Na_2Co_3 (2.67 M)
$ZnSO_4$ (2.67 M)
Column elution buffers: 0.1 N HCl; H_2O
Column regeneration sequence: 10 ml of 1.25 N NaOH; 10 ml of H_2O; 10 ml of
1.7 N HCl; 10 ml of H_2O
Materials:
Ion exchange resin: Dowex 50-H +, AG 50W-X2, 200 to 400 mesh*
Columns: plastic disposable (0.8 × 20 cm)*
Multiwell trays: 24-well flat bottom wells*
Centrifuge tubes: plastic disposable (2.0 ml) microcentrifuge tubes*
Scintillation vials (20-ml capacity)
Scintillation fluid for aqueous samples*
Erlenmeyer flasks (25- or 50-ml capacity)
Equipment: Racks for columns; Microcentrifuge

Procedure

1. Harvest cells (about 10 million cells from two 75-cm^2/250-ml flasks) as described under "Harvesting Cells for Assay," and resuspend them in 2.0 ml of
   solution III. Use a proportionately larger volume of solution III for a larger
   number of cells. Remove an aliquot (e.g., 20 μl) for enumeration of cells or for
   protein determination.
2. Transfer the cell suspension to a 25- or 50-ml Erlenmeyer flask, add 20 μl (20
   μCi, about 4 × 10^7 dpm) of either [^{3}H]guanine or [^{3}H]guanosine for about 10
   million cells.
3. Cover the flask with Parafilm and incubate it for 45 min at 37°C in a shaking
   water bath equipped with platform (60 to 80 oscillations/min).
4. After the incubation, transfer the cells to microcentrifuge tubes, and pellet them
   by quickly turning the microcentrifuge on and off. Carefully aspirate the medium, replace it with 2 ml of fresh solution III, triturate the cells *gently* (rough
   handling of cells can lead to high basal values and poor response to agonist) to
   resuspend the pelleted cells, and return the cells to the Erlenmeyer flask. As an
   alternative, the cells can be immediately diluted as described in the next step.
   However, removing the extracellular radioactive material greatly reduces the
   basal level of cyclic [^{3}H]GMP measured in the assay.
5. Dilute the cells to 400,000 to 600,000 cells/ml such that each aliquot of dispersed cell suspension (240 to 270 μl) will contain between 100,000 and
   150,000 cells. Dispense the cells into the wells of the multiwell tray while
   swirling the Erlenmeyer flask after every third addition to prevent the cells
   from settling to the bottom of the flask.

6. Add the antagonist, if one is to be used, in a 30-μl aliquot, and incubate it with the cells for 30 min or longer (depending upon the antagonist) at 37°C at 60 to 80 oscillations/min in the water bath to assure that equilibrium has been achieved. If no antagonist is used, allow the cells to equilibrate in the wells for at least 15 min under the conditions described above.

7. After this incubation period, stimulate the cells for 30 sec with agonist. The additions of agonist to the various wells are made every 5 sec. A different incubation time may be used for different agonists; 10 to 15 sec is usually the earliest time point that is feasibly measured.

8. Stop the reaction with the addition of 30 μl of 50% TCA. After a group of six wells has been processed, subsequent wells are treated with agonist and stopped in an identical manner.

9. Add 100 μl of the cyclic [^{14}C]GMP as an internal standard. In summary, the additions that have been made to the wells are:

Addition	Volume	Component	Length of Incubation
	μl		
1	240	Cell suspension	
2	30	Antagonist or buffer	30 min
3	30	Agonist	30 sec
	300	(Total volume)	
4	30	50% TCA	
5	100	Cyclic [^{14}C]GMP	

Note that the final volume of the assay is 300 μl and that the agonist and antagonist solutions are prepared as 10-fold stock solutions in solution III. If any additional treatments are necessary in addition to those described above, the volume of the cell suspension added can be adjusted downward accordingly.

At this point, the assay may be interrupted either for several hours or for several days by placing the trays in a 0 to 4°C refrigerator or a freezer. The material is stable in this latter environment for at least 2 months.

The next series of steps describes the conditions in which the cyclic [^{3}H]GMP is isolated from the precipitated cellular material and other labeled nucleotides [GTP, guanosine 5'-diphosphate (GDP), guanine, and guanosine] present. The columns used in the isolation are filled to a height of approximately 8 cm with a slurry of the Dowex resin, previously washed or regenerated by the column regeneration sequence described above. Columns used on a regular basis can be repeatedly regenerated for a year or more without significant deterioration of performance as measured by both the recovery of the internal standard and the elution profile of standard materials applied to the columns.

1. Equilibrate the regenerated columns with 5.0 ml of 0.1 N HCl, and discard the eluate.

2. Remove the contents of each well, and apply it to its respective column. Then add 500 μl of 0.1 N HCl to each well as a rinse; apply this to the column. The eluate is discarded.
3. To each column add 4.4 ml of 0.1 N HCl, and discard the eluate.
4. Add 1.0 ml of H_2O, and again discard the eluate.
5. Add 1.5 ml of H_2O to each column, and collect the eluate in 2.0-ml microcentrifuge tubes.
6. To eliminate a significant amount of residual contamination, add 30 μl of 2.67 M $ZnSO_4$ and 30 μl of 2.67 M Na_2CO_3 to each solution in the microcentrifuge tubes. Cap each tube, vortex each vigorously, and centrifuge them at 10,000 to $12,000 \times g$ for 2.5 min to pellet the precipitate, which contains a large percentage of the remaining contaminants.
7. Transfer the supernatant to scintillation vials to which 7 ml of scintillation fluid is added, and measure the radioactivity using a dual-isotope program that corrects for the recovery of the cyclic [^{14}C]GMP internal standard.
8. Analyze the data, preferably by a computer program that first calculates dpm corrected for 100% recovery. For dose-response curves, the data may be fit to a logistics function by iterative least squares regression arriving at the best estimates of the EC_{50}, the maximum response, K_D, and an exponent describing the steepness of the slope of the curve (21).

Comments

Routinely, an assay comprising 48 to 96 wells can be run and processed in 4 to 6 hr. The upper limit on the size of an assay may well be a function of the viability of the cells in the buffer. Viability of N1E-115 cells remains constant for about 2 hr. Therefore, from the time that the cells are harvested, all manipulations with the cells prior to stopping the assay with 50% TCA should be completed within 2 hr. In long assays, at various times throughout the assay repeat measurements of basal (no agonist) values and the maximum response to agonist alone, as these values may vary.

MEASUREMENT OF CYCLIC AMP IN INTACT CELLS

Introduction

Cyclic AMP is well-established as a second messenger of hormone activation for a variety of receptors (reviewed in refs. 22–24) (Table 5). Hormone activation of this enzyme is tissue specific unlike fluoride (F^-). The adenylate cyclase system, an intrinsic component of the cell membrane, is a complex association of the receptor, the cyclase, and one or more guanine nucleotide-binding proteins (25). Models of intact cell systems include a variety of receptors including the glucagon (26) and the β-adrenergic receptors (27).

Clone N1E-115 cells possess several receptors that are differentially coupled to the adenylate cyclase system (Table 1). Two of these, the prostaglandin E_1 (PGE_1) receptor stimulates cyclic AMP formation (positively coupled); the M_2 muscarinic acetylcholine receptor subtype inhibits cyclic AMP synthesis (negatively coupled) mediated by another receptor (e.g., the PGE_1 receptor) with no effect on basal formation of the cyclic nucleotide. Clone N1E-115 also possesses the M_1 muscarinic subtype that mediates the formation of cyclic GMP described above and the hydrolysis of certain phospholipids to be discussed below (28, 29).

Like the cyclic GMP assay described above, this assay makes use of the prelabeling technique and measures relative changes in cyclic AMP. Intracellular stores of adenosine 5'-triphosphate (ATP) are labeled by incubating cells with [^{3}H]adenosine. Unlike the cyclic GMP assay, a phosphodiesterase inhibitor is added to prevent the degradation of the cyclic [^{3}H]AMP that is formed. Measurement of cyclic AMP formation in the absence of a phosphodiesterase inhibitor is possible, but the amount of the nucleotide isolated is less than 10% of that obtained in the presence of the inhibitor in this clone. Isolation of the labeled cyclic nucleotide is accomplished by a two-column chromatography system (cation exchange and alumina adsorption).

Supplies

Reagents:
    Puck's modified D1 solution (see Table 3)
    PBS, solution III (see Table 3)
    Agonist and antagonist solutions prepared in solution III
    [^{3}H]Adenine* (5 to 15 Ci/mmol)
    Cyclic [^{14}C]AMP* (2,000 dpm/100 μl)
    3-Isobutyl-1-methylxanthine* (IBMX) (8 mM stock solution)
    TCA [50% (w/v)]
    Column elution buffers:
        Phosphate buffer, pH 7.05 (1 mM) (mix 1 mM potassium phosphate, monobasic and 1 mM potassium phosphate, dibasic, until pH 7.05)
        Imidazole-HCl, pH 7.05 (0.1 M) (200 ml of 1 M imidazole + 100 ml of 1 N HCl in 2 liters of H_2O and adjust pH to 7.05 if necessary with 1 N HCl)
    Column regeneration sequence: 10 ml of 1.25 N NaOH; 10 ml of H_2O; 10 ml of 1.7 N HCl; 10 ml of H_2O.
Materials:
    Ion exchange resin: Dowex AG 50W-X8, 100 to 200 mesh (H^+ form)*
    Columns: plastic disposable (0.8 × 20 cm)*
    multiwell trays: 24-well disposable flat bottom wells*
    alumina: neutral, type WN-3*
    Polystyrene disposable test tubes (12 × 75 mm)
    Scintillation vials (20-ml capacity)

Scintillation cocktail for aqueous samples*
Erlenmeyer flasks (25 or 50 ml).

Procedure

1. Harvest cells (about 10 million cells from two 75-cm^2/250-ml flasks) as described above (see under "Harvesting Cells for Assay").
2. After their final centrifugation, resuspend the cells in 2.0 ml of solution III; remove a small aliquot (e.g., 20 μl) either for enumeration of cells or for protein determination, and transfer the cells to a 25- or 50-ml Erlenmeyer flask. If larger numbers of cells are required for an experiment, increase the final volume in which the cells are suspended by approximately 2 ml per 8 to 10 million cells.
3. Add 20 μl of [^{3}H]adenine (20 μCi/2.0 ml of cell suspension), to the cell suspension cover the flask with Parafilm, place in a shaking water bath with platform at 60 to 80 oscillations/min at 37°C, and incubate the cells for 45 min.
4. After the incubation, dilute the cell suspension to 350,000 to 700,000 cells/ml with solution III. The exact cell number/well may vary with experiment based on the magnitude of the response being measured. It may be possible to amplify the response by using a larger cell number if the basal level of the cyclic nucleotide does not increase equally.
5. Dispense 270 μl of cells corresponding to 100,000 to 200,000 cells to the wells of a multiwell tray. Swirl the cell suspension after every three additions to prevent the cells from settling to the bottom of the flask so as to ensure a consistent cell number/well.
6. Add 50 μl of 8 mM IBMX, and incubate the cells for at least 5 min. After this time, an antagonist can be added in a 40-μl aliquot and incubated an additional 30 min.
7. Stimulate cells with agonist (40 μl) in solution III, PGE$_1$ for example, for 10 min. This is a routine time point established in our laboratory, but other time points can be used as well. Additions of the agonist are made at 5-sec intervals.
8. Stop the reaction with 30 μl of 50% TCA.
9. Add 100 μl of cyclic [^{14}C]AMP to each well as an internal standard.

In summary the additions that have been made to the wells are:

Addition	Volume	Component	Length of Incubation
	μl		*min*
1	270	Cell suspension	
2	50	IBMX solution	5
3	40	Antagonist or buffer	30
4	40	Agonist	10
	400	(Total volume)	
5	30	50% TCA	
6	100	Cyclic [^{14}C]AMP	

The assay can be suspended for several hours, if the material is refrigerated at 0 to 4°C or for longer periods of up to several weeks if it is frozen. Isolation of the cyclic AMP can be divided into several operations summarized below. Initially, the columns over which the samples are applied must be regenerated and equilibrated under the proper conditions. The pH of the solutions in the wells must be adjusted and the volume increased. Finally, the cyclic nucleotide must be isolated by a two-column ion-exchange procedure.

Preparation of Columns

Two columns are used in this assay. The first, a Dowex resin as described above under "Supplies" is capable of being used repeatedly after a simple regeneration sequence of washes. Prepare the set of columns by adding approximately 4 cm of Dowex resin in a slurry and washing the columns using the regeneration sequence given above. Prior to the application of the samples, equilibrate these columns with 1 mM phosphate buffer. The second column is an alumina column. The material from these columns is discarded after each use by removing the tips of the columns and rinsing the columns with water. The plastic column itself can be reused. Weigh about 1 g of alumina or measure out this amount by volume, and add it as a slurry in 0.1 M imidazole-HCl buffer to each plastic column just prior to use. Then equilibrate these columns in a small volume of the same buffer.

Sample Preparation

Add to each well 200 μl of 1.0 M [tris(hydroxymethyl)aminomethane] (Tris) followed by 500 μl of water to raise the pH and increase the volume, respectively.

Isolation

Apply the contents of each well to the Dowex columns with the use of a disposable pipette, and discard the eluate. Next, add 5 ml of 1 mM phosphate buffer to the column, and discard the eluate. Before the addition of the next buffer, position the alumina columns directly under the Dowex columns such that when you add the next buffer to the Dowex columns to elute the cyclic AMP, the eluates will pass onto and through the alumina columns, which will retain the cyclic AMP. Once the columns are positioned, apply 6.0 ml of H_2O to each Dowex column, and discard the eluate from the alumina columns. Move the Dowex columns to the side for future regeneration and use, and apply 1.0 ml of 0.1 M imidazole-HCl directly to the alumina columns, and again discard the eluate. Add an additional 3.0 ml of 0.1 M imidazole-HCl buffer to elute the cyclic AMP, and collect the eluate either directly in scintillation vials or in 12- $\times$ 75-mm polystyrene tubes and subsequently transfer to scintillation vials. Add counting cocktail (16 ml) to each vial, and count the samples using a dual-isotope program in a liquid scintillation counter.

Comments

Most difficulty from this assay arises in the isolation of the cyclic AMP. Make sure that the Dowex and alumina columns are well packed and do not contain large air bubbles. In addition, the pH and the concentration of the elution buffers are critical. Any significant deviation from the values given can have a drastic impact on the elution profile of the nucleotides.

The data analysis is accomplished by first correcting for recovery of the internal standard and converting cpm to dpm. For dose-response curves, the data are fitted to a logistics model using an iterative least squares regression as described under the assay for cyclic GMP formation.

MEASUREMENT OF INOSITOL PHOSPHATE FORMATION IN INTACT CELLS

Recently, much attention has been focused on the role of polyphosphoinositide metabolites as possible second messengers in cells (reviewed in refs. 30–32). Agonist-induced phospholipase C-dependent hydrolysis of phosphatidylinositol 4,5-bisphosphate (PIP_2) produces both diacylglycerol (DAG) and inositol triphosphate (IP_3). DAG has been shown to activate certain protein kinases, and IP_3 has been implicated as a second messenger, causing the release of calcium from intracellular stores. Receptors that mediate the formation of IP_3, which is sequentially dephosphorylated to inositol bisphosphate (IP_2) and then inositol monophosphate (IP_1) by specific phosphatases, may be influenced by yet another guanine nucleotide-binding protein.

Clone N1E-115 cells possess a number of receptors that mediate the formation of inositol phosphates (Table 1). Interestingly, all of the receptors on clone N1E-115 which mediate the release of inositol phosphate also stimulate the production of cyclic GMP. For cells of nervous tissue origin, to date, intact cells are needed to measure receptor-mediated polyphosphoinositide turnover.

The following is a convenient assay for measuring the amount of total inositol phosphates (IP_3, IP_2, and IP_1) following the addition of an agonist or other agent that is suspected of influencing the system. The method involves prelabeling the intracellular pool of phospholipid of which a small percentage ($<10\%$) is the inositol-containing phospholipid of interest and isolating total inositol phosphates, about 90% of which is IP_1. Although optional, preincubation with lithium ion (Li^+) is also part of the technique. Once inside the cell, this ion prevents the degradation of the IP_1 by inhibiting the associated monophosphatase. Thus, the levels of labeled inositol phosphates are greatly elevated in the presence of Li^+, improving the signal-to-noise ratio. The final steps of this procedure involve organic extraction of the lipid material followed by isolation of the inositol phosphates via ion-exchange chromatography.

Supplies

Reagents:
  Puck's modified D1 solution (see Table 3)
  PBS, solution III (see Table 3)
  Agonist and antagonist solutions prepared in solution III
  myo-[^{3}H]Inositol* (8 to 15 Ci/mmol)
  [^{14}C]Inositol 4-phosphate* (1200 dpm/250 μl of H$_2$O)
  LiCl stock solution in solution III (100 mM)
  Chloroform
  Chloroform/methanol (1:2)
  Column elution buffers:
    Sodium tetraborate (5 mM) + ammonium formate (60 mM) (Buffer A)
    Ammonium formate (1.0 M) + formic acid (0.1 M) (Buffer B)
  Column regeneration sequence: 10 ml of 1.25 N NaOH; 10 ml of H$_2$O; 10 ml of
  1.0 M formic acid; 10 ml of H$_2$O
Materials:
  Ion-exchange resin: Dowex 1-X8, 200 to 400 mesh (formate form)*
  Columns: plastic disposable (0.8 × 20cm)*
  Glass test tubes (12 × 75 mm)
  Polystyrene test tubes (12 × 75 mm)
  Erlenmeyer flasks (25 or 50 ml)
  Microcentrifuge tubes with caps (2 ml)
  Scintillation vials (20-ml capacity)
  Scintillation cocktail designed for aqueous samples*
Equipment: Low-speed centrifuge, capable of 500 × g

Procedure

Assay

1. Harvest the cells as described under "Harvesting Cells for Assay," and resuspend them in 2.0 ml of solution III per 8 to 10 million cells.
2. Remove a small aliquot (e.g., 20 μl) for enumeration of cells or for protein determination.
3. Transfer the remaining cells to an Erlenmeyer flask, add 20 to 50 μCi of *myo*-[^{3}H]inositol/2.0 ml of cell suspension, cover the flask with Parafilm, and incubate for 60 min at 37°C in a shaking water bath set at 60 to 80 oscillations/min. This method of labeling the intracellular phospholipid pools is sufficient if Li$^+$ is used to inhibit the monophosphatase activity.
4. After the 1-hr labeling incubation, transfer cells to 2-ml microcentrifuge tubes and centrifuge them for several seconds to pellet the cells. The method we employ is to turn the microcentrifuge on and off very quickly.

5. Resuspend the pelleted cells in the original volume of solution III by gentle trituration, and transfer them back to the Erlenmeyer flask.
6. Dilute the cells to 400,000 to 900,000 cells/ml with solution III. The density chosen will depend on the efficacy of the receptor-mediated response being measured.
7. Dispense 210 μl of cells (240 μl if no antagonist or inhibitor is present, 270 μl if, in addition, no LiCl is to be added) to each 12- × 75-mm glass test tube, gently swirling the cell suspension after every third addition to maintain an even suspension.
8. Next, add 30 μl of the 100 mM stock soltuion of LiCl to each tube, and incubate the cells for 30 min at 37°C in a shaking water bath at 60 to 80 oscillations/min. (Optionally, either the time of incubation can be reduced to a minimum of about 10 min, or the Li$^+$ treatment can be excluded altogether.) If the effect of an antagonist or inhibitor is to be measured, add this compound in 30 μl immediately after the Li$^+$ and coincubate for the same amount of time.
9. Stimulate the cells with agonist (30 μl) for a predetermined time. Routinely we use a 10-min stimulation with agonist. The accumulation or release of inositol phosphates can be measured as early as 5 to 15 sec. However, the quantity of [^{3}H]inositol phosphates measured at these early time points will be very small and will depend on the efficacy of the particular agonist-mediated response.
10. Stop the reaction by the addition of 750 μl of ice-cold chloroform/methanol, vortex the samples vigorously, and place the tubes on ice.
11. Add 250 μl of a solution of [^{14}C]inositol 4-phosphate, as an internal standard, and 250 μl of chloroform. Vortex the samples vigorously.

In summary, the additions that have been made to the test tubes are:

Addition	Volume	Component	Length of Incubation
	μl		*min*
1	210	Cell suspension	
2	30	LiCl solution	30
3	30	Antagonist or buffer	30
4	30	Agonist	10
	300	(Total volume)	
5	750	Chloroform/methanol	
6	250	[^{14}C]Inositol 4-phosphate	
7	250	Chloroform	

Extraction

1. Centrifuge the samples at $500 \times g$ for a minimum of 5 min to separate the phases.

2. Transfer 600 µl of the upper (aqueous phase) to another 12- × 75-mm glass or polystyrene tube containing 2.0 ml of H_2O, leaving behind a small amount of the aqueous phase to prevent contamination from the organic phase.

Isolation

1. Apply the 600 µl of aqueous phase to Dowex columns, containing about 1.5 cm of regenerated resin (approximately 1-ml bed volume).
2. Elute and discard the [³H]glycerophosphorylinositol and free [³H]inositol with 20 ml of column elution buffer A.
3. Then elute total [³H]inositol phosphates with 8 ml of column buffer B. Usually, the radioactive material is collected in 4-ml fractions. Either count each fraction separately, and sum the results or pool the fractions, and determine the radioactivity in an aliquot (e.g., 4 ml). We have found that the first 4-ml fraction contains more than 95% of the [³H]inositol phosphates. Therefore, it may be unnecessary to obtain the second fraction.
4. Transfer the samples to 20-ml scintillation vials. The maximum amount of aqueous sample which can be added to each scintillation vial is approximately 4 ml when the fluor is water accepting. Add 16 ml of scintillation cocktail, and measure the radioactivity in a counter with a dual-isotope program.
5. Correct the data for the recovery of internal standard. Fit dose-response data to a logistics model utilizing an iterative least squares regression algorithm (21).

Comments

The most difficult aspect of this assay is that unlike those for cyclic nucleotides detailed above, the amount of [³H]inositol phosphates measured can be quite low in this clone, as well as in tissue slices from brain. Agonist-stimulated accumulation of inositol phosphates can range from 10 to 200% above basal. Thus, it is important to exercise considerable care when performing this assay. In addition, the number of replicates/condition may need to be increased to three to six.

To increase the measured responses, consider the use of very high specific activity *myo*-[³H]inositol.* This material is adequate but needs to be first purified by diluting it in a small volume of H_2O and applying this sample to one of the regenerated columns described above. The eluate is collected and, if necessary, dried under a stream of N_2 gas while at 4°C to reduce the volume. In our laboratory, we have had the greatest success with the inositol that is labeled to 10 to 15 Ci/mmol from the vendor listed in the "Suppliers" section at the end of this chapter.

SUPPLIERS

Radioligand Binding

[³H]Neurotensin: Du Pont-New England Nuclear, Boston, MA
GF/B filters: Whatman, United Kingdom

Scintillation cocktail: Safety-Solve; Research Products International (RPI), Mount
  Prospect, IL
Filtration: Cell Harvester; Brandel, Gaithersburg, MD.

Cyclic GMP

[^{3}H]Guanosine (5 Ci/mmol): ICN Radiochemicals, Irvine, CA
Cyclic [^{14}C]GMP: Amersham Corp., Arlington Heights, IL
Dowex resin 50-H$^+$ or AG 50W-X2, 200 to 400 mesh; Bio-Rad Laboratories, Rich-
  mond, CA
Plastic columns: Disposable Chromaflex columns, no. K-420160; Kontes, Vine-
  land, NJ
Multiwell trays: catalog no. 76-033-05; Flow Laboratories, McLean, VA
Microcentrifuge tubes (2-ml capacity): Walter Sarstedt Inc., Princeton, NJ
Scintillation cocktail: Safety-Solve; Research Products International (RPI), Mount
  Prospect, IL.

Cyclic AMP

[^{3}H]Adenine: Amersham Corp., Arlington Heights, IL
Cyclic [^{14}C]AMP: Amersham Corp., Arlington Heights, IL
3-Isobutyl-1-methylxanthine (IBMX): Aldrich Chemical Company, Milwaukee,
  WI
Dowex resin 50-H$^+$ or AG 50W-X8, 100 to 200 mesh; Bio-Rad Laboratories, Rich-
  mond, CA
Alumina: neutral chromatographic, activity grade 1, type WN-3; Sigma Chemical
  Company, St. Louis, MO
Plastic columns: disposable Chromaflex columns, No. K-420160; Kontes, Vine-
  land, NJ
Multiwell trays: catalog no. 76-033-05; Flow Laboratories, McLean, VA
Scintillation cocktail: Safety-Solve; Research Products International (RPI), Mount
  Prospect, IL.

Inositol Phosphates

myo-[^{3}H]Inositol (15 Ci/mmol): American Radiolabeled Chemicals, St. Louis, MO
myo-[^{3}H]Inositol (40 to 50 Ci/mmol): Du Pont-New England Nuclear Corp., Boston
  MA
[^{14}C]Inositol 4-phosphate (50 Ci/mmol): Amersham Corp., Arlington Heights, IL.

Other

DMEM: GIBCO, Grand Island, NY; or Cellgro, catalog no. 50-013-PB; Mediatech Inc., Washington, DC

Calf serum (fetal or newborn): GIBCO, Grand Island, NY; or HyClone Laboratories, Logan UT

Filtration apparatus:
  Media preparation: model 316 (142 mm); Millipore Corp., Bedford, MA
  Binding assay: Cell Harvester; Brandel, Gaithersburg, MD
  Solutions: (0.22-μ filter): Nalgene; Nalge Comapny, Rochester, NY.

All other reagents and materials are the highest grade available.

Acknowledgments

This work was supported by United States Public Health Service Grant MH27692 and the Mayo Foundation. The authors thank Mrs. Carol Cooper for preparation of this manuscript.

REFERENCES

1. Bottenstein J. In: Murakami H, ed. *Proceedings of the international symposium on growth and differentiation of cells in defined environment.* New York: Springer-Verlag, 1985;25–30.
2. Carlson J, Smith A, Richelson E. *In Vitro* 1982;18:175–178.
3. Wilson SH, Schrier BK, Farber JL, et al. *J Biol Chem* 1972;247:3159–3169.
4. El-Fakahany E, Richelson E. *J Neurochem* 1980;35:941–948.
5. McKinney M, Stenstrom S, Richelson E. *Mol Pharmacol* 1984;26:156–163.
6. Pfenning M, Mackey S, Richelson E. Submitted, 1989.
6a. Yamamura HI, Enna SJ, Kuhar MJ, ed. *Neurotransmitter Receptor* Binding. 2nd ed. New York: Raven Press, 1985.
7. Kitabgi P, Carraway R, Van Rietschoten J, et al. *Proc Natl Acad Sci USA* 1977;74:1846–1850.
8. Lazarus LH, Brown MR, Perrin MH. *Neuropharmacology* 1977;16:625–629.
9. Uhl GR, Bennett JP Jr, Snyder SH. *Brain Res* 1977;130:299–313.
10. Quirion R, Gaudreau P, St-Pierre S, Rioux F, Pert CB. *Peptides* 1982;3:757–763.
11. Goedert M, Pittaway K, Williams BJ, Emson PC. *Brain Res* 1984;304:71–81.
12. Gilbert JA, Moses CJ, Pfenning MA, Richelson E. *Pharmacology* 1986;35:391–397.
13. Munson PJ, Rodbard D. *Anal Biochem* 1980;107:220–239.
14. Greengard P. *Cyclic nucleotides, phosphorylated proteins, and neuronal function.* New York: Raven Press, 1978.
15. Goldbert ND, O'Dea RF, Haddox MK. *Adv Cyclic Nucleotide Res* 1973;3:155–223.
16. Schultz G, Hardman JG, Schultz K, Baird CE, Sutherland EW. *Proc Natl Acad Sci USA* 1973; 70:3889–3893.
17. Matsuzawa H, Nirenberg M. *Proc Natl Acad Sci USA* 1975;72:3472–3476.
18. Deguchi T, Ohsako S, Nakane M, Ichikawa M, Yoshioka M. *J Neural Transm [Suppl]* 1983; 18:369–378.
19. Rapoport RM, Murad F. *J Cyclic Nucleotide Protein Phosphor Res* 1983;9:281–296.
20. Waldman SA, Rapoport RM, Murad F. *J Biol Chem* 1984;259:14332–14334.
21. Figge J, Leonard P, Richelson E. *Eur J Pharmacol* 1979;58:479–483.
22. Robison GA, Butcher RW, Sutherland EW. *Annu Rev Biochem* 1968;37:149–174.
23. Ross EM, Gilman AG. *Annu Rev Biochem* 1980;49:533–564.
24. Limbird LE. *Biochem J* 1981;195:1–13.

25. Rodbell M. *Nature* 1980;284:17–22.
26. Rodbell M, Lin MC, Salomon Y, et al. *Adv Cyclic Nucleotide Res* 1975;5:3–29.
27. Stadel JM, DeLean A, Lefkowitz RJ. *Adv Enzymol* 1982;53:1–43.
28. McKinney M, Richelson E. *Annu Rev Pharmacol Toxicol* 1984;24:121–146.
29. Nathanson NM. *Annu Rev Neurosci* 1987;10:195–236.
30. Michell RH. *Biochem Biophys Acta* 1975;415:81–147.
31. Berridge MJ. *Mol Cell Endocrinol* 1981;24:115–140.
32. Nishizuka Y, Takai Y, Kishimoto A, Kikkawa U, Kaibuchi K. *Recent Prog Horm Res* 1984;40:301–345.
33. Schneider EL, Stanbridge EJ, Epstein CJ. *Exp Cell Res* 1974;84:311–318.
34. Ho TY, Quinn PA. In: Johari OM, Becker RP, eds. *Scanning electron microscopy*, vol 2. Chicago: IIT Research Institute, 1977;291–300.
35. Chen TR. *Exp Cell Res* 1977;104:255–262.
36. Patrick J, McMillan J, Wolfson H, O'Brien JC. *J Biol Chem* 1977;252:2143–2153.
37. Simantov R, Sachs L. *Proc Natl Acad Sci USA* 1973;70:2902–2905.
38. Gossuin A, Maloteaux JM, Trouet A, Laduron P. *Biochim Biophys Acta* 1984;804:100–106.
39. Burgermeister W, Klein WL, Nirenberg M, Witkop B. *Mol Pharmacol* 1978;14:751–767.
40. Fishman PH, Finberg JP. *J Neurochem* 1987;49:282–289.
41. Weyhenmeyer JA, Hwang CJ. *Brain Res Bull* 1985;14:409–414.
42. Neuser D, Bellemann P. *FEBS Lett* 1986;209;347–351.
43. Snider RM, Richelson E. *J Neurochem* 1984;43:1749–1754.
44. Greenberg DA, Carpenter CL, Messing RO. *J Pharmacol Exp Ther* 1986;238:1021–1027.
45. Hollenberg MD, Cuatrecasas P. *Proc Natl Acad Sci USA* 1973;70:2964–2968.
46. Carpenter G, Lembach KJ, Morrison MM, Cohen S. *J Biol Chem* 1975;250:4297–4304.
47. Carpenter G, Cohen S. *J Cell Biol* 1976;71:159–171.
48. Billestrup N, Martin JM. *Endocrinology* 1985;116:1175–1181.
49. Murphy LJ, Vrhovsek E, Lazarus L. *Endocrinology* 1983;113:750–757.
50. Grunberger G, Lowe WL Jr, McElduff A, Glick RP. *J Clin Invest* 1986;77:997–1005.
51. Branca AA, Baglioni C. *Nature* 1981;294:768–770.
52. Charness ME, Gordon AS, Diamond I. *Science* 1983;222:1246–1248.
53. Charness ME, Gordon AS, Diamond I. *Ciba Found Symp* 1984;105:73–84.
54. Blume AJ, Shorr J, Finberg JP, Spector S. *Proc Natl Acad Sci USA* 1977;74:4927–4931.
55. Chang KJ, Miller RJ, Cuatrecasas P. *Mol Pharmacol* 1978;14:961–970.
56. Hazum E, Chang KJ, Cuatrecasas P. *Life Sci* 1979;24:137–144.
57. Miller RJ, Chang KJ, Leighton J, Cuatrecasas P. *Life Sci* 1978;22:379–388.
58. Chang KJ, Cuatrecases P. *J Biol Chem* 1979;254:2610–2618.
59. Huang JS, Huang SS, Kennedy B, Deuel TF. *J Biol Chem* 1982;257:8130–8136.
60. Richelson E, Stenstrom S, Forray C, Enloe L, Pfenning M. *J Pharmacol Exp Ther* 1986;239:687–692.
61. Snider RM, McKinney M, Richelson E. *Semin Thromb Hemost* 1986;12:253–262.
62. Messing A, Kim SU. *Brain Res* 1981;208:479–486.
63. Frick W, Hefti F, Citherlet K, Dravid A, Gmelin G. *Neurosci Lett* 1983;40:45–50.
64. Siman RG, Klein WL. *Brain Res* 1983;262:99–108.
65. Seagar MJ, Deprez P, Martin-Moutot N, Couraud F. *Brain Res* 1987;411:226–230.
66. Raizada MK, Yang JW, Phillips MI, Fellows RE. *Brain Res* 1981;207:343–355.
67. Feldstein JB, Sumners C, Raizada MK. *Brain Res* 1986;370:265–272.
68. Laribi C, Legendre P, Dupouy B, Vincent JD, Simonnet G. *Brain Res* 1985;347:94–103.
69. Walker CR, Peacock JH. *Brain Res* 1981;227:565–578.
70. Mehta AK, Ticku MK. *J Neurochem* 1987;49:1491–1497.
71. Bender AS, Hertz L. *Neurochem* 1984;43:1319–1327.
72. Vaccarino FM, Alho H, Santi MR, Guidotti A. *J Neurosci* 1987;7:65–76.
73. Talwar D, Sher PK. *Dev Neurosci* 1987;9:183–189.
74. Checler F, Mazella J, Kitabgi P, Vincent JP. *J Neurochem* 1986;47:1742–1748.
75. Stamatos C, Fine RE. *J Neurosci Res* 1986;15:529–542.
76. Dichter MA, Tischler AS, Greene LA. *Nature* 1977;268:501–504.
77. Greene LA, Rein G. *Brain Res* 1977;138:521–528.
78. Chalazonitis A, Greene LA, Shain W. *Exp Cell Res* 1975;96:255–238.
79. McKinney M, Stenstrom S, Richelson E. *Mol Pharmacol* 1985;27:223–235.

80. Wastek GJ, Lopez JR, Richelson E. *Mol Pharmacol* 1981;19:15–20.
81. Large TH, Lambert MP, Cohen NM, Klein WL. *Neurosci Lett* 1986;66:31–38.
82. Nathanson NM, Klein WL, Nirenberg M. *Proc Natl Acad Sci USA* 1978;75:1788–1791.
83. Traber J, Fischer K, Buchen C, Hamprecht B. *Nature* 1975;255:558–560.
84. Elfman L, Lindgren E, Walum E, Fredholm BB. *Acta Pharmacol Toxicol (Copenh)* 1984;55:297–302.
85. Stenstrom S, Richelson E. *J Pharmacol Exp Ther* 1982;221:334–341.
86. Sabol SL, Nirenberg M. *J Biol Chem* 1979;254:1913–1920.
87. Weiss S, Kemp DE, Lenox RH, Ellis J. *Brain Res* 1987;414:390–394.
88. Myers PR, Blosser J, Shain W. *Biochem Pharmacol* 1978;27:1173–1177.
89. Fishman PH, Finberg JP. *J Neurochem* 1987;49:282–289.
90. Neve KA, Barrett DA, Molinoff PB. *J Pharmacol Exp Ther* 1985;235:657–664.
91. Maguire ME, Wiklund RA, Anderson HJ, Gilman AG. *J Biol Chem* 1976;251:1221–1231.
92. Gilbert JA, Pfenning MA, Richelson E. *Biochem Pharmacol* 1984;33:2527–2530.
93. Buonassisi V, Venter JC. *Proc Natl Acad Sci USA* 1976;73:1612–1616.
94. Reiser G, Walter U, Hamprecht B. *Brain Res* 1984;290:367–371.
95. Osugi T, Imaizumi T, Mizushima A, Uchida S, Yoshida H. *Eur J Pharmacol* 1987;137:207–218.
96. Knapp AG, Dowling JE. *Nature* 1987;325:437–439.
97. Weiss S, Sebben M, Garcia-Sainz JA, Bockaert J. *Mol Pharmacol* 1985;27:595–599.
98. McEachern AE, Margiotta JF, Berg DK. *J Neurosci* 1985;5:2690–2695.
99. Propst F, Moroder L, Wunsch E, Hamprecht B. *J Neurochem* 1979;32:1495–1500.
100. Richelson E. *Science* 1978;201:69–71.
101. Ohsako S, Deguchi T. *Biochem Biophys Res Commun* 1984;122:333–339.
102. Oakes SG, Taylor S, Richelson E. *Fed Proc* 1983;42:906.
103. Gilbert JA, Richelson E. *Eur J Pharmacol* 1984;99:245–246.
104. Snider RM, Forray C, Pfenning M, Richelson E. *J Neurochem* 1986;47:1214–1218.
105. Amar S, Kitabgi P, Vincent JP. *J Neurochem* 1987;49:999–1006.
106. Murphy MG, Moak CM, Rao BG. *Biochem Pharmacol* 1987;36:4079–4084.
107. Gilbert JA, Knodel EL, Stenstrom SD, Richelson E. *J Biol Chem* 1982;257:1274–1281.
108. Gwynn GJ, Costa E. *Proc Natl Acad Sci USA* 1982;79:690–694.
109. Law PY, Koehler JE, Loh HH. *Mol Pharmacol* 1982;21:483–491.
110. Traber J, Fischer K, Latzin S, Hamprecht B. *Nature* 1975;253:120–122.
111. Sharma SK, Nirenberg M, Klee WA. *Proc Natl Acad Sci USA* 1975;72:590–594.
112. Christian CN, Nelson PG, Bullock P, Mullinax D, Nirenberg M. *Brain Res* 1978;147:261–276.
113. Gilman AG, Nirenberg M. *Nature* 1971;234:356–358.
114. Hamprecht B, Schultz J. *FEBS Lett* 1973;34:85–89.
115. Myers PR. *J Cell Physiol* 1979;98:11–16.
116. Bockaert J, Dumuis A, Bouhelal R, Sebben M, Cory RN. *Naunyn Schmiedebergs Arch Pharmacol* 1987;335:588–592.
117. MacDermot J, Higashida H, Wilson SP, Matsuzawa H, Minna J, Nirenberg M. *Proc Natl Acad Sci USA* 1979;76:1135–1139.
118. Traber J, Glaser T, Brandt M, Kelbensberger W, Hamprecht B. *FEBS Lett* 1977;81:351–354.
119. Snider RM, Richelson E. *Science* 1983;221:566–568.
120. L'Allemain G, Paris S, Magnaldo I, Pouyssegur J. *J Cell Physiol* 1986;129:167–174.
121. Vittet D, Berta P, Mathieu MN, Rondot A, Travo P, Cantau B, Chevillard C. *Biochem Biophys Res Commun* 1986;140:1093–1100.

BIBLIOGRAPHY

Richelson E. In: Goldberg AM, Hain I, eds. *Biology of cholinergic function*. New York: Raven Press, 1976;10.

Methods in Neurotransmitter Receptor Analysis,
edited by Henry I. Yamamura, et al.
Raven Press, Ltd., New York © 1990.

7

Receptor Autoradiography

*Michael J. Kuhar and **James R. Unnerstall

*Neuroscience Branch, Addiction Research Center, National Institute on Drug Abuse,
Baltimore, Maryland 21224; and **Departments of Neurology and Pharmacology,
Case Western Reserve University School of Medicine and The Alzheimer Center,
University Hospitals of Cleveland, Cleveland, Ohio 44106

The autoradiographic localization of drug and neurotransmitter receptors is a powerful technique for the study of receptors, particularly in complex tissues in which anatomical information is desirable. One can quantifiably localize receptors in very small pieces of tissue; depending on the situation, this approach can be three to five orders of magnitude more sensitive than biochemical methods. It is, therefore, not surprising that receptor autoradiography is widely used and applied to a great variety of biological problems. Several reviews have been written on the topic (1–5).

The goal of this chapter is to provide the reader with practical information so that he or she can produce autoradiograms with a minimum of help from others. It is intended to be a laboratory companion, particularly for the beginner but also for the more experienced. This chapter is also intended as a supplement to the one in the second edition of *Neurotransmitter Receptor Binding* (4), and it is recommended that the latter be read as well.

Finally, if you find this chapter deficient in any way or if you have suggestions on how to improve it, please write and let us know. We would especially like to hear from students.

Good luck with your experiments!

PRINCIPLES

Receptor autoradiography is dependent on biochemical studies of receptors, and the principles that apply to basic biochemical studies also apply here. The criteria for identifying a physiologically relevant receptor are especially important, and practical issues such as the proper generation of a blank can be critical. Very often, the most fundamentally reliable autoradiographic studies are those that are built upon extensive biochemical studies; therefore, preliminary biochemical studies of the receptor of interest are always recommended.

Since most available ligands bind reversibly rather than irreversibly, diffusion of and loss of ligand from the receptor site is a critical issue. Fortunately, pioneering work of Roth and Stump (6) and others has addressed this issue, and techniques for the use of diffusible substances have been incorporated into our experiments. Allowing ligands the opportunity to diffuse from the vicinity of the receptor can be disastrous, and diffusion must be eliminated or minimized.

Since receptor ligands are radiolabeled, autoradiography has been the obvious method of choice for localizing receptors. This is fortunate since autoradiography is a very well studied and precise technique. Knowledge of use of emulsions and film is obviously essential. These skills are just as critical as those mentioned in the two paragraphs above; there are many useful general publications on autoradiography (7–10).

Very often, it is necessary to quantify autoradiograms. Autoradiography is a precise and quantifiable process. The fundamentals of quantification should be known; again, there are many useful publications on the topic (8–10).

SUPPLIES

The following is a list of some needed supplies, and their sources where appropriate.

1. NTB-3 emulsion no. 165-4441 (4 oz): Kodak Special Products, 2400 Mt. Read St., Rochester, NY 14650; tel.: 716-722-2930.
2. Corning coverslips no. 0 or 1 (25 × 77 mm): catalog no. 60-4861-26; PGC Scientific, Gaithersburg, MD 20877.
3. ^{3}H-Ultrofilm no. 2208-190 (10 sheets): Cambridge Instruments, 111 Dear Lake Rd., Deerfield, IL 60015.
   ^{3}H-Hyperfilm: Amersham Corp., 2636 S. Clearbrook Dr., Arlington Heights, IL 60005; tel.: 800-323- 9750.
   Hyperfilm-B_{max}: Amersham Corp.
4. Chromerge no. 480-616 vials (6 × 1 oz): Fisher Scientific Co., 711 Forbes Ave., Pittsburgh, PA 15219; tel.: 412-562-8300.
5. Sulfuric acid.
6. "Wolf" x-ray film cassette (10 × 12 inches).
7. Open end glassine envelopes no. 119 (11 × 14 inches): Wolf X-Ray Corp., 420 Hempstead Pike, W. Hempstead, NY 11552; tel.: 1-800-356-9729.
   Brown x-ray envelopes.
8. Toluidine blue 0 3W143 Baker (25 g).
   Pyronin Y 2-U 724 Baker "analyzed" (10 g).
9. Clothespin racks.
10. Binder clip racks and small binder clips.
11. Staining dishes.
12. Flat wooden toothpicks.

13. Wooden slide boxes no. 3-451 (package): Fisher Scientific Co., 711 Forbes Ave., Pittsburgh, PA 15219; tel.: 412-562-8300.
14. Black plastic slide boxes (hold 25).
15. Duro Superglue (0.1 fluid oz, 3 g).
    Superglue pen.
16. 3M Scotch Black Opaque Tape, 235-3M (1 inch × 60 yards).
17. White Teflon $^1/_{16}$ inch thick (odd size sheets): Commercial Plastics and Supply, 1130 E. 30th St., Baltimore, MD 21218; tel.: 301-889-6640.
18. Dri Caps Type II no. 19953: Jed Pella, Inc., P.O.B. 51, Tustin, CA 92681; tel.: 1-800-237-3526.
19. Double-stick Scotch 3M Tape ($^1/_2$ inch × 36 yards).
20. Dektol D19 Rapid Fix.
21. Tupperware bread boxes.

PROCEDURES FOR *IN VITRO* LABELING AUTORADIOGRAPHY

In vitro labeling autoradiography is the procedure in which tissues are labeled *in vitro* rather than *in vivo*. It is the most popular method and has many advantages (11). The following procedures have proven helpful.

Preliminary Procedures

Preparation of "Subbed" Slides

Clean slides should be used in this procedure. It may be necessary to acid wash the slides before subbing. To help the tissue remain fixed to the slides during various procedures, the slides are precoated with a freshly made gelatin-chrome alum mixture. It is prepared in the following way. Gelatin (0.5 g) (J T Baker no. 1-2124) and 50 mg of chrom alum (chromium potassium sulfate, J T Baker no. 1624) are added to 100 ml of distilled water. The mixture is heated and stirred until dissolved. The hot solution is cooled on ice to about 20°C and then filtered. Slides (1 mm thick) are dipped in this solution and allowed to dry.

In order to facilitate subbing several slides at once, the frosted end of clean microscope slides (CMS no. 267-088; 25 × 75 mm) are placed in Peel-aways or plastic slide holders (VWR no. 48440-002) or racks for 25 to 30 slies. The slides are sequentially dipped into two separate batches of the solution so that the first dip can serve as a wash to remove dust and other fine debris. The dipped slides are allowed to stand on the absorbent surface so that excess subbing can drain. It is best to cover the drying slides so that room dust will not adhere to the surface. When the subbed slides are dried, they can be stored in a slide box at room temperature.

The subbing solution is discarded and not reused.

Preparation of Emulsion-coated Slides or Coverslips

The slides or coverslips (Corning cover glasses, no. 0 or no. 1 thickness, 25 × 77 mm) are first cleaned by soaking overnight in a sulfuric acid/dichromate (Chromerge) mixture. The following morning, they are rinsed profusely in tap water for 1 hr followed by about a 3-hr rinse with distilled water. The cleaned slides and coverslips are then dried in an oven at about 100°C for 45 min. They are then stored in a clean, closed slide box.

The emulsion is prepared for dipping as follows, which is a more or less standard procedure. With Kodak NTB-3 emulsion, a red no. 2 safelight is used, and the emulsion expiration date should be well ahead of the date by which you plan to complete your experiment. The emulsion is melted at 41 to 43°C in a circulating warm-water bath. A quantity of the emulsion is then diluted 1:1 with distilled water at the same temperature. After stirring the warm emulsion mixture gently with a clean glass slide, a slide can be dipped into the emulsion and withdrawn gently to test for surface bubbles that would produce an uneven coating. One can test for the presence of these bubbles by holding the slide up to the safelight. Usually, bubbles can be seen quite readily. Some investigators add a very small quantity of detergent (0.01% Dreft) to avoid these bubbles. In our laboratory, we usually dip the cleaned coverslips one at a time and then hang them on a clothespin rack to dry for approximately 2 hr. The rack is simply a series of clothespins strung on a wire, and each clothespin hangs one coverslip or glass slide. After drying, the slides or coverslips are stored in a light-tight black slide box with silica gel capsules at refrigerator temperatures (2 to 4°C). The edges of the box are sealed with electrical tape to form an airtight and lightproof compartment.

"Brain Paste"

Some investigators have found it useful to embed their samples in a material that has the same cutting consistency as their tissue. This can be particularly helpful when your area of interest is at the edge of the tissue or surface of the organ. Adding a similar material to the surface of the tissue can improve the cutting and subsequent histological quality of the section.

A brain paste has been useful in experiments with brain. The brain paste is used by placing a quantity of it on a microtome chuck and then gently pressing the tissue into the paste. The paste can be used to support or orient the tissue if necessary, and then the entire assembly can be frozen in powdered dry ice or liquid nitrogen.

The simple procedure for making brain paste is to use excess brain—possibly brain from a slaughter house, cow or pig—and place it in a homogenizer and mix until it is thoroughly smooth, and all of the particulate pieces have been eliminated. At this point, it is possible to add some dye and further blend or homogenize so that the boundary of the paste can readily be recognized and distinguished from the tissue. We have prepared such a brain paste and frozen and thawed it as needed many times.

Tissue Preparation

Tissue should be frozen so as to avoid or minimize fracturing, to facilitate a convenient sectioning plane (usually one that corresponds to a useful atlas), and to include regions of interest.

Usually, animals are killed, and the brain is removed rapidly but very carefully. Even slight damage during dissection and removal can result in serious interpretation problems several weeks later when the autoradiograms are developed. Since autoradiographic experiments can be so long, especially with tritium, it pays to practice and to use only the samples in which you have confidence.

After removal from brain, regions of interest are cut with a sharp razor blade. We find it convenient and helpful to place the tissue into some ice-cold saline; this makes the brain tissue firmer and easier to handle and cut.

The region of interest is then mounted on a microtome chuck by first placing a layer of brain paste on the chuck and gently sinking the tissue into the paste. Then the whole assembly can be frozen in powdered dry ice, liquid nitrogen, or isopentane cooled in liquid nitrogen or dry ice. If your region of interest is on the surface of the brain, you may wish to try placing some brain paste along this surface so that there is less distortion and curling during sectioning. Some investigators prefer to avoid brain paste completely since it is somewhat unsightly when taking photos for publication. When we wish to avoid it, we simply mount the tissue (actually just place it) in a little distilled water (or other mounting preparation) on the chuck and then freeze. Another method to improve tissue morphology is to perfuse animals first with 150 to 200 ml of 50 mM phosphate-buffered saline (PBS, pH 7.4) followed by approximately 500 ml of a 50:50 (v/v) mixture of PBS/10% sucrose. The tissues can then be frozen on dry ice, which minimizes the chance of cracking or shattering. A 13-gauge blunt needed is used to perform the intraaortic perfusion.

Tissue Sectioning and Storage

Precision sectioning is important, and therefore adequate equipment is a must. We have used cryostats from the Harris Corp. and from Hacker Instruments. Both have been reliable. Thinner sections are important for quantitative analysis of serial sections and to maintain resolution when using iodinated ligands (8 to 10 μm). This is explained further under "Quantitation of Autoradiograms." If it is necessary to cut thicker sections to get better quality, then it is worth doing so. Usually, 12- to 25-μm sections are cut. If anatomical resolution is extremely important, then thinner sections should be used. We have used 2- and 4-μm sections successfully.

After the frozen block of tissue is securely mounted in the microtome, sectioning can proceed by standard means. Antiroll bars are very useful and highly recommended. The temperature of sectioning can be critical; for brain, we find -15 to $-18°C$ useful.

When a tissue section is cut and sits on the knife, it can be straightened and flattened with a soft brush, then picked up on a subbed slide by taking a cold slide (same temperature as the tissue) and lightly pressing it against the tissue. The tissue usually adheres with little difficulty. The slide with section can then be taken out of the cold environment of the cryostat into the room air and the section thawed onto the slide by rolling the thumb under the slide upon which the section sits. The thawing can usually be controlled so that it proceeds from one side of the section to the other. At this point, the section is usually wet, and it can be examined nicely in a dark-field dissecting scope.

These mounted moist sections are then placed in a slide box at room temperature until they are very dry. It can take up to a couple of hours. Other laboratories use more vigorous conditions such as desiccation, but we have found these to be of no real advantage and more trouble. When the sections are dry at room temperature conditions, we store them in slide boxes at $-20°C$ for months.

Do these preparation conditions that involve freezing and thawing affect the binding? This question must always be kept in mind. At some point, you have to convince yourself that your procedure itself is not creating problems. Usually, you check out your results by comparing them with results obtained in biochemical studies with fresh (unfrozen) tissue.

Also, should you fix the tissue? We have found that fixation can destroy binding sites (11), and there is no real need for it. In some cases, a slight fixation can be advantageous; but the effects of fixation on binding should be studied directly in that case (11). It is also important to study the effects of fixation on the biochemistry and modulation of ligand-receptor interaction.

Preliminary Biochemical Studies with Slide-mounted Tissue Sections and the Selection of Optimal Incubation Conditions

Selection of Initial Conditions

The most reliable autoradiographic studies are those built on extensive biochemical studies with tissue homogenates. The grind-and-bind approach, although it has no real anatomical resolution and limited sensitivity, is proven in that it can characterize a ligand or receptor site thoroughly with speed and accuracy. Therefore, if the ligand of interest is not characterized completely, it is worth doing so in preliminary biochemical studies. Typically, for the very first incubation of some ligand for autoradiography, it is helpful to choose incubation concentrations that are about the K_D value reported in biochemical studies.

The buffer selected should be compatible with the known binding requirements of the ligand. If sodium is required, then it obviously should be included in the appropriate concentrations. We have been partial to using osmolarities that are similar to physiological saline, but hypotonic incubation buffers have been used with no apparent problem.

The incubation time should be selected so that you expect equilibrium has been reached. Usually 1 hr is in the ballpark.

The incubation temperature is usually room temperature, but again, preliminary

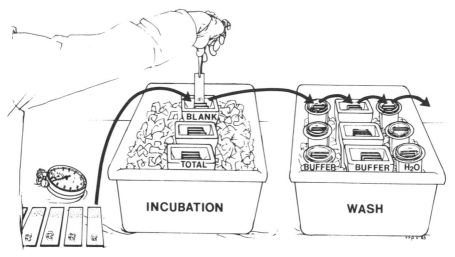

FIG. 1. Receptor labeling in slide-mounted tissue sections. Sections are incubated in Coplin jars to label the receptors and then washed in buffer to remove nonspecific binding. A final quick in-out dip in distilled water is used to remove buffer salts (which can cause auto-radiographic artifacts) from the slides. Sometimes, preincubation is used, and the incubation is often at room temperature; the wash is often at ice bath temperatures. See text for additional details. (From Kuhar, ref. 4, with permission.)

biochemical studies can provide important clues. If degradation of or active uptake of ligand is a potential problem, perhaps 0°C is the right choice. If maximal binding is achieved with 37°C, then that may be the best choice. In our experience, room temperature is a convenient and reasonable selection.

Finally, the choice of an appropriate competitive drug to define nonspecific binding is critical. Biochemical grind-and-bind experiments and publications will provide this information.

Our incubations are typically carried out in Coplin jars, and washes are made by transferring these slide-mounted tissue sections from jar to jar (Fig. 1). All data points are obtained from triplicate measurements. In order to measure radioactivity in the slide-mounted tissue sections, the sections are wiped from the slide while wet with filter paper circles (Whatman GF/B or Schleicher & Schuell no. 30) as shown in Fig. 2. All of the following studies are carried out by these simple procedures.

As an example, some of our published data on localizing the γ-aminobutyric acid (GABA) receptor in the rat cerebellum with [³H]muscimol will be presented (12). Muscimol was chosen as a ligand because it has been shown in biochemical binding studies to be an effective, reasonably high-affinity GABA receptor ligand.

First, a Washout Curve

In this example, of localizing GABA receptors, cerebellar tissue was used because GABA receptors in this tissue had been well characterized. Accordingly,

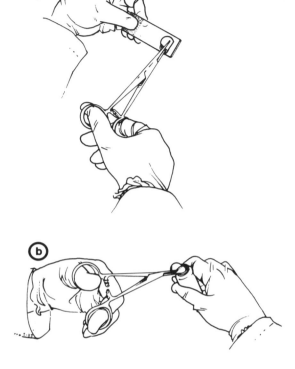

FIG. 2. Biochemical studies with slide-mounted tissue sections. After incubation and washing, wet sections can be wiped from the slide with filter paper (**a**) and placed in scintillation vials (**b**) for counting. If the sections are dry, they can be scraped from the slide with a razor blade. Biochemical studies with slide-mounted tissue sections usually must be carried out before autoradiographic studies. (From Kuhar, ref. 4, with permission.)

cerebellar sections were cut and thaw mounted onto subbed slides. They were stored for as long as 3 weeks at $-20°C$ with no detectable loss in receptor binding.

After storage, slides with mounted tissue sections were brought to room temperature and preincubated in an ice bath for 20 min in 0.31 M [tris(hydroxymethyl)aminomethane] (Tris) citrate buffer, pH 7.1. An ice bath was used because it was thought that optimal binding was obtained under these conditions for this ligand, even though many other ligands are used at room temperature. In this particular case, the slides were preincubated to remove endogenous ligand (see the next step below). The preincubation was for 20 min, at which time the sections were transferred to jars containing radiolabeled ligand ([^{3}H]muscimol, 5 nM). Parallel incubations were carried out with 0.2 mM GABA added to obtain blank values.

In general, the first experiment attempted is a washout curve. The goal of these experiments is to identify washing conditions such that high-specific to nonspecific binding ratios can be obtained without losing a large quantity of specific binding. Sections were incubated with 5 nM muscimol for 40 min to obtain total binding and other sections with the same mixture but also containing 0.2 mM GABA for nonspecific binding. Various time points were utilized in the experiment. After incubations, the slide-mounted tissue sections were transferred to Coplin jars containing

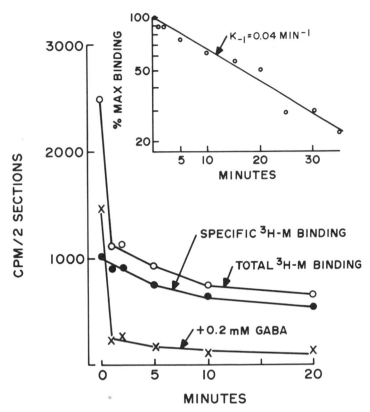

FIG. 3. Time course of dissociation of [³H]muscimol (*³H-M*) from slide-mounted tissue sections. The 0.2 mM GABA plot (*x*) is the nonspecific binding curve. The specific binding curve (●) was obtained by subtracting nonspecific from total (○) binding. The points are the average of three determinations with less than 10% difference among the samples. *Inset*, dissociation of specific binding $K_{-1} = 0.04$ min⁻¹. (From Palacios et al., ref. 12, with permission.)

buffer for various times to examine the washout of radioactivity from the tissue sections. After being rinsed in the buffer for various times, the sections were always given an "in-out" dip in distilled water to remove salts from the slide. After this in-out dip, they were wiped from the slide as described above. The data are shown in Fig. 3. Nonspecific binding rapidly decreased to very low levels, and it was only slightly decreased additionally with longer washing times. The specific binding in the sections was reduced about 50% over the duration of the wash curve (20 min). However, after only 1 or 2 min of washing, there was only about a 10% loss of specific binding. At this time point, the specific to nonspecific ratio was about 5:1. A further analysis of the rate of loss of specific binding revealed a rate constant of 0.04 min⁻¹.

Because a 1-min washing time reduced nonspecific binding to very low levels, maintained high-specific to nonspecific ratios, and did not result in a large loss of specific binding, a 1-min time point or wash time was used in all of the following experiments. Be aware that multiple washes in separate baths can produce lower nonspecific binding and that wash temperature can be varied to improve the results.

Preincubation Test for Endogenous Ligand Interference

Some ligands or endogenous substances are found in very high concentrations in tissue. This is true for GABA, which can be found in millimolar concentrations. Accordingly, we preincubated the tissue sections before incubations with radioactive muscimol. When preincubation time is varied and a 1-min wash time is used, specific binding is as shown in Fig. 4. It is demonstrated that preincubation significantly increases specific binding, and a 20-min preincubation time point was used because the increase in specific binding was maximal at this time.

Hence, all of the following experiments are done with a 20-min preincubation time and a 1-min wash time.

Next, an Association Curve

The rate of association of radiolabeled muscimol with GABA receptors was examined. Sections were preincubated for 20 min, incubated with 5 nM ligand for varying amounts of time, rinsed for 1 min, and then dipped in-out in water and assayed for radioactivity. The resulting data are shown in Fig. 5. Specific binding increased up to 20 min but did not significantly increase beyond that point.

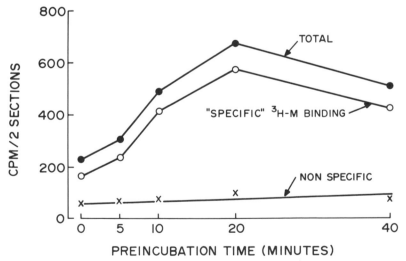

FIG. 4. Preincubation of tissue sections depletes endogenous GABA and increases specific binding of [³H]muscimol (³H-M). Preincubation time was varied, and optimal preincubation appears to be about 20 min. (Courtesy of Drs. Palacios and Kuhar.)

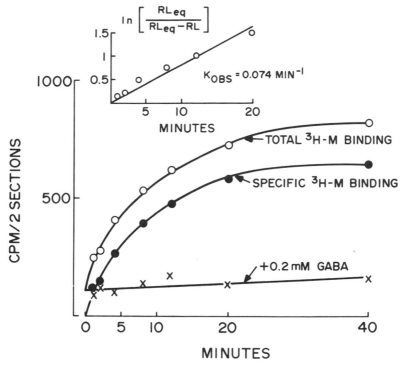

FIG. 5. Time course of association of [³H]muscimol (*³H-M*) to slide-mounted tissue sections. The 0.2 mM GABA plot (*x*) is the nonspecific binding curve. The specific binding curve (●) was obtained by subtracting nonspecific from total (○) binding. The results are the average of three determinations that differed by less than 15%. *Inset*, binding kinetics. $K_{obs} = 0.074$ min⁻¹. (From Palacios et al., ref. 12, with permission.)

Because there was no further increase in the specific binding after 40 min, this incubation time was selected for all further experiments. Thus, we have systematically determined preincubation time, incubation time, and wash time. This systematic determination is highly recommended.

Pharmacological Characterization of Binding

To be sure that the [³H]muscimol binding in the tissues is to a relevant GABA receptor, the pharmacological specificity was examined. Slide-mounted tissue sections were incubated with radioactive ligand along with different concentrations of displacing drugs. After washing, the sections were wiped from the slides and subjected to scintillation counting. The relative displacing potencies of the various drugs studied in these experiments are shown in Fig. 6. The pharmacological specificity is such that it is possible to conclude that authentic GABA receptors are being studied.

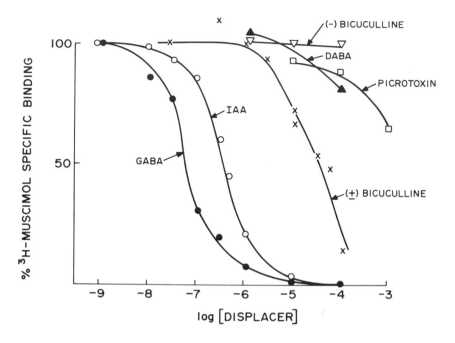

FIG. 6. Pharmacological specificity of [³H]muscimol binding. The points are the average of three to six determinations. ●, GABA; ○, imidazole acetic acid (*IAA*); *x*, (±)bicuculline; ▽, (−)bicuculline; □, picrotoxin; ▲, diaminobutyric acid (*DABA*). (From Palacios et al., ref. 12, with permission.)

Saturation Analysis

By using different concentrations of radiolabeled muscimol in incubations, it was possible to carry out a saturation analysis. The data shown in Fig. 7 indicate that the binding saturates with an apparent K_D of 13 nM. This K_D is slightly higher than (but within reasonable agreement with) biochemical experiments.

You Are Ready to Go

At this point, all of the optimal incubation and preparation conditions for generating very specifically and selectively labeled receptors in slide-mounted tissue sections have been elucidated. First, the washout conditions were optimized; then the necessity for a preincubation was tested; then an association curve was generated so that binding was carried out at equilibrium. Having obtained the proper incubation time and wash time, the pharmacological specificity of the binding and a saturation analysis were carried out to test whether or not the binding had the appropriate characteristics. If all of these preliminary biochemical data are acceptable and the receptor of interest has in fact been labeled satisfactorily, then one can proceed to

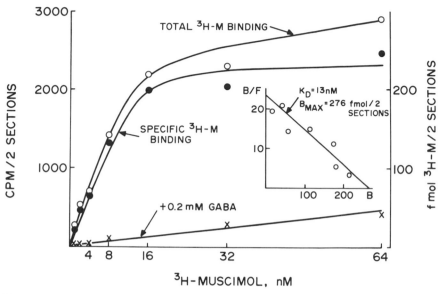

FIG. 7. Saturation kinetics of [³H]muscimol (*3H-M*) binding. The 0.2 mM GABA plot (*x*) is the nonspecific binding curve. The specific binding curve (●) was obtained by subtracting nonspecific from total (○) binding. The experiment was repeated five times with essentially identical results. *Inset*, Scatchard plot of saturation data. $K_D = 13$ nM; $B_{max} = 276$ fmol/two sections. (From Palacios et al., ref. 12, with permission.)

carry out autoradiographic studies. Keep in mind that [³H]muscimol and GABA receptors are only examples and the steps and procedures are the important things. This systematic and step-by-step approach is highly recommended. Now on to more general topics.

Generation of Autoradiograms

Incubation, Drying, and Storage of Tissue

Following incubation and washing, tissues are now not wiped from the slides and subjected to scintillation counting, but rather the slide-mounted tissue sections are dried for autoradiography as shown in Fig. 8. Rapid aspiration of water around the section with a Pasteur pipette attached to vacuum helps to remove the drop of water on the section; this facilitates drying and minimizes diffusion. The sections are dried by passing a stream of cool, dry air over the slide-mounted tissue sections. It is important that the sections be dried quickly so that the ligand has minimal opportunity to diffuse from the binding site. With low-affinity ligands or ligands whose wash times have proven to be very short, this could be a very critical step because diffusion may be a serious problem with these ligands. We have found that passing a stream of air through Drierite and through a liquid nitrogen or a dry ice-acetone

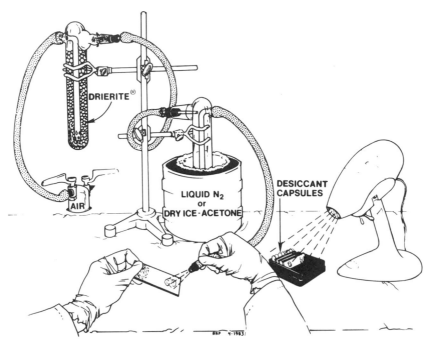

FIG. 8. Drying slide-mounted tissue sections for autoradiography. After incubation and washing, sections are dried under a stream of cool, dry air and are stored with desiccant before apposing to emulsion to generate autoradiograms. (From Kuhar, ref. 4, with permission.)

trap produces a cool, dry stream of air which is two or three times more rapid in drying sections than simply room air from a compressor. After drying, the slide-mounted tissue sections are stored with desiccant capsules in an airtight taped slide box at 4°C to be sure the tissues are appropriately desiccated. If the sections are to be stored for more than a couple of days, it is best to store them at −20°C. When you are ready to use these sections, it is important to allow the boxes to come to room temperature before opening so that moisture does not condense on the section.

It is critical that these radiolabeled slide-mounted tissue sections do not get wet or otherwise be given an opportunity for diffusion of ligand to occur. Dry storage and dry handling until the autoradiographic images are produced is critical. However, it has been shown that some ligands can be covalently cross-linked into the tissue sections by using, for example, formaldehyde vapor (13) as described below.

Cross-linking Ligands with Formaldehyde Vapor

After one produces slide-mounted tissue sections with specific receptors radiolabeled, the apparent simplest thing would be to dip these slide-mounted tissue sections into molten nuclear emulsion. We have done this (14) but with very, very minimal success. Unless the ligands are irreversibly bound to the receptors, placing these slide-mounted tissue sections into aqueous environments results in loss and diffusion of ligand (6, 15). Thus, fixation of ligand or creation of an irreversible bond between ligand and receptor can be desirable and can eliminate certain problems that arise when ligands might diffuse. Thus, it has been shown that it is possible to treat the labeled slide-mounted tissue sections with formaldehyde vapor so that an irreversible bond between the ligand and receptor is formed.

The procedure that we have used (after ref. 16) is as follows. Slide-mounted tissue sections are prepared as described above. Receptors are then labeled with various ligands according to procedures described above. After receptor labeling and drying of the slides, the slide-mounted tissue sections are then placed in a large closed jar containing paraformaldehyde (Fisher) (10 g/liter) equilibrated previously to 50% humidity. The jar is then heated for 2 hr at 80°C in an oven. After cooling, the jar is carefully opened in a vented hood. These treated slide-mounted tissue sections can then be transferred to solutions of ethanol or xylene and dried again. Ascending concentrations of ethanol [70, 90, 95, and 100% (v/v) in distilled water] and 100% xylene (5 min each) can be used to defat the sections. This defatting is important for reducing tritium quenching as described below. As mentioned above, there is some loss of ligand in the defatting solutions because the cross-linking with paraformaldehyde is not 100% efficient (see Table 1), and retention of ligand after defatting should be examined carefully. For example only 6% of $N[^3H]$methylscopolamine remained after soaking. The improvement in quenching after defatting has been shown for brain but may not be found with other organs. Thus, when using tritium with other tissues, quenching should be tested directly.

Sometimes, ligands can be prepared which can be covalently linked to the receptor by other means. For example, mustards (17) or photoaffinity labeling compounds can be used.

TABLE 1. *Loss of ^3H-ligand in 70% ethanol solution*

Ligand	Receptor	Specific binding remaining
		% control
$[^3H]$Naloxone	Opiate	65
$[^3H]$Dihydromorphine	Opiate	22
p-$[^3H]$Aminoclonidine	α_2-Adrenergic	35
$[^3H]$Prazosin	α_1-Adrenergic	33
N-$[^3H]$Methylscopolamine	Muscarinic cholinergic	6
$[^3H]$Spiperone	Dopamine and serotonin	20
$[^3H]$Muscimol	GABA	66

Slide-mounted tissue sections were prepared and labeled as described in the text. They were soaked in 70% ethanol for 5 min at room temperature and air dried. The sections were scraped from the slides, and specific receptor binding was determined. The soaked sections were compared with identically prepared sections that were not soaked. Results are the average of two or three determinations that differed by less than 15% from the mean. (From Kuhar and Unnerstall, ref. 45.)

Exposure, Exposure Time, and Development

Film

After labeled slide-mounted tissue sections have been dried and prepared for exposure, they can be apposed to film as shown in Fig. 9. The slides are adhered to a sheet of cardboard by applying two-sided sticky tape to the cardboard or spraying the cardboard with Photomount (3M). After the slides are arranged on the cardboard, they can be placed into a cassette, and in the dark, tritium-sensitive film can be apposed to the tissue sections. Try to keep sections away from edge of film when arranging the slides. Usually 36 slides (4 × 9) cover a sheet of film. Sometimes, additional cardboard is placed on top of the film to ensure a snug and movement-free apposition of film to the tissues.

After exposure times (see below), the films are developed according to standard procedures. We use the following: D-19, undiluted, 17°C, 5 min; H$_2$0 stop bath, 17°C, 30 sec; rapid fix for film, 17°C, 5 min; running water wash, 17°C, 20 min; 2 drops Photo Flo in water, rinse, dry.

Emulsion-coated Coverslips

Instead of using the film, one can use another apposition technique, with flexible, emulsion-coated coverslips, described by Roth et al. (18). The advantage of the

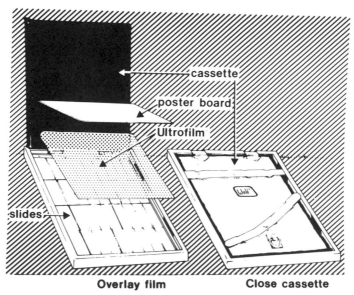

FIG. 9. Generation of autoradiograms with tritium-sensitive film. (From Kuhar, ref. 4, with permission.)

coverslips over the film tends to be that of increased resolution since the emulsion coating on the coverslips can be made thinner than it is on the film. Also, the flexible attached coverslip maintains register between the autoradiogram and the tissue. If done properly, there is never movement of image out of register from the tissue, and precise comparison of autoradiographic image and tissue can be made. Thus, the autoradiogram is viewed at the same time as the tissue is viewed. This simultaneous viewing of autoradiogram and stained tissue permits very precise identification of regions containing receptors.

Tissues and coverslips are prepared as described above. The coverslips are attached to the frosted end of the slides by "Superglue (pen or drops) in the dark. The coverslips should extend 1 to 2 mm beyond the edge of the slide so they can be pried and flexed for development. The coverslips are then firmly apposed to the tissue sections by the application of binder clips over Teflon pads in the dark. After exposure, the coverslips are gently flexed away from the tissue, and a spacer (such as a toothpick) can be placed between the slide and the coverslip for development of the autoradiogram, after which the tissue can be stained and dried and the coverslip mounted. Development conditions that we use are as follows: Dektol H_2O, 1:1, 17°C, 2 min; hardener H_2O, 1:13, 17°C, 15 sec; rapid fix for paper, 17°C, 3 min; running water wash, 17°C, 15 min; then fix, stain, dry, and mount coverslips. This procedure is shown in Fig. 10.

A useful staining procedure is as follows. The slides are immersed in, or the tissue section is covered with toluidine blue O stain (58.8 ml of 0.2 M acetic acid plus 1.2 ml of 0.2 M sodium acetate plus 0.5 g of toluidine blue O) for 2 min. After rinsing in distilled water, they are then dried on a warm plate. The sections can then be moistened with xylene and coverslipped with Permount.

Emulsion Dipping

If the ligand is *covalently* linked to the binding site, then the slide-mounted labeled tissue section can simply be dipped into molten emulsion, dried, stored, and developed by usual techniques (13, 17).

Exposure Time

The time of exposure of these autoradiograms depends on the amount of radioactivity in the tissue section. This in turn will depend upon the number of occupied receptors that one is examining and the specific activity of the ligands used. The simplest approach is to measure the radioactivity in the slide-mounted tissue sections by wiping or scraping into scintillation fluid. Once the quantity of radioactivity in the tissue section is known, then the exposure times can be estimated from the literature. Exposure time must be considered in relation to emulsion saturation. Long exposure times give pretty pictures but cannot be used for quantification (see below).

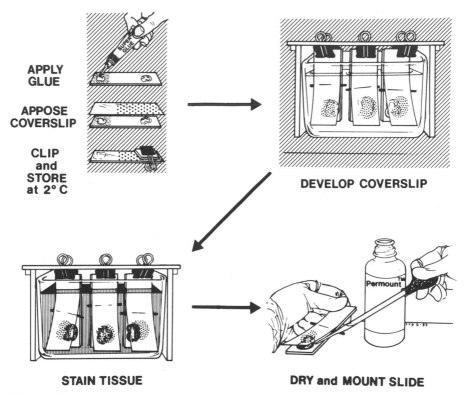

FIG. 10. Generation of autoradiograms by apposition of dry emulsion. Emulsion-coated coverslips (no. 1 or 0) are glued at one end of a labeled, slide-mounted tissue section and held against the tissue with no. 20 binder clips. After exposure at 2°C, the coverslip is bent away from the section, the emulsion is developed, the tissue is stained, and the autoradiogram (on the coverslip) is mounted to the slide and tissue section. Gluing the coverslip to the slide ensures that the autoradiogram will be kept in register with the tissue. Although [³H]Ultrofilm is easier to use than the hinged coverslips, the register of tissue and autoradiogram is lost with the film. (From Kuhar, ref. 4, with permission.)

Table 2 shows some ligands and the radioactivity content of the tissue and the resultant exposure time. Usually, the radioactivity determined in these experiments was from two tissue sections (two were used simply to get more conveniently measurable radioactivity on the slide). For iodinated ligands, the exposure times can be cut by a factor of two to three for tissues containing the same dpm.

Quantification of Autoradiograms

As stated in the first part of this chapter, autoradiography is quantitative. However, there are several important principles that must be understood and applied when quantifying autoradiograms. These will be discussed in the following pages,

TABLE 2. *Estimated exposure times for tissue sections labeled with several tritiated ligands under standard autoradiographic conditions*

Ligand (receptor)	Specific activity	Ligand concentration	Radioactivity[a]	Exposure time
	Ci/mmol	nM	cpm/slide	days
[³H]Quinuclidinyl benzilate (muscarinic cholinergic)	30–40	1	14,000–16,000	5
[³H]Flunitrazepam (benzodiazepine)	80–90	1	4,500–6,500	10
[³H]Lysergic acid diethylamide (serotonin)	25–35	5	2,500–3,000	30
[³H]Dihydromorphine (opiate)	70–80	4	2,000–2,500	35
p-[³H]aminoclonidine (α₂-adrenergic)	45–55	1	750–1,200	56
[³H]Muscimol (GABA)	10–20	5	600–1,000	70
[³H]Kainic acid (kainate)	2–6	15	100–300	112

[a]This refers to radioactivity specifically bound to two mounted 10-μm coronal sections of brain (approximately 1 mg of tissue, dry weight) that were wiped from the slides with glass fiber filters and counted using standard techniques following standardized incubation procedures. Estimates of exposure time were based on biochemical determinations listed in the fourth column. It was further assumed, based on previous experience, that radioactivity would be concentrated to approximately half the area of the tissue rather than being uniformly distributed over the surface. (From Kuhar, ref. 4.)

and examples of the practical application of these principles used by one of us (JRU) will be given. Important issues are the nonlinear response of nuclear emulsions to varying concentrations of radioactivity (hence, the need to use autoradiography standards), and the interaction between low-energy β-emissions and tissue (the problem of tritium quenching). Finally we have used an image analysis system to measure optical density (OD) values and perform some calculations in subsequent examples.

Use of Standards

To quantify autoradiograms, the accurate measurement of either grain density or optical density is essential. Grain densities can be measured by counting individual grains at moderate to high magnification with a light microscope. OD is determined with a calibrated device using Fick's law as a basis. The former is done with slide-mounted sections and emulsion-coated coverslips, whereas the latter is typically done with film images.

To relate grain density or optical density accurately to concentrations of radioligand and densities of binding sites, standards must be exposed along with the experimental tissue sections. Since the relationship between tissue radioactivity and grain density or optical density is not linear, standards containing a range of radioactivity must be used, and the equation best relating autoradiographic signal and tissue radioactivity must be derived. This equation is then used to analyze grain densities or OD obtained from regional analysis of the tissue autoradiograms.

Standards can be either made or purchased. The advantage of homemade standards is that you can select radioactivity levels to meet your needs and select tissue so that is has the same physical and quenching characteristics as your experimental tissues. The disadvantage is the time and effort needed to produce quality standards. Descriptions for producing standards from brain paste, for example, have been published (19). Procedures for making standards from tissue sections "soaked" with radioactivity will be described below. The advantage of purchased standards is the obvious savings in effort. They are usually made from a polymer, and their quality and uniformity are high. The disadvantage is that with tritium, the physical and quenching characteristics are not the same as brain, and this must be taken into account using tissue equivalence factors. (The importance of using tissue equivalence factors will be made apparent in a following section on tritium quenching.) You should probably read next two sections together before you attempt to quantify data.

Analysis of Autoradiographic Data: Generation of a Standard Curve

Once all the theoretical issues of quantitative autoradiography have been addressed, the actual measurement process, although tedious, is trivial. After coexposure of samples and standards and measurement of ODs, the standard data must be curve fitted to find the best relationship between tissue radioactivity and OD. Third-order polynomials, rectangular hyperbolas, power functions or other functions have been used to fit the curves. Theoretically, the third-order polynominal should provide the best fit over the entire range of film sensitivity. Sometimes, however, when data fall over certain ranges, the power function provides a better fit. Be sure that the ODs in the tissue samples are bracketed on both sides by ODs from standards. Choose a curve based not only on the correlation coefficient but also on how close each calculated value comes to the actual radioactivity value for each standard (root mean square error). Also, keep in mind that determination of radioactivity concentrations is less accurate when ODs are low (under 0.2) or high (over 1.2). This is due to the response characteristics of the film. If your data fall predominantly into these ranges, it may be better to reexpose your film to bring the data into a more workable range of ODs.

For tritiated ligands, methacrylate standards calibrated to tissue equivalents are now generally used (see next section). For ^{125}I-ligands, standards are usually homemade, although Amersham Corp. has recently begun to market ^{125}I-methacrylate standards. For tissue standards, a useful practice is to use soaked tissue sections rather than brain paste mixed with radioactivity. This procedure is less cumbersome and avoids contamination of the cryostat with radioactivity-laden tissue fragments.

To prepare soaked tissue sections, bovine caudate or internal capsule is used. In contrast to the situation with tritium, section thickness is very important with ^{125}I, and the standard thickness should be the same as the sample thickness for the simplest handling of the data; otherwise, additional corrections for thickness must be made. With ^{125}I, white matter tissue is considered by some to cut better, and it is sometimes preferred over gray matter since quenching (see next section) is not an issue.

One approach for generating a standard curve is shown in Fig. 11 and Table 3. More details of the procedure are given in the next section. Sections are soaked with increasing concentrations of iodinated ligand (e.g., iodopindolol), rinsed briefly,

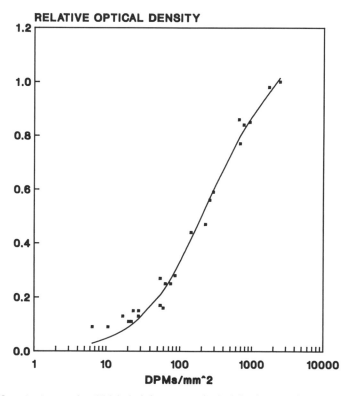

FIG. 11. Standard curve for ^{125}I-labeled tissue standards following a 1-day exposure. The actual data used to generate this curve are shown in Table 3. The line drawn here is a rectangular hyperbola in the form

$$OD = [A*X/(B + X) + C*X/(D + X) + E*X] - 1$$

where $X = dpm/mm^2$, $A = 1.018774$, $B = 208.631$, $C = 0.998369$, $D = -1.107E-9$, and $E = 0.315E-4$. The coefficient of determination was 0.989. A third-order polynomial fit these data equally well. However, note that with the function shown here, values at low OD readings (near film background) do not really fall close to the curve. With the polynomial function, more error was seen at high OD readings (above 0.8 OD). The hyberbola was chosen for this example since most of the data to be analyzed were well above 0.2 OD units. This illustrates the complexity involved in calibrating autoradiographic data and the empirical nature of the process. Although the relationships between OD and exposure are lawful, it is still difficult to control all the variables. Thus, a commonsense approach needs to be employed in analyzing autoradiographic data. See the text and Table 3 for more details.

TABLE 3. *Production of a calibration curve using* [125]*I-labeled tissue standards*

dpm/100 μl	cpm	dpm	Area	dpm/mm^2	Experimental OD	Calculated OD
			mm^2			
4,500,000	65,597	130,393	53.24	2,449.16	1.00	1.0143404
	50,061	99,512	57.87	1,719.58	0.98	0.9611005
1,500,000	24,870	49,437	53.24	928.56	0.85	0.8595103
	19,624	39,008	51.38	759.20	0.84	0.8214708
	17,065	33,922	50.18	676.01	0.77	0.7981980
	18,980	37,728	57.87	651.95	0.86	0.7907234
450,000	7,440	14,789	51.38	287.84	0.59	0.5981235
	6,470	12,861	50.18	256.30	0.56	0.5680866
	6,528	12,976	57.77	224.62	0.47	0.5336653
250,000	3,402	6,763	47.86	141.32	0.44	0.4142620
	2,475	4,920	57.77	85.16	0.28	0.2964035
	2,071	4,116	55.50	74.16	0.25	0.2679056
150,000	1,886	3,749	59.89	62.59	0.25	0.2354966
	1,635	3,251	55.40	58.68	0.16	0.2238882
	1,543	3,067	57.03	53.78	0.17	0.2089027
	1,290	2,564	47.86	53.58	0.27	0.2082691
45,000	785	1,560	55.60	28.12	0.15	0.1202873
	686	1,363	48.87	27.89	0.13	0.1194388
	715	1,421	59.89	23.73	0.15	0.1032101
	620	1,232	55.40	22.25	0.11	0.0972787
25,000	585	1,163	57.03	20.39	0.11	0.0897607
	514	1,022	60.43	16.92	0.13	0.0753661
15,000	260	517	48.87	10.58	0.09	0.0478992
	195	388	60.43	6.41	0.09	0.0290062

In this example, tissue sections (10-μm-thick sections from blocks of bovine internal capsule) were incubated with increasing concentrations of ^{125}I-pindolol in PBS (2 hr at room temperature), rinsed with two quick dips in ice-cold distilled water, and dried (more details are given under "The Tritium-quenching Problem and Standards with Tissue Equivalents"). The approximate concentration of radioactivity in the incubation solutions is given in the first column (dpm/100 μl of incubation solution; this volume was pipetted onto each section). The autoradiographic exposure was 24 hr. The counts in the second column were obtained 30 days after the initial exposure of film to the standards by scraping the sections from the slides and counting on a γ-counter at 72% efficiency. The third column dpm were calculated by dividing the cpm by the counting efficiency (cpm/0.72) and then correcting for radioactive decay using the equation provided in the text. The fourth column represents the measured area of each standard; the fifth column is simply column 3 divided by column 4. The sixth column represents the average OD *measured* over the entire standard. The final column is the OD *calculated* from the equation fitted to the empirical data and obviously compares well with the empirical data except at lower OD values. The curve and equation used to fit the data are shown in Fig. 11.

and exposed along with the samples. After exposure, the tissues serving as standards are scraped from the slides and counted in a γ-counter. The cpm are corrected for both counting efficiency and decay back to the time when the autoradiographic exposure was initiated. The area of the standard is measured, and the average OD is determined for the entire section. The initial dpm in the entire standard are divided by the area to obtain dpm/mm^2. The best equation for relating ODs to dpm/mm^2 is then estimated by curve fitting (see legend to Fig. 11).

Now, treat the experimental tissues. OD measurements obtained from regions of interest in the experimental tissues are plugged into this equation to determine radioactivity concentrations in these regions (Table 4). Again, this assumes that the radioactivity is uniformly distributed in the measured region. Finally, bound/mm^2 are determined by dividing dpm/mm^2 by the specific activity of the ligand times 2.22. This is derived from the following relationship in which the second term is the conversion of Curies to dpm, and the third term represents the specific activity of the ligand:

$$\frac{(dpm)}{(mm^2)} \times \frac{(1\ pCi)}{(2.22\ dpm)} \times \frac{(fmol)}{(pCi)}$$

Again, the specific activity of the ligand should be corrected to the point at which exposure was initiated. For correcting standard and ligand specific activity, the usual exponential decay function is used:

$$N = N_O \times \exp\left(-\ln2 \times t_{t1/2}\right) \tag{1}$$

where t is the time from the beginning of exposure to when the radioactivity was measured in the tissue standards (for the ligand, t is the time from the date of

TABLE 4. *Regional analysis of ^{125}I-peptide-YY binding by quantitative autoradiography*

Region	Total binding		Nonspecific		Specific binding		
	OD	dpm/mm^2	OD	dpm/mm^2	dpm/mm^2	fmol/mm^2	fmol/mg protein
CA3 LM	0.48	121.20	0.15	55.00	66.19	0.0149	86.13
CA3 OR	0.41	130.60	0.15	51.50	79.16	0.0178	102.89
CA1 LM	0.32	147.20	0.16	63.40	83.80	0.0189	109.25
CA1 OR	0.39	135.00	0.15	57.10	77.88	0.0175	101.16
DG	0.16	75.80	0.14	38.50	37.30	0.0084	48.55

The data illustrate the steps in the processing of autoradiographic data from raw OD measurements to concentrations of bound ligand. These data were generated from sections through the rat ventral hippocampus which were labeled with saturating concentrations of ^{125}I-peptide-YY (^{125}I-PYY), an analogue of neuropeptide-Y (NPY). [^{3}H]Ultrofilm was exposed to these sections for 1 day, and the data were calibrated using the standard curve shown in Fig. 11. The first column identifies the hippocampal regions analyzed. The second column shows the average OD reading obtained from these regions. The standard curve was used to convert these values to dpm/mm^2 as listed in column 3. Columns 4 and 5 represent the measured OD values and converted dpm, respectively, obtained from a serial section labeled with ^{125}I-PYY in the presence of excess NPY, i.e., nonspecific binding. Column 5 was subtracted fronm column 3 to generate the values for specific binding in dpm/mm^2 shown in column 6. *Never subtract OD measurements before transforming the data!* Then, dpm/mm^2 were converted to fmol bound/mm^2 by dividing dpm by the specific activity of the ligand at the time exposure was initiated (for this example, 2,000 Ci/mmol) × 2.22. The value 2.22 represents the conversion factor from Ci to dpm and has been adjusted to provide units in fmol. The last column is an estimate of fmol bound/mg of protein based on the assumption that protein concentrations are constant in gray matter regions (as determined by protein determinations in caudate tissue sections). Finally, dpm/mm^2 were converted using the factors 3.46 µg of tissue (dry weight) per mm^2 and 50 µg of protein per mg tissue, as explained in the legend to Fig. 12. Although these assumptions simplify calculations, they may not always be warranted. Other methods for determining regional protein concentrations have been suggested (29). The OD measurements were obtained using the RAS-1000 image analysis system (Amersham Corp.). See the text for more discussion on these procedures.

manufacture to the time of exposure), and $t_{1/2}$ is the half-life (in this example) of ^{125}I, which is 58 days. For the standards, since the radioactivity is measured after the experiment is over, N (final radioactivity concentration) is known rather than N_O. Thus, the equation must be rearranged to solve for N_O (divided the known dpm by the exponential). If needed, the binding can be calculated in terms of fmol/mg of protein as explained in Table 4.

One final note may be useful. In Table 3, approximate concentrations of radioactivity in the solutions used to create the ^{125}I tissue standards are given in column 1. In this example, these concentrations of ^{125}I-pindolol produced standards that gave OD readings ranging from film background to 1.0 relative OD units following a 24-hr exposure. Within this range of ODs, we have been able to produce characteristic curves using exposure times up to 14 days which do not deviate from the reciprocity law; i.e., 2,000 dpm/mm^2 times a 5-day expsoure produces the same relative OD as 1,000 dpm/mm^2 times a 10-day exposure (20). Thus, the concentrations shown in the first column of Table 3 can be used to determine the approximate radioactivity concentrations needed to produce standards for your particular experimental situation. For example, if you know that optimal exposure time for your sections labeled with an iodinated ligand is 10 days, then the values shown in Table 3 can be reduced by a factor of 10 to produce standards that will give the same range of OD readings shown in the table in 10 days instead of 1. Note that this information was dervied using ^{125}I-pindolol and that the values may differ if other ligands such as Bolton-Hunter reagent are used to produce the standards since penetration and absorption may be different. These values will also need to be adjusted for tissue sections of different thickness. Linearity of exposure can be assumed for tissue sections up to 20 μm thick. In other words, a 20-μm-thick section will have twice as many receptors as a 10-μm section, twice as much radioactivity, and will produce a much darker autoradiogram.

The Tritium-quenching Problem and Standards with Tissue Equivalents

Tritium nuclei emit β-rays of a sufficiently low energy such that the tissues containing the tritiated compounds will absorb a significant fraction of the β-rays, particularly if the emitting nuclei are deep within the tissue. The relative self-absorption of the tissues is dependent upon the relative density of the tissue; i.e., tissue mass/unit measure of surface area (21). In brain tissue, differences in tritium absorption can be related to the degree of myelination in a particular area, i.e., the amount of white matter (16, 20). In practical terms, this means that if white matter and gray matter contain the same quantity of tritiated compound, the autoradiogram will be less exposed over the white matter because there will be fewer β-rays reaching the emulsion due to autoabsorption in the tissue. This is the gray/white quenching problem that occurs with tritium. It does not occur with atoms whose emissions are of greater energy, including carbon 14, sulfur 35, and apparently iodine 125 (20).

Because of this quenching problem, care must be taken when comparing grain densities over regions or tissues of different composition. It has already been mentioned that when constructing standard curves for tritium using plastic standards, one must use tissue-equivalent conversion factors to adjust the autoradiographic signal artificially to be comparable with that which would be obtained from tissue that has a density different from the plastic. Similarly, if one is comparing autoradiographic data in different structures—for example, white matter versus gray matter, brain versus muscle, or kidney versus muscle—then one must be able to determine the relative autoradiographic efficiencies in the tissues of interest. These efficiencies have been determined for brain and plastic, and tissue equivalent factors have been identified and are commonly used when working with plastic standards (22–26). Tissue-equivalent factors are radioactivity values that are assigned to methacrylate plastic standards and are the values they would have if they were tissue and not plastic.

When you first purchase a set of plastic standards, it will be a useful exercise to calibrate them to the tissue you will be primarily studying, even if tissue equivalents are provided. A short example of the determination of tissue equivalents follows. We generally use ^{3}H microscales (Amersham Corp.) for calibrating autoradiograms that were generated from tritiated ligands. However, other commercial sources (e.g., American Radiochemical Corporation, St. Louis, MO) offer equally reliable products. When calibrating methacrylate standards, it is important to have a tissue in which the tritium signal is minimally quenched. For this purpose, we use blocks of tissue dissected from the tail of bovine caudate. From this region, uniform gray matter sections can be obtained, and the sections are usually large enough so that radioactivity absorbed into the tissue can be easily counted after scraping the tissue from the slide.

In this example (see Table 5), the gray matter tissue standards were made from sections of bovine caudate which were cut to the same thickness as the methacrylate standards (30 µm). We space three sections, each approximately 1 cm^2, on each slide. Before incubating the sections with radioactivity, we use a PAP Pen (Kiyota International, Chicago, IL) to draw a circle around each section, which places a small barrier around it. This step is not necessary, but it helps to keep the different concentrations of radioactive solutions segregated on the slides. The sections in this example were incubated in increasing concentrations of [^{3}H]dihydroalprenolol in phosphate-buffered saline. This is accomplished by laying the slides on a flat surface and pipetting 50 to 100 µl of radioactivity solution on each section. The sections were incubated for 2 hr at room temperature in these solutions. The drop of solution over each section was then aspirated, and the slides were rapidly rinsed first in a solution of ice-cold buffer, then ice-cold distilled water (1-sec dips), and then dried using standard procedures. Our interest was not in the amount of specific equilibrium binding but in the amount of total radioactivity "absorbed" into the tissue sections (using dihydroalprenolol helped to ensure that the radioactivity was uniformly distributed through the section of caudate tissue because there are large numbers of dihydroalprenolol-binding sites in this tissue).

TABLE 5. *Determination of tissue equivalents for commercial standards*

Standard	Equivalent Tissue Radioactivity dpm/mm²					Equivalent dpm/mg tissue dry weight	
	44 day	90 day	127 day	Average	S.E.	Average	S.E.
1a	198.6	195.7	206.7	200.36	3.29	57,907.43	950.11
2a	187.7	152.6	181.3	173.86	10.78	50,248.74	3,116.76
3a	153.8	131.7	149.0	144.82	6.72	41,854.30	1,943.20
4a	104.3	93.0	111.7	103.00	5.42	29,769.53	1,567.54
5a	78.1	68.6	92.2	79.63	6.86	23,013.56	1,981.87
6a	39.0	43.9	57.0	46.64	5.38	13,479.31	1,555.38
7a	22.3	28.5	34.9	28.54	3.63	8,249.57	1,049.50
8a	6.6	6.8	6.7	6.72	0.04	1,941.24	12.90
1b		46.6	41.0	43.82	2.81	12,664.37	811.53
2b	23.0	24.1	23.6	23.56	0.32	6,808.96	93.49
3b	14.3	14.3	14.3	14.32	0.02	4,137.72	5.28
4b	5.6	5.9	5.2	5.56	0.22	1,607.39	64.14
5b	4.3	3.6	2.8	3.57	0.45	1,030.54	130.58
6b	3.4	2.7	1.5	2.51	0.54	724.11	156.03
7b		2.0	1.2	1.57	0.41	452.44	118.74
8b		1.7	0.8	1.28	0.44	369.98	128.32

The equivalent dpm/mm² values for the commercial standards (^{3}H microscales) were calculated using the tissue exposure curve shown in Fig. 12. OD measurements (not shown) were taken from each methacrylate standard for each exposure time, and tissue-equivalent exposure values were determined by interpolation of the tissue curve. These values were then divided by exposure time to determine the dpm/mm² for each time point. These values (columns 2 through 5) are shown in the table above. dpm/mg of tissue, dry weight, were determined using the value 3.46 +/− 0.13 µg of tissue/pmm². This value was determined by weighing and measuring tissue standards and comparing the weights with the measured area of the autoradiogram. The *a* and *b* attached to the numbers refer to the high and low specific activity sets of ^{3}H Microscales, respectively. These values apply to the original lots of these standards and are not necessarily applicable to preparations that are currently being sold. See the text and Fig. 12 for more details.

Autoradiograms from these tissue standards and from the ^{3}H microscales were generated for varying lengths of exposure. After the films were developed, the tissues were scraped from the slides onto tared glass fiber filters, weighed (requires a steady hand, a stable and sensitive balance, and several replicates), and counted by standard liquid scintillation techniques.

Using the RAS-1000 image analysis system (Amersham Corp.) to analyze the autoradiographs, we measured the area of each tissue standard image and the average OD values over the entire standard image. From these measurements, we constructed exposure curves relating OD to dpm/mm² (Fig. 12) and dpm/mg of tissue, dry weight (by pooling the data for the entire set of tissue standards, we calculated a relationship of 3.46 +/− 0.13 µg of tissue/mm²). OD measurements were taken from the methacrylate standards (exposed in triplicate along with the tissue standards), and dpm/mg of tissue and dpm/mm² of tissue were calculated using the tissue exposure curve. The exposure value for each standard was divided by the length of the exposure to produce dpm/mm² and averaged (Table 5).

It is important to point out the rationale for expressing radioactivity concentra-

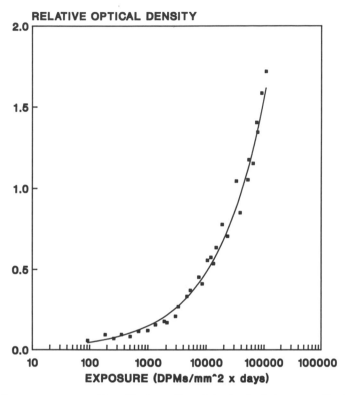

FIG. 12. Exposure curve used to calibrate methacrylate standards to gray matter (bovine caudate) equivalents. Sections through the tail of the caudate (30 μm) that were soaked in varying concentrations of [³H]dihydroalprenalol were exposed to [³H]Ultrofilm for 44, 90, or 127 days. Following exposure, the sections were scraped from the slide and weighed. Radioactivity concentrations were determined by liquid scintillation counting using [³H]toluene as an internal standard. Each point represents an individual tissue section in which the dpm/section were standarized to the area of the tissue section. For these sections, we calculated 3.46 μg of tissue, dry weight/mm² and approximately 50 μg of protein/mg of tissue. Protein concentrations were determined after tissue incubation. To combine these data, radioactivity concentrations were expressed in exposure units (on the abscissa) that represent the radioactivity concentration times the length of exposure. A semilog plot is shown to demonstrate the characteristic shape of an exposure curve. The curve shown is a power function in which $OD = 0.0795 \times dpm^{0.5089}$. Both the power function and a cubic function fit these data equally well with coefficients of determination greater than 0.98. Methacrylate standards were exposed along with these tissue standards. The ODs measured from each standard were used to calculate dpm/mm² using this tissue-derived function. The determinations from each exposure time were averaged, and the values obtained were used to assign gray matter equivalent values to each standard (Table 5). Standard errors were always less than 5% of the mean except for those standards containing less than 5 dpm/mm². The increase in error at low radioactivity concentrations can be attributed to two factors: low film sensitivity at low exposures, and the difficulty in measuring accurately small amounts of radioactivity in thin tissue sections. Although exposure curves such as these could be used to calibrate all autoradiograms, the procedure is valid only when the experiments are carried out under *exactly* the same conditions. This is especially true for film development and OD measurements. Since these film development condition factors can vary from film to film or experiment to experiment, it is far more reasonable to expose standards on each film and use these to develop standard curves for that film. See text and Table 5 for additional details. Compare this curve with the ¹²⁵I standard curve shown in Fig. 11.

tions in terms of unit area. This derives from the initial observations of Maurer and Primbsch (21) on the effects of tissue density on the autoradiographic efficiency of tritium (for English language description of their experiments, see refs. 9 and 10). In some initial quantitative studies (19), radioactivity concentrations were expressed in terms of tissue mass (dpm/mg of tissue) or protein concentration (dpm/mg of protein) in order to compare rationally autoradiographic data with homogenate-binding data. However, these values are not quantitative. Expressing tritium concentrations in terms of mg of tissue "masks" regional variations in quenching since both the numerator and denominator in the expression can vary (20), whereas using protein concentrations determined from a single set of tissues does not account for regional variations in protein concentration. Thus, using these procedures makes all determinations relative to a particular set of tissue equivalents (for example, the values provided with ^{3}H microscales are standardized to caudate equivalents). If the tissue equivalents are initially biased by some tissue-specific factor such as tissue mass or protein concentration, then any corrections for tritium quenching which are performed subsequently will be similarly biased and will not be equivalent to measures made in homogenate assays. The use of a tissue-independent measure such as area avoids this problem and provides a baseline for correcting the efficiency of the tritium signal in other regions of interest. When ^{125}I- or ^{35}S-labeled ligands are used, if the concentrations of these isotopes are calculated in terms of dpm/mm^2, the measured values will be proportional to the actual radioactivity concentration within uniformly labeled regions of interest. In all these cases, the measured radioactivity values can stand alone or can be related accurately to other biochemical or anatomical measures such as regional protein concentration or regional cell density (27, 28). For example, procedures for determining relative protein concentrations in anatomical regions of interest have been described (29).

When using tritiated ligands, you may need to correct for differential quenching depending upon your experimental question. For example, you cannot necessarily state that there is an absolute difference in receptor density between two brain regions unless you know the relative quenching in those regions. In a similar vein, you cannot necessarily compare relative receptor concentrations between normal and pathologic tissue, whether the pathology was experimentally induced (e.g., lesion) or natural (neurodegenerative diseases), unless you know the relative quenching in the tissues.

Many investigators have examined the relative quenching in different brain regions and have published quenching factors that can be used to correct autoradiograms generated by tritiated ligands (e.g., 23). Several procedures have been used. Some investigators have used animals treated with bolus injections of 3-O-[^{3}H]methylglucose to measure regional quenching (30). Since methylglucose distributes evenly through neural tissue, regional OD readings from brain sections taken from treated animals will reflect the relative amount of quenching in a region when compared with some standard region (e.g., caudate). Others have used [2-3H]deoxyglucose injections to perform the same function (23). In the procedure, autoradiograms are generated from labeled tissue sections before and after the application of defatting procedures. Since 2-deoxyglucose is insoluble in organic solvents, the label will precipitate and cannot be washed from the tissues. Regional ODs are measured before and after the defatting procedure, and the ratios generated are used as correction factors (23). Note that when either of these procedures is utilized, OD readings should be transformed to radioactivity levels by equations derived from autoradiographic standards. The use of tissue equivalents is unnecessary since the correction factors are unitless ratios.

These procedures are impractical to use in large animals and impossible to perform when studying postmorten human tissues. A variant of the [2-^{3}H]deoxyglucose procedure has been suggested which may be more universally applicable (16). Unlabeled tissue sections are incubated in the presence of tritiated protein-modifying reagents (e.g., N-[^{3}H]succinimidyl propionate) that acylate tissue proteins. Autoradiograms are generated before and after tissue-defatting and quench correction factors are generated. When using this procedure, it is best to preincubate the tissue to wash out soluble proteins. Further, you need to convince yourself that there is no differential extraction of membrane proteins from various regions due to the defatting procedure. This was tested by Henkenham and Sokoloff (16) by incubating serial sections with the chemically similar Bolton-Hunter reagent N-succinimidyl 3-[p-hydroxyphenyl]propioniate. Finally, as with the other procedures, relative ODs determined from autoradiograms generated by fresh and extracted tissues need to be transformed to radioactivity levels by using equations derived from autoradiography standards *before* deriving correction factors. An advantage of this technique is that these procedures can be applied to any tissue section, regardless of the source. Further, the measurements and calculations can be easily incorporated into computer-assisted image analysis protocols.

In order to illustrate the use of correction factors, a simple example can be shown. Tissue standards were used to transform OD readings taken from autoradiograms generated from tissue sections soaked in [^{3}H]isoleucine (20). Two sets of standards were used: one from sections of bovine caudate (gray matter), and one from sections of internal capsule (white matter). Some of the data are shown in Table 6 and are taken from regions in which we were confident that the soaked tritium was distributed uniformly through the tissue section. Using gray matter standards to calculate dpm in various regions, significant differences were seen in the calculated concentrations of tritium in gray and white matter regions, even though actual concentrations were the same (Table 6, column 2). However, when white matter standards were used, the radioactivity concentrations in white matter regions were determined to be far closer to those values obtained in gray matter regions (column 3). These data encouraged us to use ratios of dpm (region) dpm (caudate) shown in column 4 to generate correction values for regions of intermediate quenching such as the ventrolateral thalamus. These correction factors can then be used for the regions in subsequent experiments.

For example, sections were labeled with saturating concentrations of either ^{125}I-[2-(β-(4-hydroxyphe-nyl)-ethylaminomethyl) tetralone] (HEAT) or [^{3}H]prazosin, two selective ligands for α_1- adrenergic binding sites. ^{125}I-HEAT autoradiograms

TABLE 6. *Derivation of correction factors for differential tissue quenching*

Region	Gray standards	White standards	Region/caudate
	dpm	*dpm*	
Caudate	8.1×10^5		1.00
Septum	8.3×10^5		1.02
Thalamus, dorsolateral	8.2×10^5		1.01
Corpus callosum	3.9×10^5	8.8×10^5	0.48
Internal capsule	3.5×10^5	7.5×10^5	0.43
Thalamus, ventrolateral	5.9×10^5		0.73

Tissue standards made from bovine caudate (gray standards) and internal capsule (white standards) were made and used as described in the text. These standards were used to estimate the radioactivity concentration in various regions using tritium-soaked sections from the rat forebrain. The final column represents the ratio of apparent regional dpm to caudate dpm (correction factors) that were calculated using the gray matter standards.

were calibrated using iodinated tissue standards produced from bovine internal capsule, whereas ^{3}H microscales and their corresponding gray matter equivalence values. Some of the data is shown in Table 7. Although values obtained in gray matter regions (e.g., cortex and dorsolateral thalamus) are comparable for the two ligands, some differences can be seen for the measurements taken in the ventrolateral thalamus (14.7 versus 11.6). When the apparent amount of [^{3}H]prazosin bound in the thalamus was divided by the corresponding correction factor listed in Table 6, the differences were reduced and more in line with experimental error (14.7 versus 15.8). Be aware that using very low or very high OD values—values in which the standard curve has large errors—can result in highly inaccurate calculations (for example, see the low OD values in Table 3).

Image Analysis

Quantification of autoradiograms can be done rapidly and accurately and even semiautomatically by the use of computerized image analysis systems. The earliest

TABLE 7. *Comparison of regional α-adrenergic-binding site densities using iodinated or tritiated ligands and use of quench correction*

Region	[^{125}I]HEAT	[^{3}H]Prazosin (uncorrected)	[^{3}H]Prazosin (quench corrected)
		fmol bound/mg tissue	
Cortex, lamina V	15.5	15.0	
Thalamus, dorsolateral	17.7	17.3	
Thalamus, ventrolateral	14.7	11.6	15.8

Sections through the rat forebrain were incubated with saturating concentrations of either ligand. Thus, the values represent maximal binding capacities for the two ligands. Quench factors listed in the previous table were used to correct the levels of [^{3}H]prazosin binding in a region in which significant quenching had been observed, namely the ventrolateral thalamus. Thus, in the ventrolateral thalamus, the amount of [^{3}H]prazosin bound was divided by 0.73 (Table 6) to obtain the value listed in the fourth column, which is much closer to the value obtained from ^{125}I-HEAT.

systems applied to analyzing autoradiograms were quite capable but also very expensive. In the last several years, many of these systems have become reasonably priced because of the use of microprocessors and personal computers. Although several brands are currently available in a wide range of prices (you can even build your own for minimal cost), we utilize the one that is currently marketed by Amersham Corp. Contact suppliers for additional information and demonstrations. If you have a large amount of work for quantifying or if you are associated with several investigators who analyze anatomical data, an image analysis system may very well be essential. Depending on the kind of experiment you are doing, enormous quantities of time can be saved by these computerized instruments. Recently published manuscripts have reviewed the principles, applications and pitfalls of computer assisted image analysis (1, 28, 31–33).

PROCEDURES FOR *IN VIVO* LABELING AR

Preliminary Considerations: Good *In Vitro* Biochemistry

By the term "*in vivo* labeling," we mean labeling receptors with a high degree of specificity *in vivo* after intravenous administration of some radioligand. In other words, after systemic administration of the drug, you can find conditions in which it is selectively localized to one type of binding site in the brain or in other organs. This approach was first used for labeling steroid hormones in the brain (6, 15) and has been extended to labeling neurotransmitter receptors in the brain. A very important key feature about carrying out autoradiography after *in vivo* labeling is that the techniques utilized must prevent or minimize diffusion of ligand away from receptor, at least until the autoradiographic image is formed. These techniques for diffusable substances are critical, and sometimes the slightest technical error can obscure all meaningful results. This, of course, has been stressed above. Also, it has been mentioned above that *in vivo* labeling is more difficult and less workable than *in vitro* labeling.

The best opportunities for success with *in vivo* labeling require a thorough understanding of the receptor of interest as well as of the ligand you are using. Hence, the best situation is one in which biochemical binding experiments have been done extensively with your receptor and with your radioligand. Having good *in vitro* biochemical knowledge greatly enhances the chances for a successful experiment and for successful interpretation of your data.

Just as with *in vitro* labeling autoradiography, you must show that the binding of your ligand *in vivo* is to a physiologically and pharmacologically relevant receptor. This involves carrying out saturation, kinetic, pharmacological, and regional experiments. Useful examples in the literature include labeling dopamine receptors with tritiated spiperone (34) or labeling muscarinic cholinergic receptors in brain with tritiated guinuclidynol benzilate (QNB) (35, 36). In both cases, extensive biochemical experiments had been carried out *in vitro*, and the receptors and the radioligands used were reasonably well characterized before these *in vivo* labeling experiments were begun.

In *in vivo* binding experiments, to assess labeling, the animals must be killed and then dissected. After dissection, regions can be dissolved and subjected to scintillation counting.

First Experiments: Regional and Time Course Information

What is the best *first* experiment to do? How do you begin? A reasonable start is to carry out a time course and regional distribution experiment; but you need to know in advance the regional distribution of your receptor in brain. For example, it is known that the $D2$-dopamine receptor is highly concentrated in the striatum and is not found in the cerebellum in appreciable quantities. Therefore, after administering your radioligand, it should be found predominantly in the striatum and not in other brain areas such as the cerebellum. An additional factor is time; you may find an appropriate regional distribution only at certain times, and therefore, a time course is essential. Again, a useful example is labeling $D2$-dopamine receptors in brain with tritiated spiperone. In these experiments, 25 µCi of tritiated spiperone was injected into rats via the tail vein. Groups of animals were killed at different times after injection. Figure 13 shows that at times greater than 3 min, radioactivity began to accumulate selectively in the striatum as compared with the cerebellum. This preferential localization of radioligand to the striatum is consistent with the view that there is a preferential labeling of $D2$- dopamine receptors. However, additional experiments are necessary to establish this.

Pharmacological Specificity and Saturation

Having established an appropriate regional distribution in brain—in other words, having shown that the distribution of the radioactivity in your intact tissues parallels the distribution of receptor as determined from biochemical *in vitro* binding assays—you now need to show that you have pharmacological specificity. For our example with $D2$-dopamine, it must be shown that excess administration of other $D2$-dopamine receptor-blocking drugs can prevent the accumulation of radioactivity in the striatum, whereas non-$D2$-dopamine receptor drugs cannot. In these experiments, animals are pretreated with other drugs such as neuroleptics, and striatal levels of radioactivity are measured. If the striatal accumulation of radioactivity is associated with $D2$-dopamine receptors, then pretreatment of animals with $D2$-dopamine receptor-blocking drugs should prevent this accumulation of radioactivity. In fact, this is the case (34).

Since receptors are found in finite concentrations, injecting increasing concentrations of drugs should result in a "saturation" of binding. Therefore, injecting increasing quantities of tritiated spiperone into the tail veins of rats should result in an

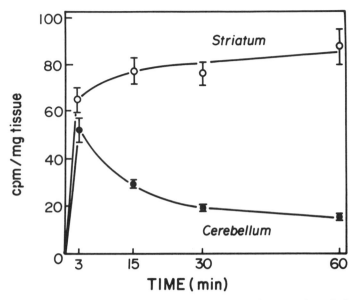

FIG. 13. Time course of [³H]spiperone accumulation in the striatum and cerebellum. Animals were injected with 25 μCi of [³H]spiperone. Note that the level of [³H]spiperone in the striatum is maintained, whereas that in the cerebellum decreases. The striatum has very high concentrations of dopamine receptors, whereas the cerebellum, by comparison, has negligible levels. These and other data are indicative of *in vivo* labeling of dopamine and other neuroleptic related receptors with [³H]spiperone. (From Kuhar et al., ref. 34, with permission.)

increase in binding *in vivo*, but only up to a point, after which there should be no further increase because of the saturation of available drug receptors. Again, this is in fact what one observes (34).

In summary, preliminary studies with *in vivo* labeling ligands are essential. After injections of the ligand, its concentration must be determined directly by dissection and scintillation counting. After you are convinced that your ligand is behaving as though it were bound to a specific receptor, then you can proceed with autoradiography.

Generation of Autoradiograms

Assuming that you have carried out preliminary studies so that you are confident you can prepare animals under conditions such that the bulk of the radioactivity in some brain regions behaves as if it is bound to specific receptors, then you can go on to generate autoradiograms. For example, injecting of 125 μCi of tritiated spiperone and then waiting 1 hr results in a fairly selective labeling of dopamine receptors in the rat striatum. After the injection and time delay, the animal can be killed and the brain dissected. If one chooses to localize receptors in coronal sections, then we recommend taking a several-mm-thick slab of the rat forebrain containing the striatum and freezing it onto a microtome chuck. Sections obtained from this slab will then yield coronal sections through the area of interest (34).

Therefore, the general plan is to identify conditions under which receptor labeling occurs, dissect the tissue, mount it on a microtome chuck, and freeze it so that it can be sectioned in a cryostat microtome. The tissue can be frozen in a little mound of brain paste or it can be frozen to the microtome chuck with a bit of distilled water. If the microtome chucks with tissues are to be stored, they can be wrapped in aluminum foil and stored at perhaps − 80°C or lower temperatures.

The cutting of these specimens is the same as the cutting of unlabeled tissues that you might be preparing for *in vitro* labeling autoradiography. These are three general approaches to cutting the radiolabeled sections and generating the autoradiograms of them.

One way is to thaw-mount the sections directly onto emulsion-coated slides (15, 36–39). Since the sections are being adhered directly to an emulsion-coated surface, the procedure must be carried out in the dark under safelights. Although this requires care, it can be done relatively easily with practice and the proper setup. A very useful arrangement is to have a red safelight directly over the cryostat. When the tissue section is on the knife blade, one can then find the section in the dark, since it appears as a shadow on the otherwise shiny knife blade under the safelight. Under these conditions, as emulsion-coated microscope slide can be removed from a lightproof container and touched to the tissue section. If the emulsion-coated microscope slide is at room temperature, the tissue section will be immediately thaw-mounted onto its surface. If the emulsion-coated microscope is kept in a lightproof container within the cryostat and is therefore cold and at the same temperature as the tissue, it will have to be pressured mounted (very light pressure) in the cryostat and brought into room temperature where it will thaw directly onto the slide. This latter procedure, using cold slides, might be a bit more dangerous than the former since bringing the cold slide into room temperature will inevitably result in condensation of moisture onto the emulsion-coated slide with a significant possibility of diffusion of ligand in the wetted surface. Although this procedure sounds difficult, in practice it is not really so. The sections can be cut with the lights on and one need only turn the lights out when working with the emulsion-coated microscope slides. Once the tissue section is adhered to the emulsion-coated microscope slide, it is stored in a desiccated light-tight container for the duration of its exposure. Although it has been mentioned several times, it is worth repeating that since the bulk of the ligands that we are using are diffusable, procedures must be used which prevent or minimize diffusion of ligand away from its binding site. Thus, until the autoradiographic image is formed, the sections cannot be exposed to any aqueous environment or indeed any environment that would permit diffusion of the ligand.

A second procedure is to desiccate the frozen tissue sections before mounting them onto an emulsion-coated microscope slide. This is done by simply taking the frozen sections and placing them in a desiccator in the cryostat (they must not thaw). Once a series of sections is cut and placed gently into a vacuum desiccator in the cryostat, the vacuum can be turned on to remove moisture from the sections. The desiccator can then be brought to room temperature while the vacuum is maintained. After the vacuum desiccator has reached room temperature, the vacuum can gently be reduced and the desiccator opened so that the tissue sections can be handled. The tissue sections can be transferred to Teflon squares (a 1/8-inch-thick Teflon sheet can be cut into squares of 1 to 2 inches per side). After the desiccated tissue sections have been placed on the surface of the Teflon square, it can then be pressed against an emulsion-coated slide in the dark. This pressure will push the tissue section into the surface of the emulsion where it will adhere and produce the autoradiographic image. This overall procedure is very safe in the sense that there is little or no opportunity for diffusion of the ligand from its binding site. However, it is technically tedious, and the tissue sections can be quite fragile in the desiccated state. Hence, handling and generating an autoradiogram are more challenging than using the other procedures. It may be that this procedure needs not only to be done once or with a few sections or with only a part of your experiment. In our experience, generation of autoradiograms by this more rigorous procedure results in autoradiograms that are identical to those prepared by the less complicated procedure described in the previous paragraph (38).

A third procedure, and maybe the simplest and most advantageous, is to thaw-mount the sections onto a subbed microscope slide. The slides can be kept at room temperature so that there is almost an immediate thawing of the tissue section as it is touched to the slide. Drying of the mounted tissue section can then be aided by a stream of cool, dry air. After you prepare these slide-mounted tissue sections that have been labeled *in vivo*, you can appose them to an emulsion-coated surface. This could be an emulsion-coated coverslip that is attached to the frosted end of the slide with Superglue, or it could be a sheet of film in a large cassette. Obviously, apposing the tissues to emulsion must be done in the dark.

After a timed exposure, the emulsion is developed by usual procedures. In the first two cases, in which the tissue is embedded in or adhered to the emulsion directly, you can usually proceed and ignore the tissue section. It is best to treat the slides gently in the developer, fixer, and wash so that the tissue sections do not float away. Loss of pieces of tissue sections can be a difficulty with this approach. After the emulsion is developed, the tissue can be stained as described previously (38). The sections can then be mounted and coverslipped, and the autoradiogram and the tissue can be viewed simultaneously through the microscope.

The last case, in which the tissue was not mounted directly onto the emulsion, can be handled somewhat differently. The emulsion can be developed without including the tissue in the process. In the case of using sheet film, the tissue and autoradiogram can be viewed separately. In the case of using the flexible attached coverslip, they can be viewed simultaneously.

The quantification and interpretation of these autoradiograms are as described above for *in vitro* labeling procedures.

EXAMPLES

In Vitro Labeling Autoradiography

Some examples of conditions for *in vitro* labeling autoradiography are shown in Table 8. A recent extensive literature review has been published (5).

In Vivo Labeling Autoradiography

In vivo labeling autoradiography, although not as currently popular as *in vitro* labeling, is becoming important again. A list of examples has been published recently (5).

Examples of autoradiograms from both approaches are shown in Figs. 14 through 16.

PRECAUTIONS, PITFALLS, AND PROBLEMS

There are several precautions and problems that you have to keep in mind when working in this area. A major issue is the specificity of labeling with your ligand. Even well-characterized ligands can later be shown to cross-react with unsuspected and new sites so that caution in interpretation is required. For example, when radiolabeled spiperone was first utilized, it was assumed that it bound selectively to $D2$-dopamine receptors. However, it was later found to bind with a somewhat lower affinity but yet significantly to serotonin receptors. Also, spiperone can label a

TABLE 8. *Examples of in vitro labeling autoradiography*

Receptor	GABA	β-Adrenergic
Preincubation	20 min	None
Incubation Ligand conc. buffer	[^{3}H]Muscinol (5 nM) 0.31 Tris-Citrate (pH 7.1)	^{125}I-Cyanopindolol 0.05 nM 50 mM Tris-HCl (pH 7.7) with 0.01% ascorbate and 5 mM MgCl$_2$
Temperature	4°C	Room temperature for 2 hr

Wash
  Buffer
  Temperature
	1 min
	0.31 Tris-citrate (pH 7.1)
	4°C
		30 min
		Same buffer
		4°C

Blank	200 μM GABA	10 μM Propranolol
Reference	Palacios et al. (12)	Zarbin et al. (42)

Many other examples can be found in the literature. A recent review listing various receptors, ligands and references has been produced (5).

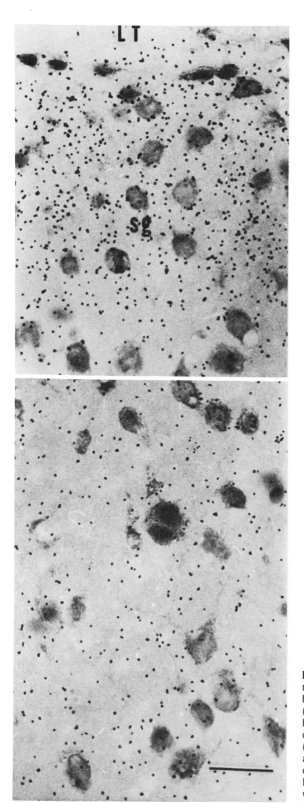

FIG. 14. Localization of opiate receptors in rat spinal cord dorsal horn. This bright-field high-power (oil, × 40) autoradiogram shows higher concentrations of grains over the substantia gelatinosa (*sg*). Specimens were produced after *in vivo* labeling of opiate receptors with [³H]diprenorphine. LT: Lissauer's Tract. (From Atweh and Kuhar, ref. 38, with permission.)

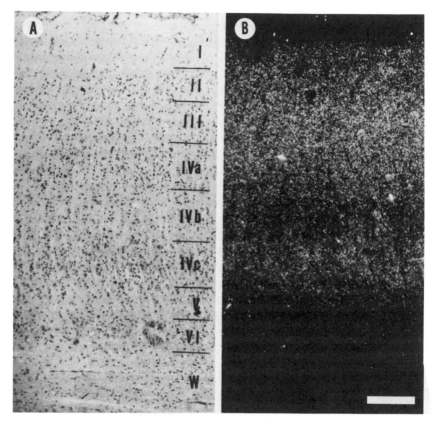

FIG. 15. Benzodiazepine receptors in human calcarine cortex. Nissl-stained section in **A** shows the various layers of cells; the autoradiogram in **B** was produced by apposing an emulsion-coated coverslip to the section shown in **A**, which was labeled *in vitro* with [³H]flunitrazepam. This is one of the first receptor maps in human brain made possible by *in vitro* labeling techniques. (From Young and Kuhar, ref. 46, with permission.)

totally nonspecific site in brain which is unrelated to receptors but appears to be a site related to its chemical structure (40).

Another issue that has been mentioned several times is the danger of diffusion of ligand. Obviously, where possible, it seems advisable to use irreversibly bound ligands. In this case, direct dipping into molten emulsion can be used. If this is not possible, then the procedures described above must be used with practice, patience, and skill.

Although quantification is quite readily done in autoradiography, it must be done under appropriate conditions. Excessively long exposure of autoradiograms will result in regions of the emulsion being saturated, and therefore precise quantification in these regions will not be possible. Inclusion of appropriate standards with each experiment is most helpful in avoiding these problems.

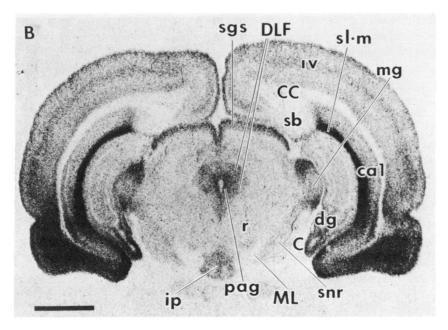

FIG. 16. α_2-Adrenergic receptors in rat brain. Slide-mounted tissue sections were labeled *in vitro* with *p*-[³H]aminoclonidine and apposed to sheets of Ultrofilm. A lower-power bright-field photo of the film image is shown. The overall procedure of using *in vitro* labeling and sheets of film for autoradiography is quite popular. (From Unnerstall, ref. 28 and ref. 28A, with permission.)

Another issue is that of chemography. Although it has not been discussed, controls for both positive and negative chemography probably should be done under the conditions of your experiments (7). Positive chemography is the production of autoradiographic grains due to some type of chemical interaction between the emulsion and some tissue constituent. In other words, autoradiographic grains are produced without radioactivity. Negative chemography is the opposite; it is the loss of autoradiographic grains due to some chemical interaction. You can test for positive chemography by taking tissues that do not contain radioactivity and carrying them through your experimental process. Negative chemography can be assessed by using tissues that have no radioactivity content along with emulsions that have been partially exposed to light so that a significant measurable grain density has been induced uniformly in the emulsion. Although chemographic artifacts have not been studied in extreme detail, enough has been done probably to say safely that they are not major difficulties in usual experiments with brain tissue. Nevertheless, the best designed experiment tests for chemographic artifacts.

Does light microscopic autoradiography really meet the needs of your experiment? If you intend to localize receptors to specific membranes, then light microscopic procedures in general are inadequate. Ultrastructural methods must be utilized. The light microscopic approach described here provides magnificent sensitivity and anatomical resolution, yet has its limitations in resolution and sensitivity. In this regard, ultrastructural studies have an important place in this discipline. There have already been many important and useful electron microscopic studies of receptors, and procedures related to these are not covered here. Also, be aware that autoradiography with the electron microscope may not be the technique that meets your needs. Immunocytochemical approaches with the electron microscope provide higher resolution, and there are several examples of its successful use in the literature (41).

APPLICATIONS

The procedures described here can be applied to a wide variety of situations. The two fundamental advantages that one obtains by these radiohistochemical approaches are sensitivity of measurement and anatomical resolution. If you need to localize receptors to small structures, then this is very possibly the best approach for you. For example, we have shown that receptors undergo axonal transport in small ligated nerves (42).

Receptor autoradiography has also been useful in several other situations. First of all, when drug receptors are localized, the results help explain the action of drugs. Although it is important to say that there is a drug receptor in brain, it is only by know which neuronal circuits contain the receptors that one can fully understand how the drug exerts its effects.

These results also provide new information on the biochemical organization of the brain. For example, after more than a decade of receptor autoradiography, it appears reliably that there is not a precise match between nerve terminals releasing neurotransmitter and receptor sites (43, 44). Although this is a controversial area and the extent of this mismatch is not finally decided, the issue could provide some interesting information on unexpected modes of chemical communication in brain. Also, several regions of the brain seem to be receptor "hot spots." Some regions contain high densities of many different kinds of receptors. Does this happen by chance or does this mean that these regions rely on chemical communication more than other regions? These questions will require further exploration in the future.

Another use of receptor mapping is neuropathology. Although receptors are not exclusively localized to neurons, they appear to be there preferentially. Hence, changes in receptor distributions can very well imply some neuropathological change in the brain. This notion has been useful in *in vitro* labeling autoradiographs of human postmortem tissue and also in PET positron emission tomographic scanning studies following *in vivo* labeling of various receptors.

Although more can be said about the applications of these techniques, we will not elaborate any further. Presumably by coming to this chapter, you already have good reasons for carrying out autoradiographic studies, and more extensive discussion of this topic can be found in other reviews (2, 4, 5).

Acknowledgments

We gratefully acknowledge our colleagues whose work over the years has helped make this chapter possible. We thank also S. Amos and T. Pierce for help in producing this manuscript, and Drs. Robert Lew, Mark Mitchell, and Scott Young for reading it.

REFERENCES

1. Boast CA, Snowhill EW, Altar CA. *Quantitative receptor autoradiography.* New York: Alan R Liss Inc, 1986.
2. Kuhar MJ. *Trends Neurosci* 1981;4:60–64.
3. Kuhar MJ. In: Bjorklund A, Kokfelt T, eds. *Methods in chemical neuroanatomy, Vol 1: Handbook of Chemical Neuroanatomy.* Amsterdam: Elsevier Science Publishing Co, 1983;398–415.
4. Kuhar MJ. In: Yamamura HI, Enna SJ, Kuhar MJ, eds. *Neurotransmitter receptor binding,* 2nd Ed. New York: Raven Press, 1985;153–176.
5. Kuhar MJ, De Souza EB, Unnerstall JR. *Annu Rev Neurosci* 1986;9:27–59.
6. Roth LJ, Stumpf WE. *Autoradiography of diffusible substances.* New York: Academic Press, 1969.
7. Rogers AW. *Techniques of autoradiography.* Amsterdam: Elsevier Science Publishing Co, 1979.
8. Dormer P. In: *Molecular biology, biochemistry and biophysics,* vol. 14. Berlin: Springer-Verlag, 1973;347–393.
9. Perry RP. In: Prescott DM ed. New York: Academic Press, 1969;305–326.
10. Przybylski RJ. In: Wied GL, Bahr GF, eds. *Introduction to quantitative cytochemistry.* New York: Academic Press, 1970;477–505.
11. Young WS III, Kuhar MJ. *Brain Res.* 1979;179:255–270.
12. Palacios JM, Young WS III, Kuhar MJ. *Proc Natl Acad Sci USA* 1980;77:670–675.
13. Herkenham M, Pert CB. *J Neurosci* 1982;2:1129–1149.
14. Young WS III, Kuhar MJ. In: Van Ree JM, Terenius L, eds. *Characteristics and function of opioids.* Amsterdam: Elsevier/North Holland, 1978;451–452.
15. Stumpf WE, Roth LG. *J Histochem Cytochem* 1966;14:274–287.
16. Herkenham M, Sokoloff L. *Brain Res* 1984;321:363–368.
17. Rotter A, Birdsall, NJM, Burgen ASV, Field PM, Hulme EC, et al. *Brain Res Rev* 1979; 1:141–166.
18. Roth LJ, Diab IM, Watanabe M, Dinerstein RJ. *Mol Pharmacol* 1974;10:986–998.
19. Unnerstall JR, Niehoff DL, Kuhar MJ, Palacios JM. *J Neurosci Methods* 1982;6:59–73.
20. Kuhar MJ, Unnerstall JR. *Trends Neurosci* 1985;8:49–53.
21. Maurer W, Primbsch E. *Exp Cell Res* 1965;33:8–18.
22. Alexander, GM, Schwartzman RJ, Bell RI, Yu J, Renthal A. *Brain Res* 1981;223:59–67.
23. Geary WA III, Toga AW, Wooten GF. *Brain Res* 1985;337:99–108.
24. Geary WA III, Wooten GF. *J Pharmacol Exp Ther* 1983;225:234–240.
25. Pan HS, Frey KA, Young AB, Penney JB. *J Neurosci* 1983;3:1189–1198.
26. Reivich M, Jehle JW, Sokoloff L, Ketz SS. *J Appl Physiol* 1969;27:296–300.
27. Hall MD, Davenport AP, Clark CR. *Nature* 1986;324:493–494.
28. Unnerstall JR. In: Swenberg CE, Conklin JJ, eds. *Imaging techniques in biology and medicine.* New York: Academic Press, 1988;217–256.
28a. Unnerstall JR, Kopajtic TA, Kuhar MJ. *Brain Res Rev* 1984;7:69–101.
29. Miller JA, Curella P, Zahnister NR. *Brain Res* 1988;447:60–65.
30. Orzi F, Kenney C, Jehlo J, Sokoloff L. *J Cereb Blood Flow Metab* 1983;3:577–578.
31. Loats HL, Lloyd DG, Pittenger M, Tucker RW, Unnerstall JR. In: Swenberg CE, Conklin JJ, eds. *Imaging techniques in biology and medicine.* New York: Academic Press, 1988;1–76.
32. Palacious JM, Niehoff DL, Kuhar MJ. *Neurosci Lett* 1981;24:111–116.
33. Rainbow TC, Bleisch WV, Biegon A, McEwen BS. *J Neurosci Methods* 1982;5:127–138.
34. Kuhar MJ, Murrin LC, Malouf AT, Klemm N. *Life Sci* 1978;22:203–210.

35. Yamamura HI, Kuhar MJ, Snyder SH. *Brain Res* 1974;80:170–176.
36. Kuhar MJ, Yamamura HI. *Brain Res* 1976;110:229–243.
37. Appleton TC. *J Microb Soc* 1964;83:277.
38. Atweh SF, Kuhar MJ. *Brain Res* 1977;124:53–67.
39. Gerlach JL, McEwen SS. *Science* 1972;175:1133–1136.
40. Palacios JM, Niehoff, DL, Kuhar MJ. *Brain Res* 1981;213:277–289.
41. Kihar MJ. *Trends Neurosci* 1987;10:308–310.
42. Zarbin MA, Palacios JM, Wamsley JK, Kuhar MJ. *Mol Pharmacol* 1983;24:341–348.
43. Herkenham M. *Neuroscience* 1987;23:1–38.
44. Kuhar MJ. *Trends Neurosci* 1985;8:190–191.
45. Kuhar MJ, Unnerstall JR. *Brain Res* 1982;244:178–182.
46. Young WS III, Kuhar MJ. *Nature* 1979;280:393–395.

Methods in Neurotransmitter Receptor Analysis,
edited by Henry I. Yamamura, et al.
Raven Press, Ltd., New York © 1990.

8

Messenger RNA Localization with the Microscope

In Situ Hybridization Using Radiolabeled Probes

George R. Uhl

*Laboratory of Molecular Neurobiology, Addiction Research Center,
National Institute on Drug Abuse, Baltimore, Maryland 21224; and the
Departments of Neurology and Neuroscience,
Johns Hopkins University School of Medicine,
Baltimore, Maryland 21205*

Information about the localization and intensity of expression of messenger RNA (mRNAs) in specific brain regions or within specific neurons is important in many circumstances. *In situ* hybridization is the method of choice for obtaining such information. In this chapter, the term refers to techniques for localizing nucleic acid sequences within tissues. This methodology has also been called histohybridization, or hybridization histochemistry, to distinguish it from work localizing sequences to chromosomal regions (1, 2).

The techniques of *in situ* hybridization are most commonly used for evaluation of the expression of mRNA products of specific genes of interest, including those for neurotransmitter receptors, within individual cells or specified cell populations. This chapter will focus on these studies, although similar approaches can be directed toward exogenous nucleotide sequences such as the DNA or RNA sequences encoding viruses and other infectious agents (3–11).

"Hybridization" refers to the recognition and noncovalent hydrogen bonding between two complementary nucleic acid sequences. This hybridization can occur between complementary DNA strands, (dA-dT,dG-dC matches), RNA strands, (rA-rU, rG-rC matches), or between DNA-RNA hybrids, (dA-rU, dG-rC matches) (Fig. 1). Random, short nucleotide segments may show some chance complementarity to each other, make several hydrogen bonds, and weakly interact. Conditions of hybridization and washing can be set, however, at high "stringency" to allow only long stretches of nucleic acids with near-perfect complementarity to remain hybridized to each other (e.g., 12). Under these conditions, the ability of a radio-

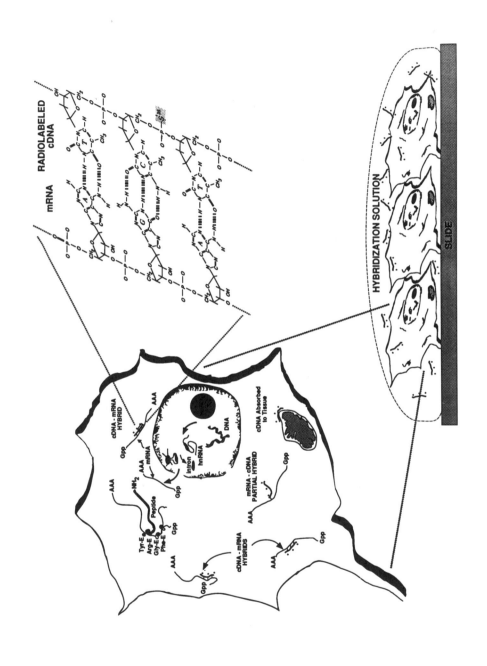

labeled complementary DNA or RNA hybridization probe to specifically recognize a hybridizing mRNA in a time section provides one significant piece of evidence that mRNA sequences complementary to the hybridization probe exist in the tissue.

The first major strength of *in situ* hybridization is thus its ability to *identify and localize* the cells expressing particular genes. In cases in which (*a*) genes are expressed at both mRNA and protein levels, and (*b*) good antibodies can specifically detect peptide or protein immunoreactivity at a tissue level, *in situ* results can supplement those obtained by immunohistochemistry. Imunohistochemical data can be ambiguous; antibodies may display cross-reactivities. In these circumstances, *in situ* detection of a mRNA in a cell can buttress the validity of observed immunoreactivity for translation products of the same mRNA in the same cell. In several cases, *in situ* results have highlighted mRNA-containing cell bodies that are poorly immunostained, perhaps due to variable processing and/or unusual intracellular distribution of immunoreactive translation products (13, 14). In addition, the presence of both mRNA and peptide or protein translation products in a cell provides evidence for local intracellular synthesis, as opposed to uptake and accumulation. The ability to make this distinction is especially important for molecules such as nerve growth factor which, for either of these two reasons, can reside inside neurons (e.g., 15).

In situ studies of the expression of receptor genes can also add significant information about the localization of receptor-synthesizing neurons (e.g., 16–18). Good antibodies that specifically recognize receptor protein in tissue sections are not available for immunohistochemical localization of most receptors. Since light-microscopic receptor autoradiography often cannot identify the cell bodies that express receptor binding sites, receptor mRNA *in situ* hybridization can provide novel information about localization of receptor-expressing cell bodies. Further, experience with acetylcholine receptor (ACHR) genes, for example, suggests that each of a number of different receptor subtype genes is expressed in a distinct individually localized pattern (16, 17). This diversity is significantly greater than the number of selective ligands currently available for ACHR receptor autoradiography.

The second sort of information that can be obtained with *in situ* hybridization techniques concerns changes in the *intensity* of neuronal expression of particular nucleotide sequences. These altered levels of mRNA can often be related to changes in the functional activities of expressing neurons (19). In many neurons that utilize peptide neurotransmitters, for example, stimuli that enhance rates of neuronal firing

---

FIG. 1. Depiction of *in situ* hybridization at three levels of resolution. **A**, *bottom right*, depiction of radiolabeled hybridization probe (*) in solution overlying tissue section, absorbed to elements within the tissue section, and hybridized to mRNA segments within individual cells. **B**, *left*, depiction of a cell synthesizing and processing RNA in its nucleus, with mRNA residing in the cytoplasm and with radiolabeled cDNA probes specifically hybridized to certain mRNAs, nonspecifically adsorbed to tissue components (mitochondrial surface, *lower right*) or partially hybridizing to a partially complementary mRNA (*middle cell*). **C**, *upper right*, depiction of a segment of hybridization of a radiolabeled ^{35}S-cDNA hybridized to segment of an mRNA.

and peptide release also augment levels of expression of the mRNAs encoding the peptides. The exact biochemical mechanisms for these changes are being actively explored in studies of several genes (19). Although the details of this coupling between gene expression and neuronal functional activity are only beginning to be understood in most instances, the "window" to greater understanding of the function of particular neurons which these techniques can provide can be of great value.

This chapter will therefore focus on studies using techniques that can be amenable to both localization and relative quantitation of gene expression. Since most of these studies use quantitative autoradiography as a detection system, the focus here is on radiolabeled hybridization probes.

PRINCIPLES: HYBRIDIZATION REACTIONS IN TISSUE SECTIONS— OVERVIEW OF THEORETICAL CONSIDERATIONS

This section will provide a brief overview to some of the specific problems faced by molecules of a radiolabeled hybridization probe in solution as they interact with tissue elements containing an mRNA hybridization target. Each of these concerns will be expanded in practical detail in subsequent sections.

Probe Distribution into Different Compartments

Molecules of hybridization probe can exist (*a*) outside of a tissue section; (*b*) within the tissue section in a manner that reflects diffusion and/or nonspecific physiochemical interactions of the probe with tissue constituents; (*c*) within the tissue associated with nucleic acid sequences to which the probe is only partially complementary; or (*d*) within the tissue associated with the appropriate nucleic acid sequence to which the probe is totally complementary (Fig. 1). Probe molecules that are associated with particular target nucleic acid sequences in tissue are thus in equilibrium with probe molecules outside the tissue. Hybridization is speeded by either increasing the concentration of radiolabeled probe outside the tissue or reducing the diffusion barrier that other tissue constituents present to stymie probe access to target nucleotide sequences. However, increasing hybridization speed by enhancing the extracellular concentrations of hybridization probe can also increase the opportunity for nonspecific interactions of probe with other tissue constituents or with cross-hybridizing nucleic acid segments. Improved hybridization *specificity* can often be obtained by use of low concentrations of hybridization probe.

The mechanisms that cause hybridization probes to "stick" nonspecifically to tissue elements that are not complementary nucleic acid sequences are largely unknown. Excess unlabeled "junk" DNAs (e.g., sheared herring sperm DNA) are often used to saturate such sites and minimize these interactions. Nevertheless, such features as the hydrophobicity of particular cDNA probes may cause anatomically specific interactions with selective brain areas which do not reflect hybridization to specific target nucleic acid sequences.

Probe Design Considerations

In designing a hybridization probe, one needs to pay attention to issues of specificity and accessibility. Long nucleic acid sequences may not penetrate into tissue sections (e.g., 20). On the other hand, longer probes may tolerate washes of higher stringency in a fashion that will allow reduced possibilities for recognition of related but nonidentical nucleic acid sequences.

Selection of the hybridization probe should take into account all known information about the structure of the target gene and of any related genes. Frequently, for example, members of "gene families" share substantial relatedness in the regions of their mRNAs which are translated to yield peptide products (21). On the other hand, they often display substantial diversity in untranslated regions. Probes directed against these sequences can be used to produce nucleic acid hybridization probes of higher specificity.

Probes displaying significant hybridization to themselves are unlikely to be as useful as those that lack this feature. Several groups have shown that single-stranded DNA probes are preferable to double-stranded DNA probes such as those resulting from nick translation or random primer labeling of double-stranded plasmids (e.g., 22). Probes that possess palindromic sequences allowing internal self-hybridization are less useful for *in situ* hybridization studies than probes free of such self-recognizing abilities.

Probe stability is also important. Since tissue elements and laboratory surfaces are notorious for their ubiquitous contamination with RNases, cRNA probes may be inherently more difficult to use than DNA probes (e.g., 23).

Features Influencing Hybridization in Solution

Studies of nucleic acid association and dissociation kinetics in solution have provided a detailed description of factors influencing hybridization (reviewed in 12). The avidity of a probe molecule in hybridizing to complementary sequences is classically described based on the initial concentrations of unassociated molecules and the time for which hybridization has occurred ($C_o t$). Hybridization itself is thought to reflect (*a*) an initial nucleation event in which a relatively short stretch of nucleic acid recognizes its complementary sequence, and (*b*) a "zippering" mechanism in which two strands aligned by the initial recognition form a long series of hydrogen-bonded base pairs (see also ref. 24). Such hybrids are more stable at lower temperatures and will eventually "melt" or dissociate as temperatures rise. Indeed, the stability of hybridization is classically described by a melting temperature (T_m). Increasing salt concentrations stabilize hybridized nucleic acid stretches, whereas increasing formamide concentrations destabilize them. G-C hybridization produces three hydrogen bonds per base pair. This interaction contributes more greatly to hybrid stability than A-T bonds (allowing two hydrogen bonds/base pair). Finally, any mismatches among incorrectly aligned or incorrectly matched sequences also result in destabilization of hybrids. Equations (such as $T_m = 81.5 + 16.6$ (log of sodium concentration) plus 0.41 (percent $G + C$) $- 675$/(probe length) $- 1.0 \times$ (percent mismatch) $- 0.65 \times$ (percent formamide) (ref. 25) are used to predict quantitatively the melting behavior of DNA-RNA hybrids in tissue sections.

The state of target nucleic acids in tissue is likely to be different from their condition in solution. In studies in which careful quantitated comparisons have been made, solution hybridization can display differences in "melting curves" in comparison with *in situ* results, suggesting that hybridization affinity in tissue sections is lower than that noted in solution (26). Conceivably, tissue constituents could block some RNA elements and thus destabilize hybrids. The next sections of this chapter examine in more detail specific elements important for maximizing accessibility and specificity of *in situ* hybridization.

SUPPLIES

In situ hybridization is a technique that has been described as "maturing" rather than completely codified (27). Alternative approaches to several procedures exist and work, as noted in the next section, in different settings. Prerequisites for the technique include appropriate tissue or cells; hybridization probe; and solutions for hybridization, washing, and pretreatments. The autoradiographic detection systems can involve film and/or emulsion, with appropriate development solutions. Appropriate approaches to each of these items can be found in the next section of this chapter.

PROCEDURES: PRACTICAL APPROACHES TO *IN SITU* HYBRIDIZATION

Tissue

A variety of cell types and tissue sources have been successful substrates for *in situ* hybridization. Tissue from the brains of numerous species, including humans, has been successfully approached with this technique (Fig. 2). In addition, several different approaches to examining the regulated expression of genes within individual neurons in culture have been developed and employed.

In selecting the species to be examined, several considerations apply. First, there are significant species-to-species differences in many regions of most genes (21). The existence of such cross-species differences provides a hybridization advantage to probes directed at gene sequences from the actual species under study. Use of sequences derived from human cDNAs on hampster tissue, for example, may result in a significant number of base mismatches and consequent reduction in hybridization affinity. Since sequences of many genes are known for the rat and for humans,

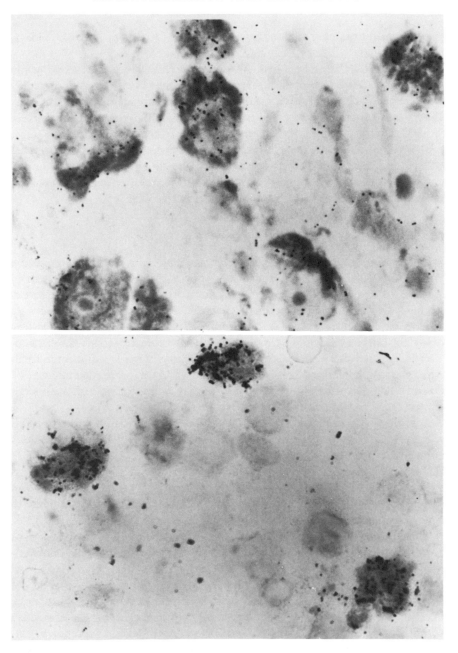

FIG. 2. Bright-field photomicrographs of *in situ* hybridization to vasopressin mRNA in supraoptic neurons from postmortem specimens. Tissue sections from immersion-fixed hypothalamic blocks were probed with ^{35}S-labeled oligonucleotide cDNAs complementary to the human prepropressophysin mRNA, and autoradiography was performed as described in the chapter.(×40 objective magnification.) (Courtesy of S. Rivkees, S. Reppert, M. Chaar, and G. R. Uhl).

these are some of the most frequently used sources of tissue for *in situ* hybridization.

Messenger RNA, the target of hybridization, is thought to be highly labile within disrupted tissue (23). Much of this instability is attributed to the activities of widely distributed and hardy RNase species. Studies of the postmortem fate of particular mRNA species coding for several neuropeptides have demonstrated a relatively surprising stability of levels of these prepropeptide mRNAs in intact tissue (e.g., 28). This stability is only relative, however, and is substantially less than that noted for the receptor binding sites themselves (29). Wherever possible, it is thus important to choose species whose tissues can be rapidly fixed and/or frozen, to preserve the maximum amount of the mRNA found in the *in vivo* state.

Fixation

Fixation speed and efficiency are major components of many *in situ* hybridization protocols (e.g., 20, 30–33). Fixation has several goals. First, it is important to maintain tissue morphology in order to allow the most accurate possible assessment of the mRNA distribution in intact cells and tissues. Second, fixation may inactivate RNase activity. This is important since residual RNase activity in tissue can destroy not only the mRNA targets of hybridization but also complementary RNA radio-labeled hybridization probes. Fixation may also serve to preserve sufficient molecular structure within the tissue section to allow the mRNA hybridization target to be retained in its appropriate site through the lengthy hybridization and wash steps characteristic of many *in situ* hybridization procedures.

An opposing consideration is also present in choosing fixatives. *Over*fixation, especially with bifunctional or cross-linking fixatives such as glutaraldehyde, may prevent large hybridization probes from reaching target mRNAs in tissue (20).

In practice, these concerns are approached by (*a*) fixing tissues as rapidly as possible, preferably by perfusion killing of animals; (*b*) use of fixative regimens that produce intermediate levels of fixation; and (*c*) careful handling of the tissue to avoid contamination with exogenous RNases (Tables 1, 2). One source of RNase, for example, can be the "brain paste" used by many laboratories to embed tissues for frozen sectioning for receptor autoradiography (GR Uhl, unpublished observations).

If hybridization to a high-copy-number mRNA is sought in studies that do not require quantitation, material preserved in a number of different fashions can be used. *In situ* hybridization has been successfully performed on parafin-embedded material, frozen sections of tissue fixed before and after sectioning, celloidin-embedded material, and even unfixed sections (1, 31, 34). Many laboratories use tissue from experimental animals that have been killed by perfusion to obtain optimal results in settings in which higher sensitivity and/or ability to quantitate may be required. We have obtained the best results in studies of human postmortem tissue that was sectioned into blocks of approximately 0.5 cm thickness, as soon as possible after the brain was removed, and immediately fixed by immersion (28).

Quantitated comparisons of the efficacies of a number of fixative types have been performed by Moench, Lawrence, Singer, Gendleman,and coworkers (20, 31). Their results are summarized in Table 1.

In our hands, as suggested by these workers, the best results have been obtained using tissue from animals that have been perfused with the combination glu-taraldehyde/paraformaldehyde fixative PLPG. Other laboratories have experienced different results in different settings, however.

Fixation is often administered as an initial period of perfusion fixation followed by a period of immersion fixation. The immersion can allow some fixation of areas that were inadequately perfused.

Residual fixative in tissue should be removed before probe application to avoid chemical trapping or cross-linking. The "soaking" procedure that removes excess fixative also can have another benefit. Ice crystal formation should be avoided as much as possible during freezing to preserve tissue morphology in frozen sections (35). This is accomplished by soaking the brains in a sucrose-containing buffer. This treatment as well as freezing quickly (at as rapid a rate as possible`without cracking the block due to internal pressure from ice) can thus minimize both resid-ual fixative and ice artifact in frozen sections.

Slide Pretreatment

Because of the affinity of several kinds of radiolabeled hybridization probes for glass, pretreatment of slides before mounting tissue or before applying cells is rec-ommended in most instances. Pretreatment regimens have evolved from the methods used to reduce nonspecific binding in blot hybridization experiments. They frequently include Denhardt's solution or acetylation, a method used to reduce backgrounds in chromosomal squash *in situ* hybridization studies (36). In addition, chrome alum/gelatin coatings often used for immunohistochemical techniques (sub-bing) are employed (35). The general requirements for slide pretreatment include

TABLE 1. *Relative in situ hybridization densities after different fixatives*

Fixative	% Maximal hybridization signal
From refs. 20, 30	
PLPG	100
Karnovsky's	95
Glutaraldehyde (1%)	48
PLP	51
Acetic acid/ethanol	20
Formalin (10%)	18
From ref. 31	
Paraformaldehyde (4%)	100
Glutaraldehyde (4%)	40
Acetic acid/ethanol	20
Carnoy's	20

TABLE 2. *Sample technique for tissue preparation*

1. Anesthetize the animal (65 mg/kg pentobarbital intraperitoneally). Check frequently for loss of nociceptive reflexes.
2. Perform Intracardiac perfusion with a bolus of phosphate-buffered saline to clear blood from the vasculature followed by PLPG (to 1 to 2 ml/g) (20, 22).
3. Remove the brain rapidly.
4. Cut the brain into 0.5-cm slabs.
5. Remove the fixative, and cryoprotect using buffered sucrose solution (22).
6. Freeze as rapidly as possible on cryostat chucks, using powdered dry ice or liquid nitrogen to minimize freeze artifact, and RNase-free synthetic mounting medium. Brains can be stored in this fashion at − 70°C for months without appreciable loss of mRNA. Loss of water from the block surface, however, will render the tissue quality less satisfactory with time.

(From Uhl, ref. 1, with permission.)

(*a*) reducing sticking of the probe to the slide material; (*b*) avoiding degradation of the probe with the procedure; and (*c*) aiding retention of sections through *in situ* procedures. One set of techniques for slide pretreatment is presented in Table 3.

It is important to note that any constituent used in handling or mounting tissue sections could also be a source of contaminating RNase or DNase activity.

Probe Considerations

Workers in *in situ* hybridization have successfully used both complementary DNA (cDNA) and cRNA probes to identify particular mRNAs in tissue (37).

TABLE 3. *Sample techniques for slide preparation: Denhardt/acetylation*

Solution: 20 × Denhardt's (1 liter); 4 of g Ficoll; 4 g of polyvinylpyrrolidone; 4 g of bovine serum albumin; distilled water to final volume of liter.
1. Heat and stir until dissolved (several hr).
2. Freeze in 50-ml aliquots and store at − 20°C.
Solution: Fix (3 parts of 95% ethanol/1 part of glacial acetic acid).

Denhardt treatment
1. Select clean glass slides.
2. Place the slides in glass staining trays (approximately 20/tray).
3. Add the slides to a solution of 1 × Denhardt's (950 ml of dH_2O; 50 ml of 20 × Denhardt's).
4. Incubate 1 to 3 hr at 65°C.
5. Dip the slides in distilled water once, and incubate them in fix for 20 min at room temperature.
6. Air dry thoroughly (at least 12 hr).

Acetylation
1. Prepare 0.1 M triethanolamine solution (74.26 ml of triethanolamine in 3915.7 ml of dH_2O).
2. pH solution to 8.0 using concentrated HCl.
3. Add 10.0 ml of acetic anhydride, and mix vigorously.
4. *Immediately* add the slides to solution, and incubate for 10 min at room temperature.
5. Dehydrate the slides by dipping them for 5 min each in solutions of ETOH: 50%, 70%, 95%, then 100%.
6. Let the slides air dry for at least 12 hr, and store them in a dustproof box at room temperature. Allow at least 24 hr before using.

(From Uhl, ref. 1, with permission.)

cDNAs can be synthesized as random primer-labeled or nick-translated double-stranded probes. In many circumstances, however, these double-stranded probes have given less satisfactory results than those obtained using single-stranded probes. The presence of a radiolabeled mRNA-sense DNA strand in these approaches provides a potential increase in background and competition for the antisense strand, with no predictable increase in the intensity of specific hybridization (but see discussions of "networking") (24). We thus prefer single-stranded hybridization probes.

In determining the optimal length for a hybridization probe, one must balance among several features. Longer sequences have the potential for increased specific activity since one can incorporate more molecules of labeled nucleotide per molecule of DNA. Higher washing stringency can be tolerated by longer probes and can reduce the potential for chance cross-recognition of a nearly identical sequence. Offsetting these advantages are the difficulties in accessibility to RNA embedded within tissue proteins found in larger probes. In practice, several studies have shown that probes in the range of 50 to perhaps 150 to 200 nucleotides may represent an optimal size. The optimal probe size can also depend on the nature of other tissue constituents and on the fixative and pretreating conditions that can hinder and enhance probe access, respectively (see below). These results are supported by studies with equivalently radiolabeled oligogonucleotide cDNA probes of increasing size and studies of cDNAs hybridized under differential conditions of nicking and size fractionation (20, 22).

cRNA probes synthesized by sp6, T7, or T3 RNA polymerases can produce single-stranded species of good length and high specific activity. Unfortunately, length constraints appear to be operative here as well; at least some investigators use basic hydrolysis to reduce the size of their cRNA probes before application to tissues (34, 38, 39). Others, however, appear to be able to rely on tissue constituents to cause sufficient degradation to reduce the probe length to an acceptable size. This procedure can create uncertainty about the size of the radiolabeled hybridization probes that actually recognize mRNA hybridization targets in tissue. Although such uncertainty can represent no great difficulty for qualitative studies, quantitating *in situ* hybridization with probe sequences of differing length can create difficulties due to (*a*) an inability to determine the relative amount of hybridized probe based on its autoradiographic signal, since the specific activities of hybridizing fragments are not known; and (*b*) a potential for selective "sieving," with admission into the tissue of shorter cRNA fragments in preference to long cRNA fragments. Each of these considerations should be addressed when using less stable cRNA probes in quantitated *in situ* hybridization studies. Nevertheless, in actual practice, data obtained using each of these approaches have been interpreted quantitatively and correlated with other measures of abundance of particular mRNAs (e.g., 40).

Tissue Pretreatment and Hybridization

Because of the difficulties with probe access noted above, several kinds of tissue pretreatment have been useful. These treatments can increase hybridization densities, presumably by allowing enhanced probe access to tissue mRNA. The treatments must be balanced with the necessity to retain the hybridization target mRNA in the tissue. Overvigorous treatments can cause loss of hybridization signal, presumably by allowing mRNA to elute from the tissue. Standard treatments developed by Brahic and Haase (26) include hydrochloric acid treatment, proteinase K treatment, and elevated temperature. In our hands, the hydrochloric acid and especially proteinase K treatments are the most effective. Protocols for these two are found in Table 4.

The conditions for hybridizing probes with cells or tissue are optimized to achieve several goals (Table 5). Specific hybridization should be maximized, with appropriate stringencies in both hybridizing and washing conditions. Stringency should be set so that nonspecific interactions of the radiolabeled hybridization probe with random nucleic acid sequences to which it is only partly complementary are minimized. Nonspecific intractions of cDNA or cRNA probes with other tissue constituents or slide material must also be minimized. Interpretation of results is facilitated if the conditions maximize stability of the probe, as noted above. Finally, the use of radiolabeled probe should be optimized so that the maximum amount of information can be derived from use of these expensive materials.

In practice, several laboratories use hybridization conditions that are of modest to moderate stringency, and washing conditions of higher stringency. We thus perform hybridizations in a mix that includes constituents to adjust the hybridization stringency (sodium chloride, formamide) and constituents to reduce nonspecific interactions (Ficoll, polyvinylpyrrolidone, bovine serum albumin, carrier DNA) in a solution that is prepared (autoclaved) and handled (with autoclaved pipettes, diethyl

---

TABLE 4. *Sample techniques for tissue pretreatment*

HCl pretreatment
1. Dry sections at room temperature.
2. Wash slides in 0.2 M HCl (16.6 ml concentrated HCl/liter) for 20 min at room temperature.
3. Wash once in water.

Proteinase K pretreatment
1. Dip slides in a solution containing 400 μl/liter stock proteinase K (final concentration, 1 μg/ml), 982 ml/liter 10 mM Tris[a] (ph 7.4 after heating), and 18 ml/liter 2 mM CaCl$_2$ for 15 min at 37°C (prewarm this solution). The solution will be at pH 7.4 after warming. *Note:* Pretreat the enzyme by warming proteinase K for 30 min at 37°C to predigest RNAse (see below).
2. Dehydrate by dipping twice in water followed by 5-min washes in: 70%, 70% and 100% ETOH.
3. Dry the slides at room temperature. They are now ready for the application of probe but can probably be stored at this step at −70°C.
4. Stock solutions for proteinase K
   a. 10 mM Tris: 1.476 g of Tris (ph 7.7)/liter.
   b. CaCl$_2$ (0.294 g/liter).
   c. Proteinase K: Prepare by dissolving it in 10 mM Tris (pH 7.7) to yield a final concentration of 2.5 mg/ml. Store in 1-ml aliquots at −20°C. Prior to use, incubate for 30 min at 37°C to predigest RNAse.

---

[a]Tris, [tris(hydroxymethyl)aminomethane].
(From Uhl, ref. 1, with permission.)

TABLE 5. *Hybridization protocol*[a]

---

1. Thaw a 1-ml aliquot of deionized formamide and add 0.2 g of dextran sulfate [a 20% (w/v) solution of dextran sulfate in deionized formamide]. Vortex and heat to dissolve (50 to 65°C).
2. Prepare mix:
   5 M NaCl (240 μl)
   2 M Tris (pH 7.4) (10 μl)
   0.2 M EDTA (5 μl)
   50 mg/ml BSA (40 μl)
        Stored frozen
   10% (w/v) Ficoll (4 μl)
   10 (w/v) PVP (4μl)
   Salmon sperm (DNA, 2 mg/ml) (1 μl)
   1 M solution of DTT (1 μl).
3. Add mix to dextran sulfate formamide, vortex, and heat until completely in solution. Add 100 μl to dry probe. Heat and vortex until the probe is in solution. If it does not go into solution, add more probe cocktail. Remove 2 μl and count. Dilute the probe to approximately 10^4 cpm/μl. Apply 25 μl to typical coronal section of rat brain and seal under siliconized coverslips with rubber cement.
4. Incubate 18 to 24 hr at 37°C.
5. Protocol for siliconizing coverslips. This procedure helps prevent tissue sticking to coverslips and RNase contamination.
   a. Place coverslips in glass beaker to maximize surface area exposure.
   b. Add 1% dimethyl dichlorosilane in CCl_4 for 30 sec.
   c. Decant the solution and wash in dH_2O for 20 min.
   d. Wash 3×5 min in dH_2O.
   e. Rinse in 95% EtOH, and spread coverslips onto Whatman paper to dry.
6. Bake in oven 80°C for 2 hr.

The abbreviations used are: EDTA, ethylenediaminetetraacetate; BSA, bovine serum albumin; PVP, polyvinylpyrrolidone; DTT, dithiothreitol.
(From Uhl, ref. 1, with permission.)

pyrocarbonate-treated and autoclaved glassware, and sialinized and autoclaved coverslips) in a way that should minimize RNase contamination and nonspecific interactions of probe with glassware (22). In addition, hybridization is performed under temperature conditions (37 to 65°C) that are important for setting the hybridization stringency.

Since the nature of probes used and the nonspecific interactions with tissue can vary from experiment to experiment, these conditions must be adapted individually for the hybridization sought. Nevertheless, we have used similar sized multiply radiolabeled cDNA probes directed against different mRNA species and in different neuronal populations in brain and in peripheral tissues. These hybridization and washing conditions have proven uniformly efficacious.

Our conditions include a material (dextran sulfate) that excludes DNA from its hydrated radius. Therefore, the radiolabeled cDNA concentration in the small amount of solution overlying the tissue is effectively enhanced, favoring the entry of the probe into tissue.

We attempt to maximize use of the probe by hybridizing in a small volume applied to the tissue under a sialinized, prebaked coverslip. Sealing the edges of the coverslip with rubber cement prevents drying during overnight hybridizations.

At the end of hybridizations, the coverslip can be gently removed, starting at a corner, using a razor blade.

Washing

Initial gentle washes in a standard salt solution (e.g., 2 × SSC) at room temperature remove the bulk of the adsorbed probe and hybridization solution. Next, washes aim to remove radiolabeled hybridization probe molecules that are (a) nonspecifically hybridized to target tissue nucleotide sequences; or (b) trapped in, adsorbed to, or otherwise interacting with other tissue constituents. Changing washing stringency requirements by adjusting temperature, formamide content, and sodium chloride content can be effective in eliminating low-complementarity hybridization (8). Longer washes can enhance removal of probe molecules that are nonspecifically trapped in tissue. Since many of the interactions that stick probes to nonnucleic acid tissue constituents are poorly understood, reducing these features may require trial and error. Since cRNA hybridization probes often display such stickiness, many laboratories use an enzymatic treatment with an RNase *following* hybridization. Such treatment spares cRNA in cRNA-mRNA double-stranded hybrids but digests unhybridized cRNA that may stick to tissue constituents. This degradation facilitates removal of unhybridized sequences (38).

For oligonucleotide cDNA probes, we typically wash at modest stringency for a relatively long period of time and then at a higher stringency for a shorter period of time. Unfortunately, washing at progressively higher temperatures can result in increasing loss of tissue sections from slides. A modest amount of agitation of the washing solution, and washing in large volumes of solution are important considerations for reducing background in these procedures.

Clues to the appropriate washing stringency can be obtained by preliminary experiments. Groups of slides hybridized under the same conditions are washed at several different temperatures with different washing stringencies. The temperature at which the specific hybridization is reduced should correlate (at least roughly) with the T_m predicted from considerations of the probe size, nucleotide content, hybridization conditions, and homology with the target mRNA (see above).

Autoradiography

Dried sections containing radiolabeled cDNA or cRNA probe are subjected to autoradiography to detect and quantitate the radioactivity residing in individual neurons or in individual brain regions. The methodologies for quantitating the autoradiographic signal are similar to those discussed in the chapters on receptor autoradiography. Film autoradiography offers low anatomic resolution but provides the opportunity to determine average hybridization densities over larger areas. These values can be conveniently quantitated with computerized digitizing and densitometric systems. One can easily coexpose autoradiographic standards of known radioactivity to the same piece of film. Film offers an additional advantage: There is no requirement for exposing tissue to the warm liquid emulsion that can provide an opportunity for dissociation of probe-mRNA hybrids and consequent loss of autoradiographic signal. In addition, the same dried slides can be exposed serially to multiple sheets of film. Autoradiographic exposures can thus be adjusted as appropriate.

Answers to many neurobiological questions, however, demand a cellular level of resolution. This resolution can only be achieved by use of emulsion autoradiography (41). The emulsion-coated coverslip technique, described elsewhere in this book, may be used to provide emulsion autoradiograms while avoiding the necessity for dipping tissue sections directly in emulsion. Unfortunately, the levels of resolution provided by this technique are not optimal for the studies at a single-cell level. Therefore, the emulsion dipping technique is most frequently used. Angerer and coworkers (38, 39) have noted a loss of hybridization signal in the low-salt conditions typical of photographic emulsions. Therefore, they and others supplement the emulsion with ammonium acetate. This volatile salt acts to prevent the substantial loss of probe-mRNA hybrids which may occur in liquid emulsion. General autoradiographic techniques as well as approaches to emulsion dilution, application to slides, and development are found elsewhere in this volume.

EXAMPLES: IMPORTANT ISSUES WITH *IN SITU* HYBRIDIZATION

Hybridization Specificity

The results of *in situ* autoradiograms reflect only the presence of radioactivity (or substances mimicking the effect of radioactivity on photographic emulsion) in particular tissue areas. A number of control experiments are necessary to allow confident assignment of the radioactivity present to specific hybridization of the probe to a complementary nucleotide sequence. None of these control experiments individually is able to rule out totally all of the possible artifacts that may appear with *in situ* experiments. As in many histological experiments, absolute biochemical certainty about the nature of the tissue elements being assessed is not possible without destroying the tissue architecture that is the reason to approach the subject in this fashion in the first place. Nevertheless, the results of several control experiments, taken together, provide a substantial body of evidence that the radioactivity viewed does in fact represent hybridization of the radiolabeled probe to target nucleotide sequences within the cells. These concerns have been reviewed in several places (e.g., 42). Important control experiments include the following.

Anatomic Distribution of Hybridization

Frequently, an expected distribution is known from studies of the distribution of immunoreactivity corresponding to the translation products of a particular gene. Thus, the match between hybridization patterns for the mRNA and the peptide immunoreactivity of the translation product provides some evidence for hybridization specificity.

Elimination of Hybridization by Pretreatment with RNase

If, in fact, RNA sequences are being sought, then pretreatment of tissue with enzymes degrading RNA should eliminate the hybridization signal.

Hybridization Stringency

As noted above, tissue elements may render the resistance of hybridization to washing in elevated temperature and low-salt conditions slightly different from those found in solution hybridization. Nevertheless a relatively close fit between the predicted melting temperature and that determined by raising the washing temperatures after *in situ* hybridization and assessing the residual radioactivity can provide evidence for hybridization specificity.

Competition Experiments

If the hybridization takes place at only a finite number of sites, the blockade of these sites by the addition of an excess amount of unlabeled hybridization probe of the same sense as the radiolabeled hybridizing species, or blockade of the hybridization by adding an excess of sequence complementary to the hybridizing species should each provide evidence that the hybridization patterns are specific. These controls are analogous to the "preadsorption controls" commonly used in immunohistochemical studies or to the "cold competition" studies used in receptor autoradiography. Although the strength of interpretations derived from success in these experiments has been criticized, (e.g., 27), failure of competition experiments should lead to significant doubts about hybridization specificity.

Multiple Radiolabeled Sequences

The use of multiple radiolabeled sequences complementary to different regions of the same target mRNA should produce similar patterns. This control should eliminate hybridization based on chance high homology between a single probe and a chance nucleotide sequence different from the authentic mRNA.

Physiological Manipulations

In cases in which physiological manipulations are known to change tissue levels of mRNA (e.g., based on studies of extracted mRNA), the *in situ* hybridization density should change similarly with the same physiological manipulations.

Controls for autoradiographic methodologies should also provide assurance for *in situ* hybridization specificity. The silver grains noted in emulsion autoradiography should not be generated or altered in ways that reflect interactions between emulsion and tissue constituents (41). Issues of negative and positive chemography, and appropriate controls for these features, are discussed in other chapters of this book.

Hybridization Qualification

Substantial additional care is necessary to convert *in situ* hybridization from a qualitative localizing technique to a semiquantitative technique. The strength of quantitative approaches is that they allow comparisons of the relative levels of cellular expression of particular nucleic acid species. Recent reviews address the differences between (*a*) examining change in *relative* levels of gene expression, and (*b*) absolute quantitation of mRNA copy number or densities/cell (43, 44). This chapter deals chiefly with issues of "relative quantitation" since these are probably the most important for answering many neurobiological questions.

In this paradigm, the relative amounts of cellular or regional hybridizable mRNA sequence are at issue, without requirements for absolute quantitation. In order for these studies to be interpretable, several conditions must be satisfied.

Determination of the Density of Radioactivity

Autoradiographic methods provide a two-dimensional record of the radioactivity in an underlying tissue volume. This record thus reflects a density of radiation (e.g., amount/area) rather than a concentration (amount/volume). Under conditions of uniform distribution of radiolabel and known tissue thickness, the conversion of radiation density to concentration can readily be made. If, however, hybridization probe access cannot be shown to be equal through the entire thickness of the tissue, radiation density is the more secure term.

A first prerequisite for quantitation of *in situ* results is that the determination of radioactivity density in the appropriate tissue area must display appropriate quantitative features. This requires demonstration that autoradiographic artifacts are not present and that the emulsion is providing an adequate record of the underlying radioactive emissions. There should be evidence that (*a*) the emulsion is not saturated and (*b*) the radioactivity in the underlying emulsion and the silver grain density in the emulsion display a definable (e.g., linear or power function) relationship over the range of values found in unknown samples (41).

The relationship between radioactivity and either grain density in emulsion autoradiograms or film optical density in film autoradiograms is thus a first issue in quantitation of hybridization. The relationship between the amount of radioactivity in tissue and the autoradiographic signal is termed the "operating characteristic" of the particular autoradiographic detection system (41). This operating characteristic can be determined by coexposing autoradiographic standards of known radioactivity along with the unknown experimental sections to the same autoradiographic detection system. These procedures, detailed in the chapter on quantitation of receptor autoradiography, allow validation of quantitative assumptions. For example, how does a twofold change in grain density over a region correlate with a change in the density of radiation in this region?

Positive and negative chemography and quenching of the emitted radioactivity by tissue elements are other concerns in interpretation of *in situ* studies as they are in tissue receptor autoradiography. Grain densities will not assess underlying radioactivity accurately if nonradioactive tissue elements falsely cause conversion of silver grains to the exposed form or falsely block ("quench") such conversion by *bona fide* radioactive emissions.

Many *in situ* hybridization probes are radiolabeled with isotopes displaying a long mean free path length. In these cases, the density of silver grains recorded in emulsion overlying a tissue with a given density of hybridized probe in each mg of tissue can vary if there are variations in the thickness of either the tissue section or the emulsion (41). Thicker tissue regions that contain the same number of dpm/mg will nevertheless have more dpm/unit area. Thicker emulsion, on the other hand, will display an enhanced number of silver grains/unit area after exposure to a given density of radiation. Careful attention should thus be paid to uniformity of thickness of both tissue and emulsion.

Another concern in using isotopes with relatively long mean free path lengths through emulsion involves the difficulty in determining all of the consequences of radioactive emissions associated with small objects such as individual neurons. In these cases, determination of the relative density of radioactivity should take into account the fact that silver grains derived from probe molecules that are localized to a single cell may be detected at a distance many microns from the emitting cell. Attention to each of these concerns can ensure that the quantitative techniques of autoradiography can describe the density of radioactivity in tissue sections or cells underlying the emulsion.

Determination of the Density of Hybridization Probe

A second set of concerns arises in relating the radiation that is associated with the tissue to the actual quantity of hybridized probe. This calculation can be performed securely under circumstances in which all of the probe in the tissue is hybridized to the appropriate mRNA target species and in which all of the radioactivity emitted from the tissue is associated with probe in a known fashion (44). In other words, both the specific activity and the exact nature of the hybridizing species must be known with some precision. When mixtures of partially hydrolyzed probes leave open the possibility for differential sieving and selective access of relatively small probe fragments to the RNA in the tissue, the specific activity of the hybridizing material may differ substantially from the specific activity of the probe mixture applied to the tissue. If a probe molecule is degraded during hybridization, similar considerations can prevail. Thus, attention to the stability and homogeneity of the hybridization probes is of great help in estimating accurately the relationship between the density of radiation detected in the autoradiographic detection system and the number of copies of hybridized probe.

Relationship between the Density of Hybridized Probe and the Density of Target mRNA in Tissue

Background

If the radiolabeled probe has significant numbers of nonspecific interactions with tissue constituents, as is almost always the case, then a background level of autoradiographic signal will be present over areas distant from cells anticipated to express the appropriate mRNA. "Background" autoradiographic estimates can be obtained from these zones and subtracted from the densities of the "specific" interactions (41). These measurements can also correct for autoradiographic method background due to ionizing atmospheric radiation. Greater assurance of quantitation can be obtained under conditions in which this background is relatively low in comparison with the specific signal being sought. The statistical basis for these background corrections is discussed by Rogers (41).

Accessibility to Probe

mRNA hybridization targets are not necessarily accessible to hybridization probes. These hybridization targets are potentially blocked, and even potentially blocked to differing degrees, by associated proteins, nascent polypeptide chains, ribosomes, and other tissue elements. The density of hybridization signal will most accurately reflect the number of molecules of mRNA in the cell if these hindrances are minimized. Several investigators use deproteinizing pretreatments (e.g., proteinase K) before *in situ* hybridization to facilitate access of the hybridization probe to the target mRNAs (26).

The relationship between the amount of mRNA hybridization target in the cell and the amount of target available for hybridization within the cell can also vary with differences in the hybridizing probes. In general, relatively shorter (e.g., 40 to *ca.* 250 bases) probes have proven of optimal effectiveness for *in situ* hybridization studies (20, 22). This may reflect the lower chance that tissue constituents could interfere with the accessibility of shorter hybridization probes to the cellular compartment at which the RNA is localized.

Attention to these considerations is potentially important. If two tissue samples under two different conditions display differential accessibility of radiolabeled probes to tissue constituents, it is conceivable that differential access to even the same number of copies of mRNA could result in differences in hybridization signal. However, demonstrating that such a mechanism actually occurs in a specific setting can be difficult.

Loss of mRNA from Tissue Sections

Pretreatments and other steps that enhance probe access to mRNA can also change the structure of tissue constituents so that otherwise hybridizable mRNA can be lost from the tissue during hybridization, washing, or autoradiographic procedures. Evidence for mRNA elution derives from examining changes in hybridization signal under different conditions anticipated to "elute" the mRNA targets from tissue sections (31). Such losses can be minimized with use of the bifunctional fixative, glutaraldehyde.

Saturation versus Nonsaturation Analyses

The relationship between the applied concentration of radiolabeled hybridization probe and the hybridization signal must be considered. Some authors feel that quantitative assessments of differential hybridization densities can be achieved only under conditions in which all of the hybridizable target RNA in the tissue is thought to be saturated with hybridization probe. In practice, use of the high probe concentrations necessary to achieve this may cause increased background due to the enhanced ability of higher probe concentrations to exhibit nonspecific interactions with the number of other tissue constituents. Use of such concentrations may also lead to an increased chance for hybridization to nucleic acid sequences with chance modest degrees of homology with the probe.

An alternative approach to determining the relationship between the density of the hybridization signal and the density of the target RNA involves construction of model hybridization targets in which known and increasing amounts of hybridization target sequence are subject to hybridization with a known, even subsaturating, concentration of hybridization probe. Using oligonucleotides partially fixed to brain paste or using sp6 product mRNA-sense RNA baked to small filter discs, it is possible to determine the relationship between known amount of hybridization targets and the density of autoradiographic hybridization signal (44, 45).

DISCUSSION AND SUMMARY

Several different issues thus need to be addressed before quantitated information can be derived from *in situ* hybridization autoradiograms.

With attention to each of these features, however, there is an increasing consensus among several laboratories active in the field that relative quantitation of *in situ* hybridization densities can be validly made. These opinions are now buttressed by numerous instances in which a change in gene expression determined by *in situ* hybridization fits well with that determined in studies of extracted mRNAs.

This chapter has approached basic features of the *in situ* hybridization technique. Developments including the use of simultaneous *in situ* hybridization and immunohistochemistry, use of nonisotopic probe labeling, electron microscopic *in situ* studies examining the subcellular localization of mRNAs, use of two separately radiolabeled probes to detect two different mRNAs in a single tissue section, use of *in situ* transcription for possible amplification of signal, and use of probes directed against intron sequences to assess the extent of expression of primary transcript hnRNAs all extend its possible usefulness (33, 43, 46–50). These studies will remain mainstays in elucidation of the molecular biology of the brain.

APPLICATIONS

The ability to define the distribution and the extent of expression of a particular mRNA within cells of a heterogeneous cell population most cogently illustrates the power of *in situ* hybridization. The major biological impact of the technique may arise from its ability to detect changes in this distribution.

Modulation of pain is an important biological problem (51). One key site in which information from peripheral afferents and signals from descending modulatory zones, drugs, and local modulating circuitry all interact is lamina I and II of the dorsal horn of the spinal cord or the equivalent area (for facial pain) of the nucleus caudalis of the spinal tract of the trigeminal. Immunohistochemical studies have shown that both of these layers contain elements, chiefly interneurons, that express the two principle brain opioid peptide genes: preproenkephalin (preproenkephalin A) and preprodynorphin (preproenkephalin B) (52, 53). (Figs. 3 and 4). In applying *in situ* hybridization procedures to studying the responses of these neurons to physiological inputs and drugs, several issues must be faced (54).

1. The mRNA regions targeted by the probes were defined. Since preproenkephalin and preprodynorphin are members of a gene family that contains many similar sequences, oligonucleotide internally radiolabeled cDNA probes were developed which recognized relatively specific segments of each of these genes. These probes, therefore, were able to avoid the regions of high homology which might allow for cross-recognition of preproenkephalin mRNA by longer cDNA or cRNA probes directed against preprodynorphin, or vice versa. Since the structures of both rat genes are known, since the rat is an animal amenable to the experimental manipulations required, and since these animals can be promptly killed by perfusion fixation, probes were constructed which were complementary to the rat preproenkephalin and preprodynorphin cDNA sequences, and only rat tissue used.

2. The specificities of probes directed against enkephalin and dynorphin were defined. Tests of anatomical specificity of hybridization, susceptibility to RNAse treatment, susceptibility to several different kinds of competition experiments, parallels between results obtained using different probes, and the results of Northern analyses with cRNA probes directed against isolated mRNA, melting temperature experiments, and RNAse digestion experiments were all consistent with specific recognition of the appropriate mRNA by each of the probes directed against preproenkephalin and preprodynorphin (45, 54). In addition, construction of several different probes recognizing each mRNA led to similar results.

3. Aspects important for quantitation were validated. Conditions were set so that emulsion saturation was avoided. Probes were used under conditions in which hybridization to synthetic mRNA, transcribed *in vitro* by sp6 or T7 polymerases from

ENK

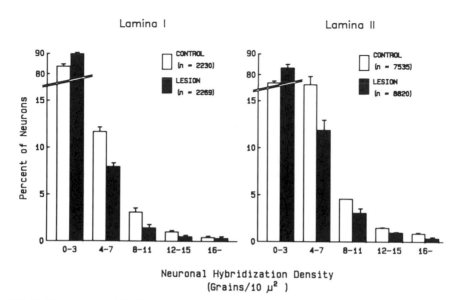

FIG. 3. Frequency distribution histograms of neuronal hybridization densities with ^{35}S-labeled oligonucleotides directed against preproenkephalin mRNA in neurons of lamina I and II of the nucleus ipsilateral (*solid bars*) and contralateral (*open bars*) to unilateral trigeminal lesions. Grains in a 10-μm area overlying each neuron in laminae I (*left*) and II (*right*) were quantitated. Background values were subtracted, and the fraction of total cells falling into each hybridization density class is noted here; n, no. of neurons evaluated. These data derive from quantitation of nine slides from the brains of three animals killed 4 days after trigeminal lesions. *Bars*, standard error of the mean; this value is essentially zero where no bar appears.

cDNAs subcloned into transcription vectors (such as pGEM) yielded a roughly linear increase in hybridization signal with linear increases in the concentration of hybridization target (42). In addition, the relative ratios of hybridization using these probes (in comparison with each other) in *in situ* hybridization studies in another brain area more amenable to mRNA extraction (the striatum) paralleled the results of quantitated Northern analyses of mRNA extracted from the same region (45).

4. *In situ* hybridization procedures using the protocols outlined in this chapter and in ref. 1 resulted in an uneven distribution of autoradiographic grains above different cells of lamina I and lamina II of the nucleus caudalis. Anatomical differences in the distribution of cells hybridizing with enkephalin and dynorphin probes were noted, in concordance with the subtle differences in the immunohisto-chemically determined distribution of peptide translation products of these two genes. Furthermore, hybridization signals over many neurons were more than four to five times background values determined from measuring grain densities over adjacent tissue devoid of preproenkephalin or preprodynorphin mRNA. It should be

ENK

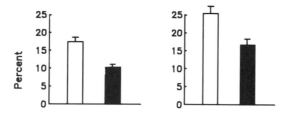

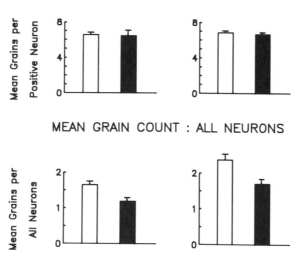

FIG. 4. Distribution of neuronal preproenkephalin mRNA hybridization densities ipsilateral (*dark bar*) and contralateral (*open bar*) to unilateral trigeminal lesions. *Top*, fraction of neurons in lamina I (*left*) and II (*right*) which display positive hybridization. *Middle*, mean grain density over positively hybridizing neurons in lamina I (*left*) and II (*right*). *Bottom*, mean grain density over all neurons. *Bars*, standard error of the mean. Values are corrected for autoradiographic background. The differences displayed in both the *top* and *bottom panels* are statistically significant (*P* < 0.01).

noted that these are pessimistic estimates of background values. Values over the slide glass adjacent to the section were significantly lower.

5. Sampling of the nucleus was important. In preliminary experiments, the rostral to caudal extent of the nucleus caudalis was assessed at 250-μm intervals. There were no large gradients in the rostro-caudal extent of expression of pre-

proenkephalin (T. Nishimori, M. Moskowicz, and G. Uhl, unpublished observations). Furthermore, right-to-left-sided variation in hybridization densities in these normal animals was quite small. We thus chose to examine routinely three different anatomical levels of the nucleus caudalis, and we feel confident that right-to-left differences observed following unilateral changes in inputs were related to these changed inputs not just to right-to-left variability in normal expression patterns.

6. Since these peptide genes are expressed principally in neurons and since neurons can be identified with fairly great reliability based on morphologic criteria, we assessed only hybridization densities over neurons. Furthermore, since partial voluming (cutting through a neuron so as to include only a thin sliver of the cell in the edge of the section) was a possibility, we sampled only neurons whose nuclei were included in the plane of sectioning.

7. Assessments of grain densities overlying neurons were undertaken. We wished to have a value that would be related to mRNA concentration more than to total mRNA content. This allowed us to sample the maximally dense grain area overlying each neuron. We used a calibrated eyepiece grid to obtain grain count information over a 10×10-μm area of each neuron examined in lamina I and II of the nucleus caudalis. Counts were performed on the right and left sides in sections taken at each of the three anatomically defined levels noted above, and background values were subtracted. We thus obtained estimates of background-corrected hybridization densities for each neuron in lamina I and II on each side of the brain. Subsequently, it became clear that sampling approximately 100 neurons/section on each side would allow biologically significant differences to be detected with less effort. Accordingly, we were able to decrease the sample size of cells assayed for each animal in subsequent experiments (54). The hybridization densities were described as frequency distribution histograms, with background values subtracted (Fig. 3). Since each value is corrected by subtraction for a background grain density of less than one grain/10 μm^2, cells displaying more than three grains/10 μm^2 are considered to be positively labeled. Changes in the entire population or changes in the population that we consider positively labeled can thus be analyzed according to these criteria.

8. Several different physiological manipulations change the expression of these genes in these neuronal populations and are reflected in alterations in the shapes of histograms that display population distributions of grain densities. We have focused on changes in afferent input. Depletion of primary afferent inputs by lesions of the trigeminal ganglia leads to a dramatic down-regulation of preproenkephalin expression. Analysis of this change reveals that it reflects chiefly a "turning off" of expression in a subpopulation of cells. Thus, the mean grain density over neurons that express preproenkephalin mRNA is virtually unchanged after deafferentation, although the fraction of positively expressing cells drops by 35 to 40% (54). Interestingly, dynorphin mRNA assayed in neighboring sections from the same animals displays increased expression. This increase is due largely to recruitment of 25 to 70% of new cells to the expressing population (54). Each of these effects is assessed by comparing the results in the control side from the same animals with results on

the side of the unilateral lesion. Control values, further, are similar to those noted in unmanipulated animals.

This application of *in situ* hybridization technology to the assessment of the dynamics of neuronal gene expression can be treated in several different statistical ways. McCabe and coworkers (55) have adapted population statistics for sophisticated comparisons. In most cases, however, the biological question to be addressed can be framed in simple terms: Is the fraction of expressing cells changed? Is the intensity of expression changed? We have obtained these values in each case and assessed their statistical significance by conventional two-sample testing.

Acknowledgments

I am grateful to Maamoun Chaar, Lisa Lloyd, Victoria Stranov, Kelly Hill, Gail Hackney, Chon Vo, Gary Garayan, and Phillip Behn for technical assistance with the studies described here; to Mrs. Debbie Button for careful assistance with the manuscript; and to Drs. Cathy Sasek, Scott Rivkes, Mark Voigt, and especially Toshikazu Nishimori for sharing in this work. Drs. E. London, M. Kuhar, M. Rattray, and J. Rao generously reviewed the manuscript. These studies from my laboratory were supported by the intramural program of the National Institute of Drug Abuse, the Howard Hughes Medical Institute, the McKnight Foundation, the Sloan Foundation, the American Parkinson's Disease Association, and the National Institutes of Health.

REFERENCES

1. Uhl GR. *In situ hybridization in brain*. New York: Plenum Publishing Corp, 1986.
2. Young WS III. *Trends Neurosci* 1986;9;549–551.
3. Cox KH, DeLeon DV, Angerer LM, Angerer RC. *Dev Biol* 1984;101:485–502.
4. Gall JG, Pardue ML. *Proc Natl Acad Sci USA* 1969;63:378–383.
5. Gee CE, Roberts JL. *DNA* 1983;2:157–163.
6. Haase AT, Stowring L, Geballe A, Blum H, Ventura P, Brahic M. *Biotechniques*, in press.
7. Harrison PR, Conkie D, Paul J. *FEBS Lett* 1973;32:109–112.
8. Hudson P, Penschow J, Shine J, Ryan G, Niall H, Coghlan J. *Endocrinology* 1981;108:353–356.
9. Kawata M, McCabe JT, Pfaff DW. *Brain Res Bull* 1988;20:693–697.
10. Lewis ME, Krause RG II, Robert-Lewis JM. *Synapse* 1988;2:308–316.
11. Terenghi G, Polak JM, Hamid Q, et al. *Proc Natl Acad Sci USA* 1987;84:7315–7318.
12. Hames BD, Higgins SJ *Nucleic acid hybridisation: A practical approach*. Washington DC: IRL Press, 1985.
13. Voigt MM, Uhl GR. *Mol Brain Res* 1988;4:247–253.
14. Segerson TP, Hoefler H, Childers H, et al. *Endocrinology* 1987;121:98–107.
15. Rennert PD, Heinrich G. In: Uhl G, ed. *In situ hybridization in brain*. New York: Plenum Publishing Corp, 1986;166–169.
16. Buckley NJ, Bonner TI, Brann MR. *J Neurosci* 1988;8:4646–4652.
17. Goldman D, Deneris E, Luyten W, Kochhar A, Patrick J, Heinemann S. *Cell* 1987;48:965–973.
18. Sequier JM, Richards JG, Malherbe P, Price GW, Mathews S, Mohler H. *Proc Natl Acad Sci USA* 1988;85:7815–7819.
19. Uhl GR, Evans J, Parta M, et al. Uhl G, ed. *In situ hybridization in brain*. New York: Plenum Publishing Corp, 1986;21–47.

20. Moench TR, Gendelman HE, Clements JE, Narayan O, Griffin DE. *J Virol Methods* 1985;11:119–130.
21. Lewin B. *Genes III*. New York: John Wiley & Sons, 1987.
22. Uhl GR, Zingg HH, Habener JF. *Proc Natl Acad Sci USA* 1985;82:5555–5559.
23. Maniatis T, Fritsch EF, Sambrook J. *Molecular cloning: A laboratory manual*. Cold Spring Harbor NY: Cold Spring Harbor Laboratory, 1982.
24. Campbell DJ In: Uhl G, ed. *In situ hybridization in brain*. New York: Plenum Publishing Corp, 1986;239–242.
25. Baldino F Jr, Davis LG. In: Uhl G, ed.*In situ hybridization in brain*. New York: Plenum Publishing Corp, 1986;97–116.
26. Brahic M, Hasase AT. *Proc Natl Acad Sci USA* 1978;75:6125–6129.
27. Watson S, Patel P, Burke S, Herman J, Schafer M, Kwak S. *In situ hybridization and related techniques to study cell-specific gene expression in the nervous system*. Toronto, Ontario: Society for Neuroscience, 1988.
28. Rivkees SA, Chaar MR, Hanely DF, Maxwell M, Reppert SM, Uhl GR. *Synapse*, 1989;3:246–254.
29. Whitehouse PJ, Lynch D, Kuhar MJ. *J Neurochem* 1984;43:553–559.
30. Gendelman HE, Moench TR, Narayan O, Griffin DE. *J Immunol Methods* 1983;65:137–145.
31. Lawrence JB, Singer RH. *Nucleic Acids Res* 1985;13:1777–1799.
32. McAllister HA, Rock DL. *J Histochem Cytochem* 1985;33:1026–1032.
33. Singer RH, Lawrence JB, Villnave C. *BioTechniques* 1986;4:230–250.
34. Angerer LM, Stoler MH, Angerer RC. In: Valentino KL, Eberwine JH, Barchas JD, eds. *In situ hybridization: Application to neurobiology*. New York: Oxford University Press, 1987:1–23.
35. Luna LG *Manual of histologic staining methods of the armed forces institute of pathology*. New York: McGraw-Hill Book Company, 1968.
36. Hayashi S, Gillam IC, Delaney AD, Tener GM. *J Histochem Cytochem* 1978;26:677–679.
37. Uhl G. In: Uhl G, ed. *In situ hybridization in brain*. New York: Plenum Publishing Corp, 1986;227–232.
38. Angerer LM, Angerer RC. *Nucleic Acids Res* 1981;9:2819–2840.
39. Angerer LM, DeLeon DV, Angerer RC, Showman RM, Wells DE, Raff RA. *Dev Biol* 1984;101:477–484.
40. Shivers BD, Harlan RE, Romano GJ, Howells RD, Pfaff DW. In: Uhl G, ed. *In situ hybridization in brain*. New York: Plenum Publishing Corp, 1986;3–20.
41. Rogers AW. *Techniques of autoradiography*. New York: Elsevier Science Publishing Co, 1973.
42. Uhl GR. In: Uhl G, ed. *In situ hybridization in brain*. New York: Plenum Publishing Corp, 1986;253–256.
43. Conn PM. *Neuroendocrine Peptide Methodology*. San Diego CA: Academic Press, 1989.
44. Uhl GR. In: Conn M, ed. *Neuroendocrine peptide methodology*. San Diego CA: Academic Press, 1989;135–146.
45. Uhl GR, Navia B, Douglas J. *J Neurosci* 1988;8:4755–4764.
46. Brahic M, Haase AT, Cash, E. *Proc Natl Acad Sci USA* 1984;81:5445–5448.
47. Fremeau RT Jr, Lundblad JR, Pritchett DB, Wilicox JN, Roberts JL. *Science* 1986;234:1265–1269.
48. Haase AT, Walker D, Stowring L, Ventura P, Geballe A, Blum H. *Science* 1985;227:189–192.
49. Lawrence JB, Singer RH. *Cell* 1986;45:407–415.
50. Lum JB. *BioTechniques* 1986;4:32–39.
51. Wall PD, Melzack R. *Textbook of pain*. New York: Churchill Livingstone, 1985.
52. Uhl G, Goodman RR, Kuhar MJ, Childers SR, Snyder SH. *Brain Res* 1979;166:75–94.
53. Watson SJ, Khachaturian H, Taylor L, Fischli W, Goldstein A, Akil H. *Proc Natl Acad Sci USA* 1983;80:891–894.
54. Nishimori T, Moskowitz MA, Uhl GR. *J Comp Neurol* 1988;274:142–150.
55. McCabe JT, Desharnais RA, Pfaff DW. In: Conn M, ed. *Neuroendocrine peptide methodology*. San Diego CA: Academic Press, 1989;107–133.

Methods in Neurotransmitter Receptor Analysis,
edited by Henry I. Yamamura, et al.
Raven Press, Ltd., New York © 1990.

9

Receptor Binding as a Method for Drug Discovery

William J. Kinnier

Nova Pharmaceutical Corporation, Baltimore, Maryland 21224

The work of Ondetti and his collaborators on captopril is the best known example of *de novo* drug design based on knowledge of the active site (1). This contrasts with the discovery of most other drugs, which required the evaluation of many compounds, serendipity, and astute observations. Often, agents made for one purpose are found to have another useful although unexpected action. Three examples of this phenomenon are imipramine, iproniazid, and mephenesin.

In 1950, the tricyclic antidepressant imipramine was originally submitted by the Giegy Company for clinical testing as an antihistamine. However, it was later found to be effective for the alleviation of depression (2).

The monoamine oxidase inhibitor (MAO) inhibitor iproniazid was designed for the treatment of tuberculosis. Although it lacked efficacy in the treatment of this disorder, it was heard to help alleviate the depression that often accompanies this disease. By 1957 it was recognized to be clinically effective in the treatment of depression (2).

Mephenesin was developed as an antibiotic for Gram-negative bacteria. During toxicity tests, researchers observed its muscle relaxant properties. The discovery of mephenesin paved the way for the identification of the anxiolytics such as diazepam and chlordiazepoxide (2).

Serendipity and experimental observation will always be fundamental requirements of drug discovery until primary, secondary, and tertiary structures of receptors have been well characterized, making it possible for computers to model active agents. Although the age of computer drug design is rapidly approaching, it is still necessary to continue to screen a variety of agents in order to identify a lead. One method to speed this drug discovery process is the receptor binding assay. The identification of a novel chemical entity using receptor binding techniques provides the chemist with the initial clue regarding the structure of a potential useful therapeutic agent. The chemical modification of this structure can then be undertaken to improve potency, selectivity, safety, and bioavailability. It must be remembered, however, that although receptor binding assays speed the drug discovery process, they do not shorten the time necessary for drug development. Nevertheless, these assays are proving to be valuable tools for identifying novel chemical structures that can be manipulated in developing new generations of drugs.

The use of binding assays to study neuronal receptor systems was popularized in 1973 (3–5). Fifteen years later, this approach has been applied successfully to more than 80 receptor systems.

The availability of so many assays makes it possible to examine the selectivity of thousands of compounds in a matter of days, as well as providing a means for discovering agents that interact at sites that have yet to be characterized in other ways. Although receptor binding assays do not improve the odds of discovery, they do speed the process in obtaining that goal. The aim of this chapter is to define the logistics, techniques, management, and pitfalls associated with the large-scale utilization of receptor binding assays in a drug discovery program.

PRINCIPLES

The underlying principles of receptor binding assays are detailed under "Methods for Receptor Binding" in *Neurotransmitter Receptor Binding*, the comparison volume of that text. The same principles apply for drug screening, which differs only in that it invokes more logistical planning and medicinal chemistry structure-activity analysis.

SUPPLIES

In addition to the standard industry equipment and supplies necessary for biochemical studies, there are some software packages that are particularly useful when performing receptor binding assays on a large scale. These include the following.

Molecular Design Limited Software for selecting compounds and performing structure activity analysis is a package available from Molecular Design Limited (MDL), 2132 Farallon Drive, San Leandro, CA 94577.

Compound Inventory System Software has many useful options for managing compound inventories, bar coding, molarity calculations, and other features. It is available from Charles Flagles Associates, Baltimore, MD.

Oracle Relational Database Management Systems is an excellent software package for analyzing binding data. It has been designed to interface with MDL software. It is available from Oracle Corporation, Belmont, CA.

PROCEDURES

The accurate analysis of thousands of compounds requires careful planning, coordination, and organization at various levels. Once therapeutic areas have been targeted and the appropriate receptor binding assays identified, test compounds must be weighed, solubilized, and analyzed. Following this, the data must be calculated, interpreted, sorted, and reported.

Compound Selection

The compounds chosen for analysis can be preselected or may be tested on a random basis. By definition, preselection introduces a certain bias, although it allows for the elimination of compounds known to be toxic or unstable (see Table 1). Prescreening can be enhanced and simplified if a general structure is placed into a database like Molecular Design Limited which enables the computer to eliminate substances based on undesirable structural characteristics. This database is most useful in selecting compounds of similar structure once a lead has been identified. With a random approach, all compounds are tested as long as they are soluble. In general, combinations of these two approaches appear to work best, with the weighting of the random selection process by 80 to 90% in the beginning and then shifting to greater emphasis on preselection as compounds with activity begin to emerge from testing.

Weighing

Once the compounds have been selected, each must be weighed to prepare a known concentration. In this step, transcriptional errors of compound identity or weights are the biggest potential errors. Bar coding each container and interfacing the analytical balance with a personal computer capable of printing the label can minimize these errors. The compound identity from the bar code reader and weight can be printed onto a label that is affixed to the sample bottle. Furthermore, software is available for calculating and printing on the label the volume to achieve a designated molarity.

Solubilization

Potential solvent that will not interfere with the receptor binding assays must first be identified before dissolving the test agents. Although there is no universal vehicle, with the success of any given solvent being largely dependent on the nature of the compounds. Certain ones have been found to be particularly useful. For example, the addition of enough dimethyl sulfoxide (DMSO) to make a 10% solution in water is a procedure that will dissolve a large percentage of most chemical libraries. It takes two individuals approximately 1 day to add vehicles to 1,000 compounds. Table 2 lists other commonly used solvents that have proven to be of value in dissolving compounds for receptor binding assays.

Inherent in screening large chemical libraries is the long sample preparation time.

TABLE 1. *Protocol for screening test agents for activity at*
β-adrenergic receptor binding sites

1. *Homogenization buffer*
   Tris[tris(hydroxymethyl)aminomethane]/HCl, 50 μM, pH 8.0, at 25°C (3 liters/100 tubes) is prepared from reagent grade materials purchased from Sigma Chemical Company.
2. *Membrane suspension preparation*
   Male Sprague-Dawley rats (150 g body weight) are killed by decapitation, and the brains are rapidly removed and chilled in ice-cold 50 mM Tris/HCl buffer, pH 8.0. The cerebral cortices are dissected and homogenized in 50 volumes of ice-cold 50 mM Tris/HCl buffer, pH 8.0, using a Polytron tissue grinder at a setting of 6 for 15 sec. The homogenate is centrifuged at $49,000 \times g$ for 15 min. The pellet is resuspended in 50 volumes of the homogenization buffer and centrifuged as before two more times. The membrane pellet is dispersed in 30 volumes of the above mentioned buffer to give a protein concentration about 1 mg/ml (referred to as membrane suspension) which should be kept on ice.
3. *Radioligand stock solution*
   $(-)$ [^{3}H]Dihydroalprenolol with specific activity >30 Ci/mmol is obtained from Du Pont-New England Nuclear and stored at $-20°C$ before use. A stock solution of 5 nM [^{3}H]Dihydroalprenolol (11 ml/100 tubes) is prepared with homogenization buffer just prior to starting the experiment.
4. *Unlabeled ligand stock solution*
   A stock solution of 10 μM $(-)$-alprenolol (11 ml/100 tubes) is prepared in homogenization buffer just prior to starting the experiment. $(-)$-Alprenolol is available from Sigma Chemical Company.
5. *Test compound stock solution*
   A stock solution for each test compound of 100 μM in homogenization buffer if possible. Addition of other vehicles maybe necessary (Table 2).
6. *Content for total tubes*
   Prepare tubes (12×75 mm; usually in triplicate) for measuring total binding by pipetting 800 μl of membrane suspension, 100 μl of radioligand stock solution, and 100 μl of homogenization buffer. A separate set of total tubes should be prepared per rack of test tubes.
7. *Content for nonspecific tube*
   Prepare tubes (12×75 mm; usually in triplicate) for measuring nonspecific binding by pipetting 800 μl of membrane suspension, 100 μl of radioligand stock solution, and 100 μl of unlabeled ligand stock solution. A separate set of nonspecific binding tubes should be prepared per rack of test tubes.
8. *Contents for test compound tubes*
   Prepare tubes (12×75 mm; usually in triplicate) for measuring test substance binding by pipetting 800 μl of membrane suspension, 100 μl of radioligand stock solution, and 100 μl of test substance stock.
9. *Incubation conditions*
   Each rack of tubes is placed in a shaking water bath at 25°C for 20 min.
10. *Termination*
    At the end of the incubation period, the rack is removed from the bath, and the contents of tube are removed using a Brandel filtration manifold with GF/C Whatman filter paper. The tubes are rinsed four times with cold homogenization buffer.
11. *Quantitation of radioactivity*
    Each filter is placed in a separate scintillation counting vial, and 4 ml of Beckman EP Ready Solv or its equivalent is added to each tube. The filter is allowed to soak overnight before counting in a scintillation counter whose settings are adjusted for counting tritium with the greatest efficacy and expressed in dpm.
12. *Results (in dpm)*
    Total binding: 1,000
    Nonspecific binding: 200
    Test compound 10001 binding: 1,000
    Test compound 10002 binding: 1,000
    Test compound 10028 binding: 204
    Test compound 10038 binding: 128

    The nonspecific dpm are subtracted from all the dpm, leaving what is defined as specific binding. Generally, these are further expressed as percent inhibition of binding when no test substance was present (i.e., total binding tube (1,000 dpm) − nonspecific binding tube (200 dpm) = specific binding (800 dpm) is defined as 0% inhibition; whereas test compound 10038 binding (328 dpm) − nonspecific binding (200 dpm) = specific test compound binding (128 dpm) when expressed as percent inhibition: $\frac{(800-128)}{800} \times 100 = 84\%$ inhibition (Table 3).

TABLE 2. *Solvents found useful for dissolving test compounds prior to receptor binding assay*

Vehicle
20% Polyethylene glycol 300
1 N HCl
1 N Acetic acid
1 N KOH
10% Dimethyl sulfoxide

During the sample selection process, compounds of limited stability should be discarded or other arrangements made for testing such agents as expeditiously as possible.

Receptor Binding Methodology

The end point of a receptor binding assay is the quantitation of radioactivity attached to a tissue fragment. The basic tools are a "hot" ligand (radioligand), receptors, "cold" (unlabeled) ligand, incubation buffer, an apparatus for terminating the receptor (centrifuge or filtration box), and an instrument for detecting radioactivity (scinitillation or γ-counter) (6–8).

The radioligand used to label the device receptor can be synthesized or obtained commercially. The selectivity, specific activity, purity, and stability of the radioligand must be known. Selectivity refers to the ability of the ligand to bind in a select manner to the receptor of interest. Typically, selectivity is characterized before a radioligand becomes commercially available, although it is wise to validate this properly before undertaking a massive screen of lead agents. Selectivity is definded by comparing the ability of a variety of unlabeled agents to inhibit the attachment of this radioligand with their known potencies to interact with this receptor in physiological assays.

Prior to the early 1970s, radioactive ligands did not possess specific activities high enough to be useful in detecting neurotransmitter receptors. Since the number of receptors is quite small in comparison with other cellular components, it is essential to utilize radioligands with specific activities >30 Ci/mmol.

A suitable unlabeled ligand is one that is selective for the receptor of interest. This substance is added to the incubation medium to compete with the labeled ligand for the receptor site being analyzed. By including a high concentration of unlabeled compound, it is possible to eliminate the binding of the radioligand to the desired site, leaving bound only those radioactive molecules that adhere to nonreceptor components on the tissue. The tissue source for receptor can be obtained from whole organ homogenates, organ subsections, tissue cultures, subcellular fractions of tissue, purified or cloned receptors. Although the preparation of a homogenate from a whole organ preparation will be described, the same principles apply for other receptor sources.

The desired tissue is disrupted by homogenization to yield cellular fragments. The receptor population is enriched usually by centrifrugation to rid the homogenate of the more soluble components, especially the endogenous neurotransmitters that may adhere to the receptor. This is accomplished by several washes using the homogenization buffer. The buffer typically has a pH and ionic strength that have been found to be optimal for labeling the receptor of interest. The homogenation procedure and all subsequent steps are routinely conducted out at 4°C to minimize receptor degradation. Furthermore, tissue concentration (mg/ml buffer) is also optimized so that the binding experiments are conducted on the linear portion of the tissue concentration versus specific binding curve. When following a published procedure, any modification in the above requires that the assay be revalidated.

The incubation conditions must also be optimized with regard to pH, ion requirements, temperature, and duration. Indeed, the choice of buffers is dependent on the buffering capacity at the optimal pH. The goal in establishing the optimal conditions is to maintain receptor binding characteristics consistent with the appropriate pharmacological profile.

Following incubation, the tissue with bound radioactivity must be separated from the incubation medium. Although centrifugation can be utilized for this purpose, filtration through glass fiber filters is the preferred method. Caution must be exercised at this step to be certain that radioactivity does not adhere to the filters. Thus, when running an assay for the first time, a set of incubation tubes should be prepared without tissue to assess whether there is specific binding to the filter paper. Also, when using filtration machines, total binding and blank values should be established for each set of tubes. Filtration cannot always be utilized if the affinity of the radioligand for the receptor is low. In this case, centrifugation must be employed to terminate the reaction.

Using either procedure, the objective is to isolate the ligand-receptor complex from free ligands. In the case of filtration, this complex is deposited onto filter paper and washed with several volumes of buffer. The filter is then placed in a scintillation vial for tritium assays or γ-vials for ^{125}I assays. For tritium, radioactivity decay is detected by capturing the electrons emitted with scintillation fluid that converts the radioactive emission to light, which is in turn detected by a scintillation counter. Although γ-emitters like ^{125}I can also be counted in a scintillation counter, a γ-counter is a less expensive approach since it does not involve the addition of scintillation fluid inasmuch as the γ-counter can detect radiation directly. In both cases, data analysis is facilitated if the results are entered into a computer file through an RS232 interface between the counter and computer.

Although the optimal conditions for each binding assay vary with different receptors, some generalizations can be made. Thus, for each assay, there is always a set of "total tubes" that contain receptor homogenate, the radioligand, and buffer. These tubes are used to measure the total amount of radioactivity that is bound under these conditions. Tubes for "nonspecific" binding contain receptor homogenate, radioligand, buffer, and unlabeled ligand. Radioactivity bound under this condition represents the amount of radioligand that attaches to sites other than the receptor since the receptor is saturated with unlabeled ligand. The difference between total and nonspecific binding represents specific binding, or the amount of radioligand that attaches to the receptor of interest. Since there is a finite number of receptors, as the radioligand concentration increases the receptors present are ultimately completely occupied or saturated. Plotting the increment of radioligand versus the amount of specific binding/mg of protein generates a saturation curve (see ref. 9). The point at which this curve plateaus is an approximation of the receptor site concentration (B_{max}). The concentration of radioligand needed to attain one-half of the B_{max} is an approximation of the affinity of the ligand for the receptor (K_D). Since it is difficult to obtain a good quantitative value from this short of plot, the data are transformed by Scatchard analysis (10–12) to give more accurate and reproducible values for the K_D and B_{max}. With all binding assays, it is important to know exactly how much radioactivity was added to the tubes. The amount of radioactivity should be determined for each concentration of radioligand so that these can be used in the Scatchard analysis. With a Scatchard analysis, the amount of specific binding/free ligand (y-axis) is plotted against specific binding (x-axis). The free ligand is calculated by subtracting the amount bound from the total amount of radioactivity added to that tube. The slope of the resultant line yields the inverse of the K_D, and the x intercept is the B_{max} if there is only one receptor class present and the ligand binds in a competitive manner. When utilizing receptor binding assays in drug screening, a single concentration of radioligand equal to or less than the K_D is employed to maximize the specific/nonspecific binding ratio and to optimize the selectivity of binding.

The objective in using a receptor binding assay for screening is to determine whether the test substance inhibits the attachment of radioligand to its receptor. If test substance binds to the receptor, it will lower the amount of hot radioligand bound to the tissue. Typically, one set of tubes is used to minimize total binding and one set to quantify nonspecific binding. Subsequent tubes contain tissue, radioligand, and one concentration of test substance, usually 10 µM. If the substance is found to be active, various concentrations (1 nM to 100 µM) are tested to determine the concentration necessary to inhibit 50% of the specifically bound radioligand (IC_{50}). Since this value varies somewhat with the radioligand concentration $([L])$ and the K_D of the radioligand, a K_i is determined using the Cheng-Prusoff (13) equation, which yields a closer apparent affinity of the text substance for the receptor.

$$K_i = \frac{IC_{50}}{1 + \dfrac{[L]}{K_D}}$$

Calculation of Data

Computerization of this process is highly desirable. The newer liquid scintillation counters generally have an RS232 interface that allows the data to be collected into a computer file. The ASCII code for the output must be supplied by the scintillation counter vendor to assure compatibility with the computer software. The Oracle software package can be utilized to reduce the data in the way required. Although this is a very simple job, it is accomplished most expeditiously by computer programmers. The program can be designed to search using the computer terminal, or hard copies (Table 3) can be generated for visual inspection and analysis.

TABLE 3. *Numeric master response list*

Compound no.	AAD	BAD[a]	DA	5-HT	BZ	EXAA	LT	ANF	SP	BDKN	NPY	CCK	AD12
10000	N[b]	N	N	N	N	N	N	N	N	N	N	N	N
10001	N	N	N	N	N	N	N	N	N	N	N	N	N
10002	N	N	N	N	N	N	N	N	N	N	N	N	N
10003	N	N	N	N	N	92	N	N	N	N	N	N	N
10004	N	N	N	N	N	76	N	N	N	N	N	N	N
10005	N	N	N	N	N	N	N	N	N	N	N	N	N
10006	N	N	N	N	N	N	N	N	N	N	N	N	N
10007	N	N	N	N	N	N	N	N	N	N	N	N	N
10008	N	N	N	N	N	N	N	N	N	N	N	N	N
10009	N	N	N	N	N	N	N	N	N	N	N	N	N
10010	N	N	N	N	N	N	N	N	N	N	N	N	N
10011	N	N	N	N	N	N	N	N	N	N	N	N	N
10012	N	N	N	N	N	N	N	N	N	N	N	N	N
10013	N	N	N	N	N	N	N	N	N	N	N	N	N
10014	N	N	N	N	N	N	N	N	N	N	N	N	N
10015	N	N	N	N	N	N	N	N	N	N	N	N	N
10016	N	N	N	N	N	N	N	N	N	N	N	N	N
10017	N	N	N	N	N	N	N	N	N	N	N	N	N
10018	N	N	N	N	N	N	N	N	N	N	N	N	N
10019	N	N	N	N	N	N	N	N	N	N	N	N	N
10020	N	N	N	N	N	N	N	N	N	N	N	N	N
10021	N	N	N	N	N	N	N	N	N	N	N	N	N
10022	N	N	N	N	N	N	N	N	N	N	N	N	N
10023	N	N	N	N	N	N	N	N	N	N	N	N	N
10024	N	N	N	N	N	N	N	N	N	N	N	N	N
10025	N	N	N	N	N	N	N	N	N	N	N	N	N
10026	N	N	N	N	N	N	N	N	N	N	N	N	N
10027	N	N	N	N	N	N	N	N	N	N	N	N	N
10028	63[c]	97[c]	N	N	N	N	N	N	N	N	N	N	N
10029	N	N	N	N	N	N	N	N	N	N	N	N	N
10030	N	N	N	N	N	N	N	N	N	N	N	N	N
10031	N	N	N	N	N	N	N	N	N	N	N	N	N
10032	N	N	N	N	N	N	N	N	N	N	N	N	N
10033	N	N	N	N	N	N	N	N	N	N	N	N	N
10034	N	N	N	N	N	N	N	N	N	N	N	N	N
10035	N	N	N	N	N	N	N	N	N	N	N	N	N
10036	N	N	N	N	N	N	N	N	N	N	N	N	N
10037	N	N	N	N	N	N	N	N	N	N	N	N	N
10038	N	84	N	N	N	N	N	N	N	N	N	N	N

[a]BAD defines β-adrenergic.
[b]N defines no response.
[c]Percent inhibition of specific binding.

Analysis

Oracle software is extremely useful in managing the enormous amount of data generated by binding assays. It can be used to sort, search, and compare with little difficulty. Oracle software, which has applications for a biological database, has been designed to be compatible with MDL software, which has greater applications for managing the chemical database. The interfacing of these computer packages allows for very effective structure-activity analysis.

EXAMPLES AND DISCUSSION

As mentioned earlier, there are more than 80 receptors and their subtypes for which there are one or more published procedures for receptor binding (Table 4).

Receptors for peptide ligands offer the greatest opportunities for discovering new therapeutic agents since nonpeptide ligands for these sites are generally not known. Past synthetic strategies centered around modifying the structure of the peptide agonist in the hopes of finding an antagonist.

To examine thousands of compounds in a binding assay, the test substances are typically analyzed at a concentration of 10 µM. This concentration is chosen since at higher concentrations noncompetition interactions are more likely to occur. Criteria are established to define a compound of interest. In assays in which it is easy to identify leads, an interesting compound would be one that inhibits more than 50% of the specific binding at 10 µM. In contrast, for those assays in which the identification of active compounds is less common, any degree of inhibition may be a clue to potential activity. Care must be taken not to expend significant synthetic efforts on developing agents that interact with the receptor in a nonselective manner. In this regard, dose-response curves should be generated to determine whether the inhibition is competitive or noncompetitive as well as to determine the potency (K_i) of the lead.

Receptor binding does not routinely distinguish between an agonist and antagonist. Consequently, compounds active in those assays must be tested using appropriate assays to measure their effect on receptor function. Some examples include isolated tissue assays or *in vivo* tests of receptor activity. The usefulness of receptor binding in accelerating the drug discovery process relies on the continuous reiteration of chemical synthesis, testing, and chemical redesign. The strategy is similar to previous screening approaches that utilize enzyme assays, *in vitro* tissue baths, or whole animal models to assess a compound's activity, except that receptor binding assays are capable of yielding data on more compounds more rapidly. Once an active agent is identified, efforts must be made to ensure that the compound has the appropriate bioavailability and safety for *in vivo* use. This normally requires the synthesis of numerous analogues that are tested *in vivo* and *in vitro* to refine the molecule further. Here again, one receptor binding assay can be used to ensure that any chemical modification does not significantly diminish the ability of the com-

TABLE 4. *Summary of receptors and ligands with assay reference and potential therapeutic target*

Receptor	Subtype	Ligand and method reference	Potential therapeutic targets	
			Agonist	Antagonist
Adrenocorticotropic hormone (ACTH)		^{125}I-ACTH(14)	Diagnostic testing of ACTH function	
Adenosine	A$_1$	[^{3}H]CHA(15)		Cardiotonic
	A$_2$	[^{3}H]NECA(16)	Antianginal	
Adrenergic	α$_1$	[^{3}H]Prazosin (17–19)		Antihypertensive
	α$_2$	[^{3}H]Idazoxan (17, 19)	Antihypertensive	Antihypertensive
	β$_1$	^{125}I-Cyanopindolol (20)		Antiarrhythmic
	β$_2$	^{125}I-Iodocyanopindolol (20)	Bronchodilator	Antihypertensive
Angiotensin II		^{125}I-Angiotensin (21, 22)	Antihypertensive	
Angiotensin-converting enzyme		[^{3}H]Captopril (23)		
Atrial naturietic factor (ANF)		^{125}I-ANF (24)	Cardiotonic	
Benzodiazepine		[^{3}H]Flunitrazepam (25, 26)	Anxiolytic	
Bombesin		[^{3}H]Bombesin (27)		Antitumor
Bradykinin		[^{3}H]Bradykinin (28)		Analgesic
Calcitonin		^{125}I-ECT (29, 30)		
Calcium channels	L	[^{3}H]Nitrendipine (31)		Antianginal, antiarrhythmic
	L	[^{3}H]D-800 (32)		Antiarrhythmic
	L	[^{3}H]Diltiazem (33)		Antianginal, antihypertensive
	N	^{125}I-Conotoxin (34)		
Chloride channel		[^{35}S]-TBPS (35)		
Cholecystokinin (CCK)		^{125}I-CCK-8 (36)		Treat irritable bowel syndrome
				Irritable bowel syndrome
Corticotropin-releasing factor (CRF)		^{125}I-tyrosine-CRF (ovine) (37)		
Dextromethorphan		[^{3}H]Dextromethorphan (38)	Anticonvulsant; cough suppressant	
Dopamine	D1	[^{3}H]SKF-23390 (39)	Shock	Antipsychotic
	D2	[^{3}H]Spiperone (39)		Antiemetic
Enkephalin convertase		[^{3}H]GEMSA (40)		
Epidermal growth factor (EGF)		^{125}I-EGF (41)		Antitumor

Ligand	Receptor subtype	Radioligand	Therapeutic use(s)
Estrogen		$[^{3}\mathrm{H}]$Estrogen (42)	Treat menopause
Excitatory amino acid	Nonselective; NMDA; Quisqualate; Kainate	$[^{3}\mathrm{H}]$Glutamate (43), $[^{3}\mathrm{H}]$CPP (44), $[^{3}\mathrm{H}]$AMPA (45), $[^{3}\mathrm{H}]$Kainate (46)	Ischemia
Follicle-stimulating hormone (FSH)		$^{125}\mathrm{I}$-FSH (47)	Induction of ovulation
Forskolin		$[^{3}\mathrm{H}]$DHF (48, 49)	Cardiotonic
γ-Aminobutyric acid (GABA)	$GABA_A$, $GABA_B$	$[^{3}\mathrm{H}]$GABA (50), $[^{3}\mathrm{H}]$Baclofen (51)	Muscle relaxant; Anxiolytic
Glucagon		$^{125}\mathrm{I}$-Glucagon (52)	Hypoglycemia
Glucocorticoids		$[^{3}\mathrm{H}]$Dexamethasone (53)	
Gonadotropin-releasing hormone (GnRH)		$^{125}\mathrm{I}$-GnRH (54, 55)	Reduce circulating testosterone in patients with prostatic carcinoma
Growth hormone (GH)		$^{125}\mathrm{I}$-GH (56, 57)	Promote growth in dwarfism; Treatment of acromeglia
Growth hormone-releasing factor (GRF)		$^{125}\mathrm{I}$-Tyr,N1E-h GRF (58)	Promote growth in dwarfism; Treatment of acromeglia
Guanosine 5′-triphosphate (GTP)		$[^{3}\mathrm{H}]$GppNp (59)	
Histamine	H-1	$[^{3}\mathrm{H}]$Pyrilamine (60)	Decongestant
Human chorionic gonadotropin (HCG)		$^{125}\mathrm{I}$-^{3}HCG (61)	
Imipramine		$[^{3}\mathrm{H}]$Imipramine (62, 63)	Antidepressant
Insulin		$[^{3}\mathrm{H}]$Insulin (64)	Treat diabetes
Interleukin 2 (IL-2)		$[^{3}\mathrm{H}]$leu,lys-1L-2 (65)	Antitumor
Leukotriene D_4	LTD_4	$[^{3}\mathrm{H}]LTD_4$ (66)	
Lutenizing hormone (LH)		$^{125}\mathrm{I}$-LH (67)	Induction of ovulation
Mineralocorticoids		$[^{3}\mathrm{H}]$Aldosterone (68)	
Muscarinic cholinergic	M-1, M-2, M-3	$[^{3}\mathrm{H}]$Pirenzipine (69), $N[^{3}\mathrm{H}]$Methyl scopolamine (69), $N[^{3}\mathrm{H}]$Methyl scopolamine (69)	Antiulcer; Treat irritable bowel syndrome; Antiinflammatory
Nerve growth factor (NGF)		$^{125}\mathrm{I}$-NGF (70, 71)	Antitumor
Neuropeptide Y (NPY)		$^{125}\mathrm{I}$-NPY (72)	Appetite suppressant
Neurotensin		$[^{3}\mathrm{H}]$Neurotensin (73)	
Nicotinic			

(*Table continues*)

TABLE 4. (Continued)

Receptor	Subtype	Ligand and method reference	Potential therapeutic targets	
			Agonist	Antagonist
Opiates	μ	[³H]DAGO (74)	Analgesic	Immunosuppressant
	δ	[³H]DADLE (75)	Shock	Appetite suppressant
	γ	[³H]U-50,488 (76)	Analgesic	
Oxytocin (OT)		[³H]OT (77)	Initiate uterine contractions	
Platelet-activating factor (PAF)		[³H]PAF (78)	Antiinflammatory	
Phencyclidine		[³H]TCP (79)		Antipsychotic
Platelet-derived growth factor (PDGF)		125I-PDGF (80)		
Prolactin		125I-Prolactin (57)		
Prostaglandin E₁		[³H]Misoprostol (81)	Cytoprotective	
Serotonin	5-HT₁ₐ	8-0-[³H]DPAT (82)		
	5-HT₁ᵦ	[³H]Cynapindolol (83)		
	5-HT₁ᵧ	[³H]Mesulergine (83)		
	5-HT₂	[³H]Ketanserin (84, 85)		
Somatostatin		125I-Tyr-somatostatin (86, 87)	Treat irritable bowel syndrome	
Substance P		[³]Substance P (88, 89)		Analgesia; treat irritable bowel syndrome
Thrombin		125I-Thrombin (90)		
Thyrotropin-releasing hormone (TRH)		[³H]TRH (91)	Treat narcolepsy	
Thyroid-stimulating hormone (TSH)		125I-TSH (92)	Antipsychotic	
Vasointestinal peptide (VIP)		125I-VIP (93)		
Vasopressin		125I-Vasopressin (94)	Treat symptoms of diabetes insipidus	

pound to interact with the receptor in a potent and selective manner. Thus, the receptor binding assay can be a powerful tool not only for discovering novel chemicals, but also in providing assistance as those chemicals are sculpted into drugs.

REFERENCES

1. Ondetti MA, Rubin B. Cushman DW. *Science* 1977;196:441–444.
2. Berger PA. In: Barchas JD, Berger PA, Ciaranello RD, Elliott GR, eds. *Psychopharmacology*. New York: Oxford University Press, 1977.
3. Pert C, Snyder SH. *Proc Natl Acad Sci USA* 1973;70:2243–2247.
4. Simon EJ, Hiller JM, Edelman I. *Proc Natl Acad Sci USA* 1973;70:1947–1949.
5. Terenus L. *Acta Pharmacol Toxicol* 1973;33:377–384.
6. Bennett JP Jr. In Yamamura HI, Enna SJ, Kuhar MJ, eds. *Neurotransmitter receptor binding*. New York: Raven Press, 1978;57–90.
7. Burt DR. In: Yamamura HI, Enna SJ, Kuhar MJ, *Neurotransmitter receptor binding*. New York: Raven Press, 1978;42–55.
8. Rodbard D. In: O'Malley BW, Means AR, eds. *Basic principles in receptors for reproductive hormones*. New York: Plenum Publishing Corp, 1973;289–326.
9. Minton AP. *Biochim Biophys Acta* 1979;558:179–186.
10. Scatchard G. *Ann NY Acad Sci* 1949;51:660–672.
11. Dahlquist FW. *Methods Enzymol* 1978;48:270–299.
12. Chamness GC, McGuire WL. *Steroids* 1975;26:538–542.
13. Cheng YC, Prusoff WH. *Biochem Pharmaco* 1973;22:3099–3108.
14. Lefkowitz RJ, Roth J, Pricer W, Pastan I. *Proc Natl Acad Sci USA* 1970;65:745–752.
15. Williams M, Braunwalder A, Erickson TE. *Naunyn-Schmiedeberg's Arch Pharmacol* 1986;332:179–183.
16. Bruns RF, Lu GH, Pugsley TA. *Mol Pharmacol* 1986;29:331–346.
17. Reader TA, Briere R, Grondin L. *J Neural Transm* 1987;68:79–95.
18. Timmermans PBMWM, van Zwieten PA. *Eur J Pharmacol* 1979;55:57–66.
19. U'Prichard DC, Greenberg DA, Snyder SH. *Mol Pharmacol* 1977;13:454–473.
20. Neve KA, McGonigle P, Molinoff PB. *J Pharmacol Exp Ther* 1986;238:46–53.
21. Bennett JP, Snyder SH. *Eur J Pharmacol* 1980;67:11–25.
22. Campanile CP, Carne JK, Peach MJ, Garrison JC. *J Biol Chem* 1982;257:4951–4958.
23. Srittmatter SM, Snyder SH. *Mol Pharmacol* 1986;29:142–148.
24. Napier MA, Vandlen RL, Albers-Schonberg G. *Proc Natl Acad Sci USA* 1984;81:5946–5950.
25. Speth RC, Wastek GJ, Johnson PC, Yamamura HI. *Life Sci* 1978;22:859–866.
26. Braestrup C, Squirer RF. *Eur J Pharmacol* 1978;48:263–270.
27. Moody, TW, Pert CB, Riveier J, Brown MR. *Proc Natl Acad Sci USA* 1978;75:5372–5376.
28. Innis RB, Manning DC, Stewart JM, Snyder SH. *Proc Natl Acad Sci USA* 1981;78:2630–2634.
29. Olgiate VR, Guidobono R, Netti C, Pecile A. *Brain Res* 1983;265:209–215.
30. Fabbri A, Fraioli F, Pert CB, Pert A. *Brain Res* 1985;343:205–215.
31. Murphy KMM, Gould RJ, Largent BL, Snyder SH. *Proc Natl Acad Sci USA* 1983;80:860–864.
32. Reynold IJ, Snowman AM, Snyder SH. *J Pharmacol Exp Ther* 1986;237:731–738.
33. Balwierczak JL, Johnson CL, Schwartz A. *J Pharmacol Exp Ther* 1987;31:175–179.
34. Cruz LJ, Olivera BM. *J Biol Chem* 1986;261:6230–6233.
35. Squires RF, Casida JE, Richardson M, Saederup E. *Mol Pharmacol* 1983;23:326–335.
36. Hennogle LP, Steel DJ, Pesrack B. *Life Sci* 1985;36:1485–1490.
37. De Souza EB. *J Neurosci* 1987;7:88–100.
38. Craviso GL, Mussacchio JM. *Mol Pharmacol* 1983;23:619–628.
39. Hess EJ, Albers LJ, Le H, Creese I. *J Pharmacol Exp Ther* 1986;238:846–854.
40. Synch DR, Strittmatter SM, Venable JC, Snyder SH. *J Neurosci* 1986;6:1662–1675.
41. Palombella VJ, Yamashiro DJ, Maxfield RF, Decker SJ, Vilcek J. *J Biol Chem* 1987;262:1950–1954.
42. West NB, Brenner RM. *J Steroid Biochem* 1985;22:29–37.
43. Slevin J, Collins J, Lindsley K, Coyle JT. 1982;249:353–360.

44. Murphy DE, Schenden J, Bochm C, Lehmann J, Williams M. *J Pharmacol Exp Ther* 1987; 240:778–784.
45. Murphy DE, Snowhill EW, Williams M. *Neurochem Res* 1987;12:771–781.
46. Simon JR, Contrera JF, Kuhar MJ. *J Neurochem* 1976;26:141–147.
47. Melson BE, Sluss PM, Reichert LE. *Anal Biochem* 1987;160:434–439.
48. Seamon KB, Vaillancourt R, Edwards M, Daly JW. *Proc Natl Acad Sci USA* 1984;81:5081–5085.
49. Schmidt K, Baier, HP, Shariff A, Ayer WA, Browne L. *Can J Physiol Pharmacol* 1987;65:803–809.
50. Enna SJ, Collins JF, Snyder SH. *Brain Res* 1977;124:185–190.
51. Hill DR, Bowery NG. *Nature* 1981;290:149–152.
52. Pingoud V, Thole H. *Biochim Biophys Acta* 1987;929:182–189.
53. Weill CL. *Dev Brain Res* 1986;27:167–173.
54. Bilezikjian LM, Seifert H, Vale W. *Endocrinology* 1986;118:2045–2052.
55. Aten RF, Ireland JJ, Weems CW, Behrman HR. *Endocrinology* 1987;120:1727–1733.
56. Leung FC, Jones B, Steelman, SL, Rosenblum CL, Kopchick JJ. *Endocrinology* 1986; 119:1489–1496.
57. Phares CK, Booth JM. *Endocrinology* 1986;118:1102–1109.
58. Bilezikjian LM, Seifert H, Vale, W. *Endocrinology* 1986;118:2045–2052.
59. Gehlert DR, Wamsley JK. *Eur J Pharmacol* 1986;129:169–174.
60. Le Fur G, Malgouris C, Uzan A. *Life Sci* 1981;29:547–552.
61. Spicer LJ, Ireland JJ. *Anal Biochem* 1986;156:25–30.
62. Raisman R, Briley M, Langer SZ. *Nature* 1979;281:148–150.
63. Kinnier WJ, Chuang DM, Costa E. *Eur J Pharmacol* 1980;67:289–294.
64. Zahniser NR, Goens MB, Hansway PJ, Vinych JV. *J Neurochem* 1984;42:1354–1362.
65. Robb RJ, Rusk CM. *J Immunol* 1986;137:142–149.
66. Cheng JB, Lang D, Bewtra A, Townley RG. *J Pharmacol Exp Ther* 1985;232:80–87.
67. Bousfield GR, Ward DNM. *Biochim Biophys Acta* 1986;885:327–334.
68. Kuhnle U, Land M, Ulick S. *J Clin Endocrinol Metabol* 1986;62:934–940.
69. Doods HN, Mathy MJ, Davidesko D, Charldorp KJ, Jonge A, Zwieten P. *J Pharmacol Exp Ther* 1987;242:257–262.
70. Woodruff NR, Neet KE. *Biochemistry* 1986;25:7967–7974.
71. Woodruff NR, Neet KE. *Biochemistry* 1986;25:7956–7966.
72. Chang RSL, Lotti VJ, Chen TB, Cerino DJ, Kling PJ. *Life Sci* 1985;27:2111–2122.
73. Goedert M, Pittaway K, Williams BJ, Emson PC. *Brain Res* 1984;304:71–81.
74. Kosterlitz HW, Lond JAH, Paterson SJ, Waterfield AA. *Br J Pharmacol* 1980;68:333–342.
75. Gillman MGC, Kosterlitz HW. *Br J Pharmacol* 1982;77:461–469.
76. Lahte RA, Mickelson MM, McCall JM, Von Voigtlander PF. *Eur J Pharmacol* 1985;109:281–284.
77. Antoni F. *Endocrinology* 1986;119:2393–2398.
78. Robaut C, Durand G, James C, et al. *Biochem Pharmacol* 1987;36:3221–3229.
79. Gundlach AL, Largent BL, Snyder SH. *Brain Res* 1986;386:266–279.
80. Nister M, Heldin, CH, Wasteson, A, Westermark B. *Proc Natl Acad Sci USA* 1984;81:926–930.
81. Tsai BS, Kessler LK, Schoenhard G, Collins PW, Bauer RF. *Gastroenterology* 1987;25:201–206.
82. Peroutka S, Snyder SH. *Mol Pharmacol* 1974;16:687–699.
83. Peroutka SJ. *J Neurochem* 1986;47:529–540.
84. Sanders-Bush E, Breeding M, Roznoski M. *Eur J Pharmacol* 1987;133:199–204.
85. Leysen JE, Niemegers, CJE, Tollenaere JP, Laduron PM. *Nature* 1978;272:168–171.
86. Epelbaum J. *J Neurochem* 1982;38:1515–1523.
87. Strikant CB, Patel YC. *Proc Natl Acad Sci USA* 1981;7:3930–3934.
88. Park JP. *Peptides* 1984;5:833–836.
89. Perrone TA. *Eur J Pharmacol* 1983;95:131–133.
90. Mc Kinney M, Snider RM, Richelson E. *Mayo Clin Proc* 1983;58:829–831.
91. Kajita S, Ogawa N, Mitsunoto S. *Epilepsia* 1987;28:228–233.
92. Bianco AC, Maron MM, Nunes MT, et al. *Rev Paul Med* 1985;103:176–181.
93. Ogawa N, Miguno A, Mori, A, Nukina I, Yahaihara N. *Peptides* 1985;6:163–169.
94. Dorsa DM, Majumdar LA, Petracca FM, Baskin DG, Cornett LE. *Peptides* 1983;4:699–706.

Subject Index